SCHOOL NEUROPSYCHOLOGY

SCHOOL NEUROPSYCHOLOGY

A Practitioner's Handbook

JAMES B. HALE
CATHERINE A. FIORELLO

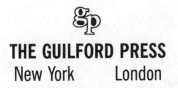

THE GUILFORD PRESS
New York   London

© 2004 The Guilford Press
A Division of Guilford Publications, Inc.
72 Spring Street, New York, NY 10012
www.guilford.com

Printed in the United States of America

This book is printed on acid-free paper.

Last digit is print number: 9 8 7 6 5 4 3 2 1

Library of Congress Cataloging-in-Publication Data
Hale, James B., 1961–
  School neuropsychology : a practitioner's handbook / by James B. Hale and Catherine A. Fiorello.
    p. cm.
Includes bibliographical references and index.
  ISBN 1-59385-011-5 (pbk.)
  1. Pediatric neuropsychology. 2. School psychology. 3. School children—Mental health
services. 4. Behavioral assessment of children. I. Fiorello, Catherine A. II. Title.
  RJ486.5.H235 2004
  618.92′8—dc22

                                                                      2003023396

To Kenneth Merrell, PhD, whose inspiration, guidance,
and perseverance led to this publicaton.

To my wife, Melissa, daughter, Helen, and son, Alex,
for their support, patience, and commitment.

—J. B. H.

To my husband, Keith, and son, Derek,
for their unflagging support during this journey.

—C. A. F.

About the Authors

James B. Hale, PhD, provides psychological and neuropsychological services to children with learning and behavior problems at the Children's Evaluation and Rehabilitation Center in the Bronx, New York. He is a faculty member in the Department of Pediatrics at Albert Einstein College of Medicine and Ferkauf Graduate School of Psychology of Yeshiva University. Dr. Hale received a BS in natural sciences/mathematics from the University of Wyoming, an MEd in special education from the University of Illinois at Chicago, and a PhD in school psychology from Loyola University Chicago, and completed a pediatric psychology fellowship at Columbus Children's Hospital and the Ohio State University College of Medicine. His presentations and publications examine the ecological validity of brain–behavior relationships in children with attention and learning problems, and can be found in several education, school psychology, clinical psychology, and neuropsychology journals.

Catherine A. Fiorello, PhD, is Associate Professor of School Psychology at Temple University, where she currently serves as program coordinator for school psychology. She received a BA in psychology from Clark University and an MS in education and PhD in school psychology from the University of Kentucky. Dr. Fiorello also completed a clinical postdoctoral fellowship at the University of Kentucky, focusing on assessment and intervention for children with attention-deficit/hyperactivity disorder. Prior to completing her doctorate, she worked as a certified school psychologist in public schools in Kentucky, and she continues to maintain a private practice in diagnostic assessment. Dr. Fiorello's specialization is in the area of cognitive assessment. She also has publications and clinical experience in the areas of learning and behavior disorders, health-related disorders, and low-incidence disabilities.

Contents

Introduction to School Neuropsychology

RECOGNIZING AND APPLYING NEUROPSYCHOLOGICAL PRINCIPLES

Studying Brain–Behavior Relationships

The study of brain–behavior relationships is remarkably compelling and at the same time incredibly overwhelming. These relationships are difficult for professors to teach, students to learn, and practitioners to implement. Applying the principles in clinical practice seems impossible at first glance. However, as when you first learned other psychological skills in your training, expertise in neuropsychological interpretation of test data requires diligent practice, a continued desire to better your interpretive skills, learning about theoretical and empirical advances in the field, and finding ways to apply this information in your daily practice of psychology. Hundreds of articles and books elucidating brain–behavior relationships are written each year. Although it is a daunting task to try to digest all of the relevant neuropsychological literature, it is a noble goal nonetheless. Moreover, applying these skills and the knowledge base to individual children requires clinical acumen—something that cannot be taught in any textbook or manual. Though the information contained in this book can help you utilize neuropsychological information in daily assessment and intervention practices, it is not a substitute for the training and supervised experience needed to become a neuropsychologist.

The goal of this book is to provide readers with a survey of the relevant brain–behavior literature and practices, but the material presented is not exhaustive. Because most training programs require at least one course in the biological bases of behavior, we presume that most of our readers will have had one or more courses in neuropsychology or the neurophysiology of behavior, but we realize that there will be considerable variability in your training and experience. Prior to reading this book, it may be helpful to review relevant neuropsychology and neuroscience textbooks from your courses, or to examine the resources listed in the chapter appendices. The neuropsychological knowledge base is growing at a phenomenal rate, so many of the concepts we learned in our neuropsychological training have now been revised or discarded. For instance, when most people think of the cognitive constructs subserved by the left and right hemispheres, they think of verbal and nonverbal skills, respectively. As we discuss in this book, this long-held dichotomous belief does not accurately reflect the true nature of hemispheric processing differences. Though not all scholars in neuropsychology would concur with our position, the theoretical and empirical advances made in recent years confirm the validity of the model we describe in the following chapters. The implications of these findings are dramatic and meaningful in daily practice, providing you with new insight into brain–behavior relationships. These novel insights form a conceptual framework for differential diagnosis and treatment of the learning and behavior disorders you encounter in your daily practice of psychology.

Making Neuropsychology User-Friendly

While most students and practitioners studying neuropsychology find the material fascinating or at the very least interesting, they typically complain that the material is inaccessible, too complex to master, or irrelevant in daily practice. We think there are four major reasons for these difficulties, and we offer possible remedies for each in an attempt to overcome these criticisms.

The first reason has to do with neuropsychology nomenclature, or—simply put—too many big words that sound medical or biological in nature. School personnel recognize that medical issues have an impact on their children, but are more comfortable leaving the diagnostic and treatment issues to the "doctors." However, medical doctors and clinic staff are counting on the school personnel; they are saying to each other, "We really need the school's input on this kid," and "The school can handle the intervention." School teams have a tendency to compartmentalize disciplines in an artificial manner. For instance, speech and language pathologists describe language processes, teachers discuss classroom behavior and pedagogy, and psychologists focus on "ability" and "personality." This artificial segregation minimizes the psychologists' knowledge and training, relegating them to specific diagnostic issues that are seldom related to intervention in a meaningful way. As is the case with physicians, who are typically outside the school system, psychologists defer responsibility for helping children if they ignore the need to use an *interdisciplinary* approach rather than a typical *multidisciplinary* one. All team members need to keep in mind that children are their primary clients. As members of the team, psychologists need to bridge the diagnosis–intervention gap, and learning neuropsychological terminology and principles can make this happen.

Learning about neuropsychological terminology is a lot like learning a foreign language, with no one to help you master the terms before they are used to describe concepts and techniques. Having taught neuropsychology to a variety of students at different levels of training, we are well aware that this hinders their acquisition and application of the material. Standing in a classroom full of students and telling them about brain structures and functions reminds me (Hale) of when I was in Central America. Spanish dictionary and tour guide in hand, I went to study Mayan ruins during my senior year of college. Getting off a bus in an unknown town, I tried to ask a man for directions to a youth hostel. During the conversation, I recall having what must have been a totally blank facial expression on my face, and nodding my head frequently in response to his detailed directions. I understood about a quarter of his words. Nodding graciously while saying "*gracias*" and "*adios*," I returned to the bus stop to try to orient myself and find my way using my resources, written in English. You may experience a similar feeling when reading the material that follows. However, don't be discouraged if you come across a term you haven't heard of when reading this book. In our neuropsychological studies, we were always amazed at how many different ways there were to convey comparable concepts or brain structures, so we attempt to use the same terminology throughout the book. We have also provided an appendix of common neuropsychology terms for you, and a list of Internet resources that provide additional information.

The second obstacle for those studying neuropsychology is related to depth of coverage. Many neuropsychology texts go into incredible detail regarding the anatomy and physiology associated with brain–behavior relationships. As with statistics, the depth of coverage can become overwhelming, especially when it is conveyed in complex terminology. We could have expanded the material presented in this book into several volumes, but instead we have chosen to highlight major structures and functions without becoming overly detailed in presentation. For instance, this book does not include a discussion of the cellular basis of behavior (as many textbooks do), and the coverage of neurochemistry is limited. Although this information is certainly important for an understanding of the psychopharmacological treatment of psychological disorders, and further study is highly recommended, the cellular basis of behavior is of limited use in daily school practice. Gender and racial issues are briefly addressed, but it is important for you to realize that the material presented is often cursory in nature. Although some additional information can be found in the In-Depth boxes in the chapters, further reading of the resources provided in the chapter appendices will help you become thoroughly knowledgeable in your areas of interest and practice.

The third difficulty learners experience has to do with the techniques used in neuropsychological research. Many think that neuropsychological principles have been derived from the study of adult patients and animal models with brain damage. This was true for most of the 20th century, but it is far from the case now. Noninvasive neuroimaging techniques, such as positron emission tomography (PET) and functional magnetic resonance imaging (fMRI), have provided us with great insight into brain–behavior relationships. PET and fMRI have been used to study mental processes both in typical children and in those with disabilities. These are children very similar to those in your classrooms. We need to recognize that typical children and those with disabilities lie along a continuum, and that the brain processes described in this book apply to all children. The brain is directly related to learning and behavior. We all knew this, but now we can measure changes in brain functioning while children perform cognitive tasks, and can visually depict these changes as they occur. However, it is important to realize that even these techniques require inferences about brain function, and that results may vary because of the tasks, methodology, and analyses used. Reviewing the literature for this book, we came across an article claiming to study episodic memory, but the research task was actually a word list learning task rather than one tapping episodic memory. We feel that when you are studying the neuropsychological literature, it is critical for you to review the participants, instruments, and procedures used in these studies. It is also important to realize that all studies have limitations, which are typically glossed over or minimized in some journal article discussions. It is essential for you to become an "informed consumer" in reading about brain–behavior relationships.

The fourth obstacle has to do with the real-world application of neuropsychological principles. Our experience suggests that many of those who study brain–behavior relationships take courses from professors of physiological psychology or neuropsychologists who work with adults. As many academics do, these professors often highlight their own research in the course, which may be irrelevant for practitioners working with children. For instance, I (Hale) remember when several school psychology students came to me to complain about their class on biological bases of behavior, which was taught by a physiological psychologist. They said they had spent the last 3 weeks discussing the structure and function of the eye in relation to visual processing. Although this was interesting and relevant, the level of detail provided was overwhelming to the students and unlikely to help them understand reading, math, and writing problems. To help overcome this obstacle, we regularly encourage psychology departments to use only licensed practitioners with knowledge of child neuropsychology to teach these courses.

We feel that neuropsychological assessment and intervention principles should become integral parts of psychology training programs. In addition to neuroanatomy and neurophysiology classes, we believe that courses in child neuropsychological assessment and intervention techniques, as well as neuropsychology practica and clerkships, should be developed. We agree with others who call for the development of a psychology subspecialty called "school neuropsychology." A school neuropsychologist is aware not only of brain–behavior relationships, but of their application in real-life settings, both for typical children and those with disabilities. The information presented here is but one step in a larger mission to bring neuropsychological principles to the forefront of educational practice. We realize that application of neuropsychological principles in school settings takes individual determination and system-level change. Many practitioners already are overwhelmed by their caseloads; adding additional measures and lengthening reports for the sake of diagnostic accuracy is laudable, but just not feasible for most. We believe that it is critical for practitioners to *intervene* so they may *assess*. The only way you are going to free up your time to do thorough neuropsychological assessments is to reduce the number of referrals for formal evaluation. To do this, you must rigorously adopt preventative intervention methods, pursue data-based prereferral interventions, and develop school-wide intervention assistance teams to assist you (and of course, each other). In an attempt to begin the change process, we provide you with a better understanding of brain–behavior relationships and of methods to apply this information when carrying out interventions for children with learning and behavior problems. You will be provided with real-life examples and Case Study boxes that highlight application of neuropsychological principles in assessment and intervention practices.

The Relationship among Cognition, Brain Function, and the Real World

During a televised New York–Philadelphia baseball game the other day, the complexity of brain–behavior relationships was revealed. The batter hit a line drive toward left center field. The quickly sinking line drive had just cleared the infield, and the left and center fielders converged on the ball simultaneously. As the ball veered slightly more toward center field, the left fielder stopped at the last second, and the center fielder dove to make an apparently spectacular catch. Although the dive was nearly perfect and the ball hit the webbing of his glove, it popped out. In the subsequent confusion, the left fielder finally picked up the ball and threw it to second base, but the runner slid safely beneath the tag.

What does this have to do with brain structure and function? Everything. One goal of this book is to help you, our readers, think about how brain–behavior relationships can be applied to real-life situations. Task-analyzing the players' actions, think about the various cognitive processes that led to the outcome. When the ball left the bat, both the left and center fielders had to visually examine the direction, velocity, and trajectory of the ball to know that it was coming their way. They might have done nothing, thinking that the ball would be caught by an infielder, but they "knew" that the probability of this happening was small. So, visually tracking the ball; they "knew" that they must run toward where it was likely to land. They couldn't walk or jog to get to the ball; they had to sprint. The left fielder had to decide, at the last minute, to yield to the center fielder. This required combining knowledge of the ball's path and the actions of the center fielder. The left fielder had to have this knowledge, plus a way to stop his actions, realizing that it was in the best interest of the team's goal for the center fielder to catch the ball and make an out. Now the center fielder was also trying a similar strategy, but he was probably distracted by the left fielders' coming at him and then stopping abruptly. Although he knew he had to dive and extend his mitt—coordinating eye, hand, and body to make a spectacular catch—the combined factors resulted in his failing to account for the impact of the ground on his mitt, and how this impact would affect his closing the mitt to catch the ball. Since there was an apparent catch, neither the left nor the center fielder had planned well for the new situation—that the center fielder had dropped the ball. The delay in planning, organizing, and carrying out the throw to second base resulted in the runner's making it safely to second—a chance the runner might have not taken, had he not seen the play unfold as he rounded first base. To summarize, there was a line drive to short left center field, the center fielder was charged with an error, and the player made it safely to second base.

Why not just say it in those few words? We all watched the play unfold, and our summary adequately reflects what happened—or does it? Recall that the center fielder was charged with an error, meaning that the official scorer thought he should have caught the ball. Without evidence, the fans would have expressed their dismay, and the two opposing factions could have erupted in conflict over it. Something similar can happen in clinical practice when you are trying to decide whether a child's attention problems are due to an attention problem, or an auditory processing problem, or even oppositional behavior. To understand brain–behavior relationships, you must analyze the task demands of any given cognitive or neuropsychological measure. This task analysis explores the *input demands, processing demands*, and *output demands* of a given task. However, as we note later in the text, making a judgment just on the basis of input or output has often led psychologists astray in their attempts to understand brain–behavior relationships. Within the last dozen years, it has become increasingly clear that the *processing demands* of a task are essential for linking assessment to intervention. With a thorough understanding of the neuropsychological basis of task processing demands, you will gain a better understanding of how children learn and behave in the classroom.

Returning to our example, let's task-analyze the missed catch. Catching a ball requires visual processes to identify where the ball is, the velocity, trajectory, and direction. A fielder must not only track the ball path, but determine the speed of his own running and whether he needs to catch it on the run or engage a diving sequence to bring the mitt closer to where the ball will land. Prior knowledge of the size, shape, and density of the ball, and of his trusty glove, helps the fielder recognize the force the ball will exert on his mitt. The tactile sensation of the hand against the leather glove helps to identify the impact of the ball. The posterior part of the brain is involved in these processes. The anterior or frontal part of the brain is critical for eye–hand coordination to track the ball into the glove. After completing the running and then diving motor sequences, the fielder must reach out his arm and grasp the ball instantaneously as it hits his glove. Given that the center fielder in our example accomplished all these activities successfully, he should have caught the ball. However, within a split second, his anterior brain manager ("brain boss") should have helped the fielder monitor his performance (running/diving) in relation to the ball's position and exerted "executive" control, allowing the fielder to modify his behavior. The executive could have provided the sensory system with direction to alter the glove's position and motor instructions to change the force of grasp to account for the glove's coming into contact with the ground before the ball arrived. And all of this might have happened if the brain boss had helped him to ignore the left fielder's actions.

This is, of course, a very difficult task to accomplish, but one that occurs regularly in professional sports and, of course, our daily lives. Think of a time you narrowly missed having an accident with another car, or bumped into someone on the street, or missed a step going down a flight of stairs. Many of the cognitive processes outlined above were required for you to avoid the accident. Examining the input, processing, and output demands required in any activity will help you apply your knowledge of brain–behavior relationships in real-life situations, including the classroom. In this book we highlight the brain structures associated with the cognitive skills described above, and help you to link cognitive and brain processes together so you may apply them in your life and psychological practice. The following chapters and materials have been organized with this purpose in mind, but deciphering how actions are related to brain functions takes regular practice and perseverance.

THE BOOK'S PURPOSE AND STRUCTURE

The purpose of this book is to provide current information on brain–behavior relationships, as well as suggestions for applying this information in daily practice. Most chapters include both content and methods, with the former emphasized initially, and the latter becoming more prevalent in the last sections. The first chapter reviews practices in school psychology assessment of cognitive processes, and provides an overview of the promises and pitfalls of early attempts to link cognitive profiles to treatment. It explores early research into the cognitive and behavioral characteristics of children with learning disorders. Chapter 1 sets the stage for an introduction of brain–behavior relationships in Chapter 2, and then this new understanding is adopted to further your assessment skills in Chapter 3. Chapter 4 provides a methodology to link assessment results to interventions, and is designed to encourage the use of brain–behavior relationships within the context of a problem-solving consultation approach to service delivery. Chapters 5, 6, and 7 provide current brain–behavior research and intervention strategies for children with various types of learning problems, all within the paradigm offered in the earlier chapters. Finally, Chapter 8 provides you with an understanding of how neuropsychological processes could be related to developmental psychopathology, and it describes interventions designed to address particular behavioral strengths and needs.

The chapters in this book are both informational and applied. The application of brain–behavior relationships in clinical practice is difficult, and some diligence will be required on your part to ensure that the patterns and relationships discussed are relevant to your daily practice, which is the ultimate goal of this book. It is designed for practitioners—individuals who have experience administering and interpreting standardized and informal measures of cognitive functioning. As such, it assumes a basic understanding of the areas of child development, learning, cognition, behavior, psychopathology, and brain–behavior relationships. It also assumes an understanding of individual, group, and system-level interventions, and of both direct and indirect service delivery models. Some of the information may be redundant with your training, but we have designed the book to meet the needs of practitioners who have varying levels of training and experience in the aforementioned areas. Given that the goal of this book is to help you develop a new way of thinking about how children learn and behave, the information and methods will help you analyze all types of data and interventions from this new brain–behavior perspective.

This book is *not* designed to provide you with the necessary information or skills to call yourself a neuropsychologist, which requires formal training and supervised experience. The Clinical Neuropsychology section (Division 40) of the American Psychological Association can provide you with additional information about neuropsychology training and credentialing. However, this book is designed to help you interpret test performance and behavior from a neuropsychological perspective—one we hope you will adopt in your educational assessment and intervention practices in the years to come. It is also about thinking and practicing psychology in a flexible and evolving manner. No book for practitioners has the answers to all your clinical questions; it merely provides new ideas and methodologies that you incorporate into your own clinical worldview. This material should not be the end of your training in neuropsychological principles applied in school settings. Instead, we hope it will fuel your desire to further your neuropsychological knowledge base and interest in rigorously applying these principles in daily practice. It is likely that much has changed since you took your first course in neurobiology, and the exponential growth of neuropsychological knowledge and practice suggests that these changes will continue in the years to come. We hope our work will open a new path for you—one that is fruitful for the children, parents, and teachers you serve in your educational or clinical setting.

CHAPTER 1

└┴┴┴┴┴┴┴┴┴┴┴┘

Assessment and Intervention Practices in Educational Settings

FOUNDATIONS OF INTELLECTUAL AND COGNITIVE ASSESSMENT

The Relevance of History

For the past century, scholars and practitioners alike have debated the merits of using psychological assessment for educational purposes. Whatever form it has taken in the past or is likely to take in the future, psychological assessment is a part of what psychologists do in educational or clinical settings. We begin this chapter with an overview of the promises and pitfalls of assessment practices in the schools. A chronological review of assessment theory and practice, test interpretation, and identification of learning disabilities culminates in an overview of our recommendations for the practice of psychology in the schools. This overview serves as an important foundation for the remainder of this book, where we integrate apparently disparate fields within psychology, including cognitive assessment, behavioral psychology, educational psychology, special education, and neuropsychology.

Why examine the history of assessment practices in the schools in a book about neuropsychology? First, a historical context helps you understand how past, current, and probable future assessment practices are related and have changed over time. Examining these trends can provide you with a conceptual continuity of service delivery that advances your practice of psychology. Second, it is important to recognize that the same brain is responsible for intellectual, cognitive, neuropsychological, academic, and psychosocial functioning. Understanding the relationship among these domains will give you the necessary template to rethink long-held assumptions about the practice of psychology in the schools, and (we hope) will provide you with the necessary motivation to incorporate new ideas and skills into your existing practice.

Historical Views of Intelligence: The Debate Begins

Although the primary purpose of this book is not historical, a brief overview of the foundations of psychological assessment will set the stage for the practice changes suggested later in the book. Like so much else psychologists do, cognitive testing in particular has always existed in a sociopolitical context. Intelligence, especially the concept of *g* or general intelligence, has been associated with notions of a person's value. Because IQ measures have been used to deny immigration, support sterilization, segregate individuals into categories, and deny educational opportunities to entire groups of people, it is only fair to ask where the tests came from and what they are being used for today. Three pertinent questions will form a framework for your examination of the following material:

- What is the relationship between early conceptions of intelligence and current models of cognitive and neuropsychological functioning?
- How have the content and process of cognitive assessment changed in relation to theory?
- What are the benefits and costs of intellectual/neuropsychological assessment as a model of service delivery?

We hope that this historical perspective will help you gain a better appreciation for the strengths and limitations of the tests we use. That is, these measures are merely tools for use in a comprehensive, multifaceted model of service delivery.

The assessment of individuals can be traced to early philosophers, but the first person who is typically associated with the systematic measurement of human abilities is Sir Francis Galton. Though his work in the late 1880s and 1890s at the University of London's Anthropometric Laboratory marked the beginning of scientific interest in testing mental ability, his notion that sensory discrimination and motor functioning form the basis of intelligence was reductionistic. Though Galton interpreted results solely on the basis of observable stimuli and responses, it is important to note that this was perhaps the last time that truly objective methods were used for assessing intelligence, because his items were least influenced by prior educational opportunity or experience. Another assessment pioneer was Lightner Witmer, usually hailed as the first "school psychologist," who founded the Psychoeducational Clinic at the University of Pennsylvania in 1896. He is credited with the first systematic attempts to link measurement of individual characteristics to specific interventions. These efforts at the end of the 19th century stimulated the ambitions of many who would follow; the pioneering work of Galton and Witmer served as a catalyst for many researchers and practitioners to examine the link between assessment and intervention.

Actual "intelligence test" development is usually credited as beginning with Alfred Binet (see Binet & Simon, 1905), who attempted to devise an instrument capable of determining the children who could benefit most from educational experiences. Binet developed his scale to measure higher-level reasoning and problem solving, but the actual items included prior knowledge and language-based questions that we would today recognize as "crystallized" items—those dependent on prior experience and education. Although Binet designed his tool to be sensitive to individual differences and thought that interpretation should be individualized for each child, his premise was dismissed when the concept of IQ was introduced several years later. Before you read further, what words do you think of when you think of IQ? Most people would think of the words "ability," "intelligence," "aptitude," or "potential," but how many would think of the word "achievement"? Ever since Binet introduced items that tapped crystallized and language skills, intelligence tests have been partly achievement tests. We *learn* things when we develop, and crystallized abilities—the abilities due to experience and education—are *learned* abilities. Unless all children have equal opportunities for learning, then differences on intelligence tests that include crystallized measures cannot be attributed solely to differences in ability. We return to this point later in the chapter.

How did Binet's test become the first "intelligence test"? Binet's original scale of hierarchically arranged items according to developmental age expectations was later adopted by Terman (1916), who added a scoring system that would change the nature of intellectual assessment. Terman's IQ, or "intelligence quotient," was originally computed by dividing the child's "mental age" (MA) by the child's chronological age (CA) and then multiplying by 100 to eliminate the decimal point. Ever since its inception, the IQ has been reified as the "true" measure of human intellect. Although some have questioned its utility, many have devoted their entire careers to attempting to validate the IQ as psychology's truly "objective" measure. However, within a few decades David Wechsler introduced another intelligence test, which was based on the works of Binet and the Army entrance exam tests. Though the Wechsler–Bellevue Scale (Wechsler, 1939) was designed to measure an individual's global capacity to act with purpose, Wechsler's Verbal and Performance subtests were thought of as clinical tools for examining individual differences in test performance (Kaufman, 1994).

Contemporary Views of Intelligence: The Debate Intensifies

It is important to realize that since the earliest days of mental testing, there have been disparate views about the structure of intelligence, and these differences continue today (see In-Depth 1.1 and Appendix 1.1). Originally proposed by Spearman (1904), the model of *g*, or general intelligence, assumes that intelligence is a single construct; IQ is seen as a meaningful measure of the brain's overall power, much like a motor's horsepower. Among modern researchers, Arthur Jensen (1998) is perhaps the most widely known of the *g* proponents. His body of work has explored the links between *g* and a variety of other measures, with fairly convincing evidence of its validity. Similarly, Linda Gottfredson (1997) contends that *g* is the best predictor of success in school, job training, and overall occupational attainment, and her arguments have been used to support conservative political agendas. In their book *The Bell Curve*, Herrnstein and Murray (1994) argue that *g* is predictive of various real-world outcomes, including educational attainment, income level, and likelihood of incarceration. However, it is important to note that this "seminal" work was flawed by the use of an *achievement* test to measure *g* (Roberts et al., 2000).

Several writers, such as Paul McDermott, Joseph Glutting, and Marley Watkins, recommend interpretation of only the global IQ derived from cognitive testing; they note the importance of *g* in predicting school learning. However, it has become clear that their methodology is also statistically flawed (see Hale, Fiorello, Kavanagh, Hoeppner, & Gaither, 2001). It is important to note that most *g* proponents do not deny the reality of other, more specific cognitive functions. They just question the utility of interpreting anything other than global IQ. The implications of these ideas are significant: No longer would practitioners need to waste time on clinical assessment or interpretation; they could simply give an intelligence test and report the global IQ. However, this argument implies that IQ is an intransient measure of innate ability, and that no intervention, whether educational or sociopolitical (such as affirmative action), can alter the likelihood of individuals' success if they have a low global IQ.

Beginning with the Thurstone (multiple abilities) versus Spearman (single ability) debate in the early 20th century, many researchers and clinicians have argued that clinically useful intelligence tests must measure a variety of functions rather than a unitary IQ (e.g., Guilford, 1967;

IN-DEPTH 1.1. Major Players in Intelligence, Test Theory, Research, and Practice

ADVOCATES OF GLOBAL INTELLIGENCE

Arthur Jensen sees general intelligence, or *g*, as the most important predictor of just about everything. In Jensen's view, selection of an appropriate test depends solely on its *g* loading, or how well it measures general intelligence.

Linda Gottfredson produces research that links general intelligence to success in a variety of learning environments, including later career and life success.

Paul McDermott, Joseph Glutting, Marley Watkins, and their colleagues have studied the use of profile and subtest analysis with a number of commonly used intelligence tests. Their conclusion, based on dubious multiple-regression techniques, is that little variance is accounted for by subtests or factors beyond global IQ.

Gregg Macmann and **David Barnett** base their objections to profile interpretation on simulation studies that show little reliability of subtest profiles on retesting.

THEORETICALLY/EMPIRICALLY ORIENTED ADVOCATES OF COGNITIVE STRENGTHS AND WEAKNESSES

John Carroll was a hierarchical theorist supporting *g*, but his true contribution to our understanding of the structure of intelligence beyond IQ has been unparalleled. His treatise synthesizes 512 databases of cognitive test data; this is great for researchers, but not for the faint of heart!

J. P. Das and **Jack Naglieri** adapted parts of Luria's neuropsychological model in their development of the Cognitive Assessment System (CAS), a measure of cognitive processes that minimizes assessment of crystallized abilities or prior knowledge, and has been used to demonstrate individualized aptitude–treatment interactions.

John Horn argues strongly against interpreting *g* and in favor of interpreting various cognitive processes and abilities. His extended *Gf-Gc* model (fluid and crystallized intelligences) is one of the components of modern Cattell–Horn–Carroll (CHC) theory.

Richard Woodcock is well known for both theory and test development. He recommends interpretation of the new WJ-III from a variety of perspectives, including the CHC clusters of abilities, specialized clinical clusters, and an integrated information-processing model (which includes consideration of the cognitive and noncognitive factors that affect performance).

PRACTICE-ORIENTED ADVOCATES OF COGNITIVE STRENGTHS AND WEAKNESSES

Colin Elliott argues for a model of both global and specific abilities, recommending interpretation of other cognitive abilities and inclusion of diagnostic subtests to analyze strengths and weaknesses.

Randy Kamphaus calls for a scientist-practitioner approach to stay abreast of the research findings and apply them to the interpretation of an individual child's performance.

Alan Kaufman and **Nadeen Kaufman** are the founders of the modern practice of research-based clinical interpretation of test performance. The methodology involves interpretation of a child's strengths and weaknesses, based on statistical information about the test and research information about what subtests actually measure.

(continued)

IN-DEPTH 1.1. *(continued)*

Kevin McGrew, Dawn Flanagan, Sam Ortiz, and their colleagues have combined Carroll's hierarchical model with Horn and Cattell's extended *Gf-Gc* model to form CHC theory. Their research-based cross-battery approach allows for comprehensive, individualized evaluations of multiple cognitive abilities.

Jerome Sattler is the author of the books "most likely to be owned" by psychologists everywhere. He compiles research and clinical information on assessment and test interpretation for comprehensive service provision.

ADVOCATES OF MULTIPLE INTELLIGENCES

Howard Gardner explores nontraditional areas such as musical and interpersonal "abilities"; although his humanistic theory is not grounded in empirical science, it compels others to value individual differences and is popular among educators.

Robert Sternberg developed the triarchic theory and measures of intelligence, with preliminary empirical support suggesting that all three aspects of intelligence (analytical, creative, and practical) are related to academic success.

ADVOCATES OF A "PARADIGM SHIFT"

Frank Gresham and **Joseph Witt** argue that intelligence testing is a waste of time, as the tests are not useful in developing interventions and are frequently disregarded during team eligibility determinations.

Dan Reschly and **James Ysseldyke** agree that intelligence tests are not useful for diagnosing mild disabilities or developing interventions; they call for a "paradigm shift" that eliminates standardized testing.

Horn & Cattell, 1967; Thurstone, 1938). Multifactor theorists focus on cognitive functions derived from test data and basic cognitive science research, although neuropsychological research has recently come to the forefront in contributing knowledge of cognitive functions (Hale & Fiorello, 2001). Guilford's structure-of-intellect model explored the diversity of cognitive skills differing in content, operations, and product—concepts similar to the input demands, processing demands, and output demands in our cognitive hypothesis-testing (CHT) model, discussed throughout this book. Another processing model—the planning, attention, simultaneous, and successive (PASS) model (Das, Naglieri, & Kirby, 1994), has demonstrated relationships between cognitive processes and educational achievement. Sternberg's (1997) triarchic theory adds creative and practical intelligences to the analytical abilities typically thought of as "intelligence." His ongoing body of research into the cognitive processes, experiences, and environmental context of intelligent behavior has demonstrated aptitude–treatment interactions at the school and university levels (Sternberg, Grigorenko, Ferrari, & Clinkenbeard, 1999).

Many current theories of cognitive ability are hierarchical; that is, they assume the existence of both an overall *g* and a variety of important cognitive processes subsumed under *g*. Recently, McGrew and colleagues (e.g., McGrew & Flanagan, 1998) have combined Carroll's (1993) hierarchical concept of intelligence with Horn and Cattell's (1967) multifactor model to yield what is known as Cattell–Horn–Carroll (CHC) theory, with the Woodcock–Johnson III Tests of Cognitive Abilities (WJ-III Cognitive; Woodcock, McGrew, & Mather, 2001) as its primary measurement tool. Taken together, the thorough analyses embodied in a cross-battery approach, and the extensive database used for linking CHC cognitive abilities to academic achievement domains, provide irrefutable evidence that our understanding of cognitive functioning has grown immensely and that practitioners should incorporate this knowledge into their daily assessment practices. Even more exciting is the convergence of neuropsychological and cognitive theory, providing the *why* for what researchers and practitioners have observed on intellectual and cognitive measures.

MEASURING INTELLECTUAL AND COGNITIVE FUNCTIONING

Is Theory Quantifiable?

You probably believe in "intelligence" and "cognition" as constructs, but these questions remain: How do psychologists measure them, and do they do it well? Accepted by many contemporary theorists (Neisser et al., 1996), the hierarchical model, with *g* at the top and several abilities underneath, is often adopted by intelligence test developers because of practical considerations. Possibly because of the important role IQ has played in differential diagnosis and eligibility determinations, a test that does not provide a global IQ score is often deemed less useful. For example, *Diagnostic and Statistical Manual of Mental Disorders*, fourth edition (DSM-IV; American Psychiatric Association, 1994) conceptions of mental retardation and learning disorders depend on an overall measure of intellectual functioning in clinical settings, and educational decision making typically requires a global score for identification of learning disabilities under the Individuals with Disabilities Education Act (IDEA, 1997) in the schools.

As noted earlier, the earliest practical intelligence tests—the Stanford–Binet (Terman, 1916) and the Wechsler–Bellevue scales (Wechsler, 1939)—yielded IQ scores, but did not dismiss the relevance of underlying abilities that should be interpreted clinically. Moving beyond the infamous Wechsler Verbal–Performance dichotomy, the Stanford–Binet Intelligence Scale: Fourth Edition (SB-IV; Thorndike, Hagen, & Sattler, 1986) was designed to measure Verbal Reasoning (crystallized ability), Abstract/Visual Reasoning (fluid ability), Quantitative Reasoning, and Short-Term Memory, and was based on a version of the CHC model. The new SB5 (Roid, 2003) has moved even further toward assessing a variety of cognitive skills from CHC theory, measuring Knowledge (crystallized), Fluid Reasoning, Working Memory, Quantitative Reasoning, and Visual–Spatial Reasoning through both verbal and limited-language tests. Another test battery derived from this theoretical model is the Differential Ability Scales (DAS; Elliott, 1990), which measures Verbal Ability (crystallized), Nonverbal Reasoning (fluid reasoning), and Spatial Ability in its core battery, and includes diagnostic subtests to test auditory and visual memory and processing speed. The PASS model led to the development of the Cognitive Assessment System (CAS; Naglieri & Das, 1997), though the relationship between the CAS and Luria's model is not always congruent with Luria's writings. The SB5, the DAS, and the CAS all provide an overall measure of *g* in addition to their measures of specific cognitive skills. The WJ-III Cognitive (Woodcock et al., 2001) is based on the hierarchical CHC theory, and measures nine different abilities in addition to providing an overall score weighted according to the *g* loading of the tests. Even the Wechsler Verbal–Performance scales have been abandoned in the Wechsler Intelligence Scale for Children—Fourth Edition (WISC-IV; Wechsler, 2003), with Verbal Comprehension, Perceptual Reasoning, Working Memory, and Processing Speed factors replacing the old Verbal–Performance dichotomy. As can be seen, intelligence/cognitive tests have moved away from single constructs such as "intelligence" to encompass more diverse cognitive abilities and functions.

Another movement in current assessment practice is the increased use of neuropsychological assessment and interpretation strategies in psychology practice. Based on the process approach, the WISC-III Processing Instrument (WISC-III PI; Kaplan, Fein, Kramer, Delis, & Morris, 1999) and its successor, the WISC-IV Integrated, extend the traditional "testing of the limits" into a formal neuropsychological assessment. The process approach, discussed in Chapter 3, is a valued hypothesis-testing practice among many psychologists and neuropsychologists. Designed as the first neuropsychological test battery for young children, the NEPSY (Korkman, Kirk, & Kemp, 1998) measures constructs traditionally thought of as neuropsychological in nature, such as executive functions, memory, and sensory–motor processes. Although the WJ-III Cognitive was derived primarily from the psychometric CHC theory (as noted above), it includes an information-processing interpretive model and explicitly provides clinical cluster scores based on neuropsychological concepts. As discussed later, several measures of memory—including the Children's Memory Scale (Cohen, 1997), the Test of Memory and Learning (Reynolds & Bigler, 1994), and the Wide Range Assessment of Memory and Learning (Sheslow & Adams, 1990)—provide practitioners with an understanding of memory encoding, storage, and retrieval (constructs essential for school learning). This merging of cognitive and neuropsychological principles in the assessment of individual differences forms the foundation of this book. A growing body of evidence suggests that neuropsychology and cognitive assessment are intimately interrelated, and that knowing about both areas leads to better assessment practices and to interventions sensitive to individual needs.

Statistical Methodologies and Conceptions of *g*

How do research methodologies regarding intellectual testing and *g* affect you? Policy issues and legislation are based on these studies, often dictating practice guidelines that may or may not make clinical sense. One of the reasons why discussions of *g* are so contentious is that intelligence researchers use a wide array of statistical methods to extract different information from the test data. An understanding of the major methodologies used in the quest for, or dismissal of, *g* may shed some light on the conclusions drawn by competing constituencies. First, it is important to understand that any task (test or subtest) assessing cognitive functioning is measuring many different brain functions at the same time. Part of the variance in scores reflects psychometric *g*, the underlying factor most equated with general intelligence and IQ scores. Part of the variance is related to other tests, and this variance can be represented by multiple factors, or it can be represented by *g*. Finally, "unique" variance—variance that is not related to other tasks—is considered specific to the subtest (its specificity). Subtests also have "error" variance, which is associated with any measure and can be related to things like test construction, items used, or administration time. Different types of analyses often favor one portion of variance over another, giving you a different picture about the meaning of the subtest scores you obtain during testing.

The most common methodology used to study cognitive test scores is *factor analysis*. Exploratory factor analysis is often used to examine the performance of many people on multiple measures. The intercorrelations of the derived scores are used to identify underlying factors that account for the common score variance, leaving the unique variance and error variance behind. When factor analysis is done on a broad array of cognitive tasks, a factor common to all the tasks, often called psychometric *g*, is typically identified. This finding of a common underlying factor on all cognitive tasks is also referred to as the *positive manifold* effect (Brody, 1997). Many theorists, starting with Spearman (1904), have considered this one underlying factor to be *g*, an overall measure of cognitive ability or mental power, since some portion of it has been common to all complex cognitive tasks analyzed.

Single-factor solutions, which many researchers label *g*, have been found for many different cognitive measures. This consistency provides convincing evidence of the construct's validity, right? Well, it is not so clear-cut as some would lead you to believe. First, it is important to note that you can take just about any measure—say, one that has anxiety and depression items—and achieve a single-factor solution. The point here is that we say the one-factor solutions of "intelligence" tests measure *g*, but in reality they merely measure a statistical construct; this construct is probably related to "true" intelligence, but to many other factors as well. In addition, there are a number of different factor-analytic methods. Some of these emphasize identifying a common factor, and some use rotated factors to emphasize finding several meaningful factors that can either be treated as related (oblique) or separate (orthogonal). Since we know that cognitive skills are interrelated, it doesn't make much sense to do orthogonal rotations, and results using these rotations are inherently misleading. Finally, choosing one or multiple factors during exploratory factor analyses often requires the researcher to use an eigenvalue cutoff of 1 to determine the number of factors, but there is no clear consensus on what eigenvalue should be used. If you set the eigenvalue cutoff high enough, you can almost always achieve a one-factor solution for a cognitive test.

Another methodology used frequently in studying cognitive test scores is *regression analysis*. Regression analyses are used to examine the amount of variance in an outcome (or dependent) variable that is explained by the independent variables. There are many ways of constructing the regression equation, depending on how the independent variables are related. In a *hierarchical regression analysis*, whatever variable is entered into the regression equation first will keep all of its own variance, plus all of the variance it shares with variables entered later in the equation. Therefore, if the independent variables are related to each other, the order in which the variables are entered can significantly affect the results of the analysis. When Glutting, Youngstrom, Ward, Ward, and Hale (1997) studied the contribution of WISC-III scores to predicting achievement and used hierarchical regression analysis, they entered the Full Scale IQ (FSIQ) into the regression equation first, and then entered the four Index (Verbal Comprehension, Perceptual Organization, Freedom from Distractibility, and Processing Speed) scores. They concluded that FSIQ explained the majority of the variance in all achievement domains, and that the Index scores should not be interpreted, since they explained so little achievement variance.

Are the Index scores really that useless? Stop and think about it for a second. First, Glutting and colleagues (1997) made the FSIQ predict the achievement measure; then they entered the four factors. Is there something wrong here? How do you compute FSIQ? How do you compute the four Index scores? FSIQ is composed of 10 of the 12 subtests that make up the Index scores (think of the WISC-III face sheet). Obviously, there is a great deal of shared variance here, and in the regression analyses the FSIQ took it all. This left a relatively small amount of variance for the Index scores to explain (although the Digit Span and Symbol Search subtests alone surprisingly contributed appreciable amounts!). If you enter the Index scores first, they take all the shared variance and leave the FSIQ appearing to be useless in predicting achievement domains (Hale, Fiorello, et al., 2001). So you enter FSIQ first and then the four factors, and FSIQ is everything; you enter the factors first, and then FSIQ becomes irrelevant. Which way is correct? *Neither* of these analyses gives a good picture of the pattern of shared and unique subtest or factor variance that makes up a factorially complex measure like the WISC-III. It is important to note that Glutting and his advocates of global IQ have published several works, but if you carefully examine their findings in these works, you will find that they used similar inappropriate methodologies to dismiss the validity of assessing factor or subtest results.

So what kind of analysis can you do with highly related scores (i.e., collinear data)? A more appropriate analysis for collinear data is called *regression commonality analysis*. In a commonality analysis, the unique variance of each task and the various combinations of common variances among the tasks are all examined separately. It is similar to the examination of main and interaction effects in analysis of variance. Instead of entering FSIQ or the factors first, and assuming that one or the other is the best measure of academic achievement, it is possible to identify how much variance is unique to each measure, and how much variance is common to all measures. We present our findings a little later, using WISC-III commonality analysis with various samples of children to demonstrate the factorial complexity of that measure (Fiorello, Hale, McGrath, Ryan, & Quinn, 2001; Hale, Fiorello, et al., 2001). Although factor analysis can provide useful information about how well tests predict outcome measures, commonality analysis provides the most information about the complexities of cognitive test performance, and it gives relevant information for individual clinical interpretation of test scores.

Another common methodology for studying cognitive tests is called *structural equation modeling*. This approach requires an a priori theoretical model of how variables are related before you conduct the analysis. Measures are combined to define a factor, or *latent variable*. For instance, the WISC-III Information, Vocabulary, Similarities, and Comprehension subtests might be combined to define the latent variable of Crystallized Intelligence. The relationships between latent and observed variables are defined via directional paths—visual representations of the causal links. For example, Crystallized Intelligence would be one cause of reading achievement, so there would be a path from the latent construct Crystallized Intelligence to an observed variable such as the WJ-III Letter–Word Identification subtest. The analysis then calculates the strength of all the paths in a manner similar to regression analysis, and goodness-of-fit indices tell you whether your model fits the data well or needs to be modified.

The Final Word: Is *g* Relevant for Psychological Practice?

Is global IQ relevant for psychological practice? In a recent special issue of the journal *Learning and Individual Differences*, we (Fiorello et al., 2001) and several colleagues recently addressed this important issue. One of the most enduring constructs in psychometrics, global IQ *is* a good predictor of school and occupational success (Buckholdt, 2001; Kranzler, 2001); it is a strong indicator of how well a child will perform in an English-speaking U.S. school with no instructional accommodations, supports, or services. It is also an excellent predictor of a child's performance on standardized achievement tests, but evidence is emerging that using a variety of cognitive skills predicts achievement domains even better (e.g., Vanderwood, McGrew, Flanagan, & Keith, 2001). Although comprehensive intelligence tests often contain strong predictors of outcomes, none measure all essential components of cognitive functioning (Bowman, Markham, & Roberts, 2001). This has led some observers to conclude that the movement away from *g* to explore the complexities of cognitive functioning will prevail in the future (McGhee, 2001).

Even if global IQ is a valuable measure predictive of important outcomes, subtest performance will affect the overall score—a fact often ignored when clinicians focus solely on IQ. Consider a child with a hearing impairment. If you administer an intelligence test in spoken English, the results will predict the child's classroom success, because the inability to hear and comprehend language will strongly influence both the test score and classroom performance. We can make similar arguments for a child with a visual, motor, or language impairment. But the same thing is also true when we are discussing a child with a sociocultural or linguistic difference, as the child's classroom performance will be limited if such a difference is not addressed and accommodated. The IQ will also predict this child's classroom performance well, but the error occurs when we assume that the child's limitations are due to a difference in intelligence. For example, an African American child typically grows up in a different culture from the dominant culture in U.S. schools. John Ogbu's (2002) research documents how "involuntary minorities," such as African Americans and Native Americans, perform poorly on IQ tests and in school not because of any inherent lack of intelligence, but because of cultural differences, prejudice, and their own resistance to being culturally assimilated. An IQ score accurately predicts school success because of a host of factors, only one of which is its measurement of cognitive functioning. Intelligence tests are statistically unbiased because they predict outcome equally well for most children. But we are less concerned with statistical bias than with the concept of *fairness* (Hale & Fiorello, 2001). Even if a test predicts outcomes well, it is not fair if it leads to misconceptions about the innate ability of certain groups of children. *A critical point here is that the fairness problem does not lie in the instrument or its construction; the problem is associated with clinicians who uniformly interpret low test scores as reflecting low global intelligence.*

As noted earlier, another major problem with intelligence tests as measures of "ability" is that most intelligence tests measure crystallized abilities—those skills acquired through formal and informal experiences and education. By definition, these skills are inseparable from prior learning or achievement, so they cannot be true measures of innate ability. Those who have enriched backgrounds and educational experiences typically score better on crystallized measures than those who come from impoverished or varied backgrounds do. Does this mean that the former children are necessarily smarter? We think not. Assessment of acquired knowledge—language development, general information, and other crystallized skills—is still extremely important to fully understand a child's current level of school functioning. However, such measures should only be used to make inferences about a child's underlying cognitive ability, or intelligence, if it can be ascertained that the child has been exposed to mainstream U.S. language and culture to exactly the same degree as the normative sample. Can you, as the clinician, make this judgment? Since it is impossible to separate out experience and directly assess the underlying brain function, we can never truly measure ability. Ever since Binet introduced the first "true" intelligence test, we have never truly measured intelligence—only a confusing blend of ability and achievement.

In conclusion, we feel that IQ overemphasis is one of the major problems in psychology practice. This overemphasis has led to inappropriate identification of impoverished and minority children as having mental retardation, to the flawed "discrepancy model" of learning disability, and to testing practices that are irrelevant for individualized interventions. Obviously, this is a big problem, so what is the solution? We recommend extending interpretation beyond the IQ in assessing a student's cognitive functioning, but ensuring that the results reflect reality and are meaningful for intervention. In the chapters that follow, we outline a neuropsychologically based approach to cognitive testing that occurs within the context of a comprehensive evaluation—one that ensures both the ecological and treatment validity of the findings.

PRINCIPLES OF EFFECTIVE COGNITIVE ASSESSMENT

Intervening to Assess

We begin this section by ironically recommending that you practice intervention. Can psychologists practicing in today's administrative climate do the sort of comprehensive evaluation that we recommend in this book? The answer is no, not if every child experiencing academic or behavioral difficulties is referred for testing and evaluated. We believe that you must *intervene to assess*. That is, systematic prereferral strategies and intervention assistance teams (IATs) must be used *first* to help a majority of children in need—not only in order to help children, but also to reduce the number of children referred for comprehensive evaluations. Rather than completing a short evaluation that is not helpful, and making a diagnostic "leap of faith" (Reschly & Gresham, 1989) based on limited test data on every child, we recommend that you design, implement, and monitor prereferral interventions on every child. Only when those interventions are not successful should a comprehensive evaluation be conducted—one that provides a thorough diagnostic description of the child to help you develop individualized interventions.

Too much of your time is probably spent administering standardized tests and writing reports (see, e.g., Sheridan & Gutkin, 2000), so our proposition that you conduct *more* comprehensive evaluations probably seems outlandish and impractical. We concur. We do not expect you to conduct comprehensive evaluations if your assessment caseload is too high. However, through the use of problem-solving consultation and IATs (see Ross, 1995), you can effectively reduce the number of children who require comprehensive evaluations. Sharing your knowledge of the brain–behavior relationships with educators and other professionals can foster the efficacy of these interventions. You can help teachers recognize behavioral manifestations of certain disorders, and can tailor interventions accordingly. Similarly, if a child does not show the neuropsychological characteristics discussed in this book, you can hypothesize that environmental contingencies are playing an important role in the problem behavior. Thorough examination of prereferral data, permanent products, and other school records can help you determine whether a formal evaluation is truly needed, because you can be more confident that the problem behavior is not just related to environmental contingencies. Obviously, this is not an "either–or" phenomenon, but careful examination of available data can help shape referral questions and determine whether formal evaluation for disability determination is needed (see Application 1.1).

Even if a formal evaluation is required after systematic prereferral interventions have been unsuccessful, you will have collected some initial data to help formulate your diagnostic hypotheses, and these data can serve as a basis for developing the formal assessment protocol. You will also have developed important relationships with teachers and parents—relationships that will serve as a foundation during implementation of subsequent assessment and intervention activities. To reiterate, you must *intervene* with a majority of children who have academic and/or behavior problems before you can adequately *assess* the few children with complex neuropsychological problems and instructional needs requiring more comprehensive evaluations.

Importance of Comprehensive Cognitive Assessment

Only psychologists are trained to administer and interpret many of the cognitive and socioemotional measures discussed in this book. Other psychologist roles, such as consultation with teachers and parents, counseling with individuals or groups, or even participating in individualized education plan (IEP) development, can be fulfilled by other professionals. It is up to you to help administrators recognize that cognitive and socioemotional assessments are essential to understanding many (but not all) children with unique needs. In addition, as the burden of mandated assessment practices has been lifted from psychologists' shoulders, the proverbial door has been opened for you to engage in innovative practices. No longer does a child need an intelligence test every 3 years—but this does not mean that cognitive, behavioral, or curriculum-based measures cannot be used to evaluate child changes over time. You must use the changes in disability law wisely to become involved in other roles and functions, so that you may provide individualized, comprehensive evaluations that have ecological and treatment validity.

You may wonder why we are adamant that cognitive assessment must remain an important component of school psychology practice. Psychologists have a wide array of tools, and cognitive

APPLICATION 1.1. Reducing Referrals through Data-Based Decision Making

Ensuring successful prereferral interventions requires adequate data collection. Some teachers may resist collecting formal data, so you must reinforce the necessity of data-based decision making, and decide collaboratively on the data collection methods that are feasible in each classroom. It does no good to have a data collection method that is so difficult that the teacher doesn't adhere to it. The data collection methods touted in training programs are great, provided you have a staff of graduate students or teacher's aides sitting around collecting data for you. The average teacher has a full classroom with students of various needs, and the last thing he or she needs is a complex data collection system. Keeping the data simple but meaningful will avoid the propensity of teachers to avoid data collection altogether or do a mediocre job at it. Some teachers refer students more often then others, and you must find these teachers and provide them with support to reduce referrals. I once consulted with a teacher who made many referrals for formal evaluation. When I asked her about her most recent referral, she said, "I wrote the three interventions on the sheet. They didn't work; he's still calling out in class. Why do you think I made the referral?" She believed she had tried "everything in the book" to overcome a problem behavior. But often the "problem" should not be seen as a deficit per se, but as a poor fit between the child and the environment (Bernstein, 2000). The three interventions attempted included moving the boy's seat (isolating and stigmatizing him), calling his mother (blaming Mom was not helpful), and sending him to the principal's office (the boy's preferred intervention—allowing him to escape classwork and get individual attention from the principal, whom he liked). Although the behavior had reportedly been going on "since the beginning of the year," the teacher had tried all of these "prereferral interventions" within a 2-week period, and no data were available to confirm or refute their efficacy. Although it was a lengthy consultation, we successfully intervened with this child, and he did not require a comprehensive evaluation. Whether you use observation methods, a scatterplot, permanent products, or some other data (see Chapter 4), collecting data is necessary to help reduce comprehensive evaluation referrals, and it is legally mandated. For many problems, a functional analysis will reveal that environmental determinants are primarily responsible for a child's poor academic performance or behavior problem. IATs can help teachers solve problems and develop ecologically sound systematic interventions before formal referrals are made.

---

measures are some of the best-made ones. We are convinced that cognitive assessment provides an abundance of valuable information about a student's functioning that cannot be obtained in any other way. A child's overt symptoms may have one or more underlying etiologies, and just treating the symptoms could have a negative effect if the wrong treatment is chosen. For instance, a child with attention problems due to a thought disorder could actually be harmed by treatment with stimulants, the most common treatment for attention-deficit/hyperactivity disorder (ADHD). Case Study 1.1 highlights how essential cognitive assessment can be in recognizing and treating children with special needs.

The implications of Charles's case are profound. Even if a majority of the childhood problems we see do not have a clear biological etiology, missing one child with acute brain deterioration is unacceptable. Will a pediatrician pick this up during a routine well-child visit? Will a teacher or behaviorally oriented psychologist recognize the changes? The answer is likely to be no, not until the condition progresses to a point when it becomes obvious that something is wrong (e.g., seizures, falling down, vomiting). You are on the "front line" of children's cognitive, learning, and socioemotional needs—the first one "on the scene" to recognize whether a child's attention problems are related to ADHD, or absence seizures, or any other number of possible causes. As the front-line intelligence expert, you must remain vigilant to ensure the mental health of the children you serve.

CASE STUDY 1.1. Saving Charles's Life

Charles was classified as having a learning disability and was receiving special education services when he came to the clinic for a second opinion. He had one "full" evaluation in second grade to determine eligibility. Subsequent team reevaluations consisted of record review and some anecdotal data provided by his special education teacher. At each reevaluation, the few team members required by law concluded that Charles still had a learning disability and needed services. Frustrated by Charles's poor progress and the team's refusal to reevaluate him more fully, his parents brought him to a private psychologist. When the cognitive results were compared to his previous results, it was revealed that Charles had experienced a severe decline in overall functioning, and that his profile had changed dramatically. Follow-up evaluation and referral to a neurologist revealed the reason for the cognitive and achievement decline: Charles had developed a brain tumor! If the team members had acceded to the parents' request for a full evaluation (as they legally should have), the cause of Charles's continued school difficulty might have been identified and treated sooner.

This front-line role certainly serves the needs of prevention and early intervention, but keeping vigilant for relationships between cognitive functioning and other sources of data can also yield new insight into a child's characteristics and needs. For instance, you may find cases when a child's history becomes critical in understanding their cognitive, academic, and socioemotional functioning. Some psychologists skip the history section or touch on it briefly, thinking that it is only important to talk about a child's current functioning. Others suggest that you should only address the "reason for referral." Limiting history and your evaluation questions, however, limits your opportunity to meet children's needs. Case Study 1.2 highlights the rele-

CASE STUDY 1.2. Donald and His Orthopedic Disability

Due to begin high school in the fall, Donald was brought to our clinic by his mother for help with vocational planning. A review of the history revealed that Donald had experienced a birth trauma (right-hemisphere cerebral vascular accident or stroke) that led to left-arm/left-leg hemiparesis, some speech impairment, and a fairly serious visual impairment. He was receiving special education services with a diagnosis of orthopedic impairment. His IEP contained some physical adaptations and accommodations, but he was enrolled in regular academic classes. Donald had never received a comprehensive evaluation. Our assessment revealed significant cognitive impairment. Although he had adequate basic skills and language development, his fluid reasoning, visual–spatial skills, and higher-level comprehension skills were all well below average. Consistent with our findings, his academic performance had showed a steady decline over the years, because the use of right-hemisphere cognitive processes increases with age. Only his extraordinary level of motivation and effort had helped him survive the higher grades.

Think of what Donald could have accomplished if his school had done a full evaluation earlier. There would have been time for intensive interventions to remediate some of his difficulties—but, considering his age and years remaining in school, we were left with trying more compensatory strategies. In both this case and that of Charles (see Case Study 1.1), the cognitive assessments revealed important information that drastically affected our interventions. In addition, both evaluations were conducted by psychologists from outside the school system and were paid for by parents. Both sets of parents sought outside help, but what if they didn't, what would have become of Charles and Donald? As front-line advocates of children's needs, we need to recognize that cognitive assessment is a valuable component of what we do as psychologists. We cannot rely on others to make judgments about children's cognitive functioning when the stakes are so high.

vance of taking a more holistic perspective when you are trying to interpret cognitive assessment information.

Intelligence Test Interpretation: Levels versus Patterns of Performance

Having a good understanding of the "cognitive" interpretation strategies of Kamphaus (2001), Kaufman (1994), and Sattler (2001) will provide you with the basis of neuropsychological interpretation discussed in subsequent chapters. Kaufman's "intelligent testing" approach moves from global (IQ) to specific (subtest profiles). He presents a detailed analysis of subtest constructs and recommends idiographic (individualized) analysis of common abilities. Sattler recommends a similar successive-level approach that culminates in a qualitative interpretation. Kamphaus emphasizes an integrative approach for combining qualitative and quantitative data about a child. He recommends a priori hypothesizing and hypothesis testing during the evaluation. O'Neill (1995) formalizes the process by providing an interpretative hierarchy, with Level 1 indicating scores and descriptors, Level 2 including conclusions based on statistical properties, and Level 3 individualizing the interpretation for high-level inferences. As these scholars do, we argue that both nomothetic (normative) and idiographic (individualized) approaches have merit and are not antithetical. In Chapter 3, we present an applied neuropsychological perspective in our CHT model—one that allows for the integration of both product (levels of performance) and process (patterns of performance), and is sensitive to a child's background, environment, and behavior.

Unfortunately, straight subtest profile or pattern analysis can be problematic for a number of reasons. Individual subtests are generally less reliable than cluster or global scores (Anastasi & Urbina, 1997). In addition, these measures are factorially complex (McGrew & Flanagan, 1998), and using a "cookbook" approach of listing all possible skills and influences on a given score is not useful. There are also several interpretations based on "clinical lore," despite strong empirical evidence that these are incorrect (Kamphaus, 1998), and measurement error is more likely to affect interpretation at the subtest level (Macmann & Barnett, 1997), leading some opponents of subtest interpretation to admonish practitioners to "just say no" (McDermott, Fantuzzo, & Glutting, 1990). It is clear that the global IQ or a level of performance interpretation is appropriate for some children. When subtest variability is limited, the IQ seems to be the most parsimonious measure of a person's level of intellectual functioning. As we have noted earlier, IQ is a strong predictor of several important outcomes (Buckholdt, 2001; Kranzler, 2001)—generally those that are equated with success in our society (Brody, 1997).

Although global IQ interpretation may be appropriate for some children, several have suggested that it should not be interpreted when factor or subtest differences are extreme (e.g., Prifitera, Weiss, & Saklofske, 1998). An examination of the pattern of performance in these cases is necessary, because the IQ score is rendered invalid by significant subtest or factor variability (Fiorello et al., 2001). This belief is not merely a philosophical one. Our work (Fiorello et al., 2001; Hale, Fiorello, et al., 2001) demonstrates that the WISC-III IQ should not be interpreted for about 80% of children. In Figure 1.1, we show the unique and shared factor variance of FSIQ for two groups of children—one with flat profiles (no significant Index score differences) and one with variable profiles (one or more significant Index differences). For flat-profile children, the FSIQ appeared to be a fairly good measure of their overall ability, since the shared four-factor variance explained about 64% of the IQ variance. For the variable-profile group, only 2% of the FSIQ variance was made up of the shared variance among the four factors. We have also completed similar analyses for children with learning disorders, children with ADHD, and clinic-referred children. In addition, the results have now been replicated with the DAS standardization

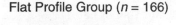

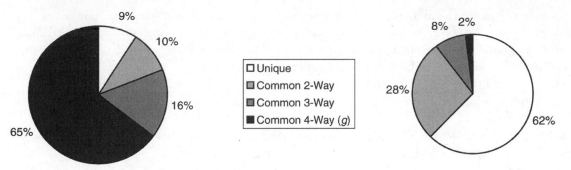

FIGURE 1.1. Comparison of variance sources in WISC-III FSIQ. From Fiorello et al. (2001). Copyright 2001 by Elsevier. Reprinted by permission.

data (Hale, Willis, Dumont, Fiorello, & Rackley, 2004). In all cases, we found that IQ (or, for the DAS, General Conceptual Ability [GCA]) were not interpretable when significant variability was present. However, we did find a variety of interpretable patterns for different subtypes of children, indicating that interpretation and recommendations must be individually tailored.

Our studies of children with learning disorders (Hale, Fiorello, et al., 2001) and replication studies using hundreds of children with and without disorders (Fiorello et al., 2001; Hale, Willis, et al., 2004) confirms that *the IQ should never be interpreted when there is significant subtest or factor variability or scatter.* In addition, even if a child has a flat profile, it is important to recall that intelligence tests may be unfair for children with linguistic or cultural differences, and that IQ scores are intimately related to prior education and experience. Even if a child shows little subtest variability, you must take into account what is actually assessed by the instrument, because no two intelligence tests use the same tasks or administrative format. The scores are not interchangeable, but should instead be interpreted in light of the content processes and content knowledge required by each test. You must remember that IQ scores are probably *related* to ability, but they are not a direct measure of, nor should they be *equated* with, ability.

Although this should provide you with convincing evidence that IQ should not be interpreted when significant factor or subtest variability is present, our research findings have additional implications. You might conclude that interpretation of Index or factor scores is appropriate, but the situation is more complex than that. Children's Index or factor performances can be explained as combinations of unique factor variance, and combinations of shared variance with other factors. This would also apply to the factor scores that are derived from subtests. Similar to IQ, this argument implies that Index or factor scores, rather than being unitary measures of only primary ability, are also factorially complex and require further analysis for each individual child. We do not want to suggest here that every child with significant subtest or factor variability has a disability. We are simply asserting that significant variability warrants the interpretation of cognitive strengths and weaknesses, and that this interpretive strategy is both clinically justified and empirically supported. In addition, because these scores are so factorially complex and interrelated, a simple "cookbook" interpretation approach cannot be employed. Interpretation must take into account not only a child's performance on the test, but also other data from testing, observations, background information, and environment.

Intelligence Test Interpretation: Idiographic Interpretation and Demands Analysis

As a majority of the children we see in clinical practice show significant subtest and/or factor variability, we have no choice but to interpret cognitive processes. Many clinicians in the field apparently agree with this conclusion, as almost 90% of school psychologists use factor scores, subtest profile analysis, or both in interpreting intelligence test results (Pfeiffer, Reddy, Kletzel, Schmelzer, & Boyer, 2000). If psychologists are analyzing intelligence test data beyond IQ, they need a methodology that is likely to lead to more reliable and valid conclusions—conclusions that have ecological and treatment validity. We have developed the CHT model's methodology with this need in mind. The CHT model allows you to form and test hypotheses about a child's performance on cognitive measures, and is designed to link those findings to intervention. Only in this way can we overcome the diagnostic "leaps of faith" (Reschly & Gresham, 1989) that have plagued idiographic interpretation for so many years.

Another problem with traditional profile analysis that must be overcome for accurate idiographic interpretation is similar to the one found for IQ: focusing on the scores instead of on children. The approach we present helps you recognize that different children may achieve the same score on the same task, but for different reasons. Just interpreting a score, without considering *how* the child approached the task, may obscure important differences. Consider the WISC-IV Block Design subtest. One child may glance at the design and put the blocks together correctly without looking at the model, clearly using the visual gestalt to solve the problem. Another may look at the design and then match one block at a time, in a methodical, step-by-step fashion. A third may use a trial-and-error approach, looking back and forth between the model and the blocks, and flipping the blocks over and over until they are in the correct position. Even if all three children obtain the same score, hypotheses about their cognitive functioning will differ, as will recommendations for intervention. This is a major reason why subtest and factor profile interpretation models can also lead to erroneous conclusions. Clinicians using scores for interpretation often assume that there are a finite number of ways to approach a task, instead of considering the process a child uses to solve the problem.

While acknowledging that factor or subtest analysis can lead to error if we are not careful, we even recommend looking at a child's performance on the subtasks within a single subtest. For example, we recently found the WISC-III Digits Forward and Digits Backward subtasks to be differentially related to attention problems: Digits Forward appeared to be a test of short-term rote auditory memory span, whereas Digits Backward seemed to be related to standardized attention, working memory, executive function measures (Hale, Hoeppner, & Fiorello, 2002). In addition, only Digits Backward performance was related to teacher ratings of attention problems. Our demands analysis provides a methodology for analyzing the input, processing, and output demands of individual cognitive tasks, so you can more easily describe a child's strengths and weaknesses in a way that will allow you to develop useful individualized interventions. By testing the hypotheses derived from the measures, and ensuring external validity, you can truly tailor an IEP to a child's needs. The CHT model and demands analysis are described further in Chapters 3 and 4, with forms and tables to assist you in the process.

Factors Influencing Intelligence Test Interpretation

Numerous additional factors can affect the conclusions you draw about a child's test performance, several of which we briefly review here—including test behavior, technical adequacy, linguistic/cultural sensitivity, and ecological validity.

In regard to test behavior, any interpretation must take into account the wide array of child behaviors displayed during testing. Although we all learn about this during graduate school, we tend not to notice the subtle variations in test performance that can affect interpretation (Hale & Fiorello, 2002). Sattler (2002) provides guidelines for observing specific behaviors that may indicate performance variability and psychological problems. These observations, combined with observations in the natural environment and input from parents and teachers, can provide important contextual information for interpreting the child's test performance.

We will assume that you are already familiar with how to assess the technical adequacy of a test—an issue that has been covered extensively elsewhere and thus is not reviewed here. Good resources include Sattler's *Assessment of Children* (2002), and Bracken's classic article, "Ten Psychometric Reasons Why Similar Tests Produce Dissimilar Results" (1988). We would like to stress, though, that no test should be administered to a child unless its reliability, validity, floor, and ceiling are sufficient to permit you to draw conclusions about the child's performance. In addition, you should consider issues of content validity and sample space, to ensure that you are not drawing conclusions about a broad area of skills based on a very small sample of actual behavior.

We have previously discussed linguistic and cultural sensitivity in interpretation, arguing that crystallized abilities or skills are related to prior experience and education. Although crystallized skills are of critical importance in a psychological evaluation, it is essential to remember that they are significantly affected by a child's language, educational experience, and sociocultural background. We have argued that tests measure different things for different children, and this is certainly the case for many children with racial, linguistic, and/or cultural differences. The questions of test appropriateness raised here allow us to review "test bias," a statistical concept that determines whether the statistical properties of a test are the same for different groups. The following questions are often used to determine whether a test or task is biased:

- Is the item difficulty the same for all children?
- Is the reliability the same for all children?
- Is the prediction of school or occupational success from the test scores the same for everyone?
- Is the underlying structure or model of the test the same across groups?

Since modern test developers examine these factors, no modern test of cognitive functioning is statistically biased. However, the absence of bias does not mean that a test is uniformly *fair* for all children. Fairness takes a child's linguistic and sociocultural background, and formal and informal educational opportunities, into account. An IQ score will not be biased as long as it equally predicts school success for all children, but it is not fair to conclude that children with linguistic, sociocultural, or experiential differences are unintelligent because they have a low IQ score.

The relationship between a child's environment and test performance is bidirectional if assessment and intervention are to have ecological validity. Comparing the conclusions about input, processing, and output demands that you draw from a child's performance to indicators of classroom performance and behavior will help establish the accuracy of your interpretations. For example, poor WISC-IV Processing Speed performance may reflect a variety of problems, including limited attention to detail, visual acuity, visual scanning, processing speed, psychomotor speed, fine motor coordination, and/or graphomotor skills. Simply listing these in a report would be a meaningless "cookbook" approach, unrelated to the child's current functioning or to needed interventions. It is your responsibility as a clinician to evaluate these as hypotheses, comparing them to results from other tests and other evaluation information (see Case Study 1.3).

CASE STUDY 1.3. Jordan's Slow and Sloppy Work

Imagine that you have a student, Jordan, who was referred for testing because he was slow to complete his written work. You found that his work samples showed messy writing, with some evidence of poor spacing and coordination. His WISC-IV results revealed poor Processing Speed performance and some difficulty with Working Memory. There are several hypotheses you would be likely to consider. Besides slow processing speed, which might also reflect attentional or affective problems, you might consider deficits in visual tracking, perception, visual–motor integration, fine motor coordination, graphomotor abilities, or executive function. What further testing and observations might you use to test these hypotheses? You might do further testing with something like the Beery Developmental Test of Visual–Motor Integration to decide whether difficulties with visual–motor integration, visual discrimination, and/or fine motor coordination were contributing to the problem. A computer-based test of attention (such as the Conners Continuous Performance Test II), or the CAS Attention or Planning scales, or the NEPSY Attention/Executive Functions subtests might help you decide whether attention or executive function problems were contributing. What behaviors might you see in the classroom that would help you evaluate these different hypotheses? Jordan might show signs of neglect of himself (e.g., appearing disheveled) or of the environment (e.g., missing information from the board). He might bump into other people or not catch baseballs well. Fine motor problems might show up in difficulties with tying shoelaces or fastening his coat. Visual–motor integration problems might lead to a tendency to use "abstract" drawings in art class, as well as the messy handwriting and poor spacing already noted. Copying from the board could be difficult for Jordan, and he might fall behind during note taking or not write the correct information in his notes. Jordan's attention during activities not involving visual–motor skills, such as listening while the teacher reads a story, might indicate whether attention is a problem. And planning and other executive function deficits might reveal themselves in difficulties with transition times (such as getting ready to leave at the end of the day), playing age-appropriate games at recess, or completing complex multistep tasks (e.g., research papers). Finally, Jordan could be depressed, so you might look for signs of mood disturbance, such as flat affect, anhedonia, and withdrawal. It is your job as a clinician to consider all of this information in deciding on a probable cause for Jordan's difficulties, and to work with the teacher to design and monitor an appropriate intervention. This will ensure the ecological validity of your findings.

Although clinical judgment and teacher impressions are important for establishing ecological validity, you should, whenever possible, use direct observation and classroom behavior rating scales to obtain objective information about a child's behavior in the classroom. Systematic observations, whether you use time sampling, interval recording, latency/duration, or event recording, can provide important ecological validity information. Several formal coding systems have also been developed, such as the Ecobehavioral Assessment Systems Software (EBASS; Greenwood, Carta, Kamps, Terry, & Delquadri, 1994), the State–Event Classroom Observation System (SECOS; Saudargas & Lentz, 1986), or the Behavior Assessment System for Children—Student Observation System (BASC-SOS; Reynolds & Kamphaus, 1992). We recommend starting with an anecdotal observation that codes a variety of child and teacher behaviors. After the informal observation, choose specific target behavior(s) and compare the child to a control peer. Sattler (2002) provides a good overview of various observation systems. Another source of ecological validity information can come from behavior rating scales, which are easy to administer and score, and usually have good psychometric properties. As opposed to direct observation methods, ratings sample behaviors over an extended time, so they are useful for both diagnosis and treatment. It important to keep in mind that parent and teacher ratings are subject to bias, due to differing expectations or tolerance for behaviors. Examples of classroom behavior rating scales that have good psychometric characteristics are the Achenbach Teacher Report Form (Achenbach, 2001) and the BASC—Teacher Rating Scale (BASC-TRS; Reynolds & Kamphaus, 1992).

Major Cognitive/Intellectual Assessment Instruments

Cognitive assessment, through the use of one or more of the major intelligence/cognitive assessment instruments, forms the basis of our CHT model. After the initial assessment instrument is administered, the next step is to develop hypotheses about a child's cognitive strengths and needs based on these initial results. The CHT model takes the interpretive process further, in that additional intellectual, cognitive, and/or neuropsychological measures are administered to examine the validity of the original hypotheses. This process continues until possible explanations for a child's classroom performance and behavior have been confirmed or refuted. In CHT, an intelligence/cognitive test can be used as the main first-step instrument, or subtests from the measures can be used to test hypotheses.

In this section, we provide you with a brief overview of the major cognitive assessment instruments we feel are useful in formulating initial CHT hypotheses. They are listed in alphabetical order, not by order of preference or utility. Your choice of instrument should be based on the referral question and on other information gained from prereferral data, observation, and interview. We provide information about the constructs and processes tapped by individual subtests, in order to allow you to begin the process of analyzing a student's strengths and weaknesses. However, further in-depth analyses of these constructs should be individualized for each child, to avoid the tendency to take a "cookbook" approach. The resources listed in Appendix 1.1, such as those by Elliott (1990), Flanagan and Ortiz (2001), Kamphaus (2001), Kaufman (1994), McGrew and Flanagan (1998), and Sattler (2001), should be helpful in understanding the constructs tapped by these measures. In addition, we provide a number of forms helpful for more fine-grained demands analysis of subtest performance in Chapter 4.

Differential Ability Scales

An adaptation of the British Ability Scales, the DAS (Elliott, 1990) is an increasingly popular cognitive assessment measure since its introduction in the United States in 1990. One important feature of the DAS is the separation of Verbal Ability, Nonverbal Reasoning Ability, and Spatial Ability tasks into cluster scores for meaningful interpretation. Another is the use of diagnostic subtests to assess rote and long-term memory and processing speed. The DAS also has a preschool version available, although we focus on the school-age version as being most useful for CHT. Several DAS subtests are useful in looking at essential cognitive processes and memory. The DAS includes brief measures of basic achievement skills, but these should really be seen as screening measures of word reading, math calculation, and spelling. Table 1.1 presents the core and diagnostic DAS subtests and the constructs they purportedly tap, which are helpful in interpretation.

The DAS was revised for the United States in 1990 and is currently undergoing revision. It was standardized on 3,475 children from ages 2 years, 6 months (2-6) to 17 years, 11 months (17-11), stratified on age, sex, race/ethnicity, region of the United States, and education level of the parents (as a measure of socioeconomic status [SES]). The sample matches the 1986 U.S. census information very well, but demographics have changed since then. In addition to the stratification variables, the sample was also monitored for appropriate representation of children with disabilities and school dropouts, as well as gifted students. An oversample of African American and His-

TABLE 1.1. Differential Ability Scales (DAS)

Subtest	Constructs purportedly tapped
Core subtests	
Verbal Ability	
Word Definitions	Vocabulary task; child defines words orally; task depends on lexical/semantic knowledge and expressive language skills.
Similarities	Child expresses the similarities among three named objects of increasing abstractness; task requires verbal knowledge, concept formation, reasoning, categorical thinking, and oral expression.
Nonverbal Reasoning Ability	
Matrices	Multiple-choice matrix reasoning task; it requires fluid abilities/deductive and inductive reasoning; multiple-choice response may foster trial-and-error approaches.
Sequential and Quantitative Reasoning	Fluid reasoning task requiring inductive reasoning; later items involve oral response to a pattern in a numerical series; task assesses both fluid reasoning and quantitative reasoning—may tap math skills if impaired.
Spatial Ability	
Recall of Designs	Child uses pencil and paper to reproduce visual designs presented for 5 seconds each; test of visual memory, visual–spatial orientation; visual–motor integration and motor skills also required.
Pattern Construction	Block Design-like task; it requires perceptual analysis and synthesis; it can be interpreted with or without time bonuses.
Diagnostic subtests	
Recall of Digits	Test of rote short-term auditory–sequential memory; no working memory component; quick aural presentation of digits to discourage rehearsal.
Recall of Objects— Immediate	Card is presented with numerous pictures, which are then named, and card is taken away; three trials to recall the objects with time limits; memory task with a learning component and both visual and verbal cues.
Recall of Objects— Delayed	The same objects are named after a delay; test of long-term memory, using both visual and verbal cues.
Speed of Information Processing	Speeded clerical task; child indicates by pencil the circle with the most boxes/highest number in a row; test of attention, visual scanning, and processing speed.

Note. Diagnostic subtests are optional.

panic children was also drawn, in order to allow for bias analyses. Reliability studies indicate that the GCA is reliable enough for individual decision making at the school-age level, with coefficients ranging from .95 to .96 across age levels. Individual subtests have average reliabilities ranging from .70 to .92. Some subtests at some ages do not have sufficient reliability for individual interpretation, most notably Recognition of Pictures for out-of-level testing above age 7 and the alternate (untimed) Pattern Construction above age 12. The floors are not adequate for low-functioning children at the youngest ages, though the core subtests have good floors starting at age 4-6. Ceilings are adequate until age 13 for all core subtests, though some of the diagnostic subtests have inadequate ceilings for high-functioning children starting at about age 7-6. The availability of out-of-level testing makes the DAS especially attractive for assessing children with disabilities.

Also helpful is the availability of the Special Nonverbal Composite—though, as we have noted before, an assessment that avoids language and crystallized abilities has limited utility in neuropsychological assessment. The DAS provides extensive evidence of validity, including concurrent validity indices with the WISC-R of .84 to .91 at different ages, and predictive validity indices of .46 to .66 with the Basic Achievement Skills Individual Screener, .40 to .76 with group achievement tests, and .45 with grade point average. Factor analyses confirm the structure of the test, which shows increasing differentiation of abilities over time.

We especially like the way the DAS uses three main factors at the school-age level; it separates the Nonverbal Reasoning Ability cluster from the Spatial Ability cluster, thereby deemphasizing the traditional verbal–nonverbal dichotomy. We also like the addition of diagnostic subtests to explore strengths and weaknesses. The technical manual is extremely complete and helpful for designing an appropriate assessment for an individual child, and it also presents information about special-group studies and bias analysis. The interpretation section is especially strong, providing a great deal of information about the cognitive processes required for subtest performance; this information makes the DAS very useful for CHT. Subtest performance should be used to generate hypotheses about functioning and subsequently examined within the context of all other information sources (Dumont, Willis, & Sattler, 2001). As with all the measures we discuss, the DAS has several drawbacks, necessitating the use of additional hypothesis-testing measures. First, it does not explore the complexity of language processes as well as some other cognitive measures do, and teasing out crystallized knowledge from language functioning is difficult. The assessment of memory is a good idea, but the DAS memory-related subtests are not sufficient for a comprehensive memory assessment. The Recall of Designs subtest is a measure of spatial skills, but interpretation is influenced by both visual memory and praxis components. Finally, the DAS does not appear to have an adequate measure of executive function, but the Nonverbal Reasoning subtests are certainly affected by executive skills.

Stanford–Binet Intelligence Scales: Fifth Edition

The SB5 (Roid, 2003), the most recent revision of the venerable Stanford–Binet, returns to the tradition of measuring high-functioning and low-functioning individuals well, while updating the content to take advantage of modern cognitive/intellectual functioning theory. The SB5 is designed to assess five basic constructs from CHC theory as described earlier (Fluid Reasoning, Knowledge, Quantitative Reasoning, Visual–Spatial Processing, and Working Memory), using both verbal and nonverbal formats. Keep in mind, though, that many of the nonverbal tasks still require the student to understand spoken directions. Table 1.2 outlines the tasks and processes involved in each subtest, summarized across age levels.

The SB5 was standardized on 4,800 people aged from 2 to over 85 years, stratified on age, sex, race/ethnicity, region of the United States, and education level of the examinee or parents (as a measure of SES); it generally matches the demographic characteristics of the 2000 U.S. census well. In addition, 6.8% of the sample were receiving special services (special education or clinical treatment), and 2% of the sample had been identified as intellectually gifted. Reliability studies indicate that the Full Scale score is highly reliable, with coefficients of .97 to .98 across all age groups. Individual subtests have average reliabilities ranging from .84 to .89, although some subtests have reliabilities below .75 at some ages. The SB5 has good evidence of validity, including concurrent validity indices of .82 to .84 with the Wechsler scales, as well as predictive validity indices of .66 to .84 with the WJ-III Achievement and .53 to .80 with the Wechsler Individual Achievement Test—Second Edition. Factor analyses confirm that the structure of the test (verbal

TABLE 1.2. Stanford–Binet Intelligence Scales: Fifth Edition (SB5)

Subtest	Constructs purportedly tapped
Nonverbal	
Fluid Reasoning	Object series/matrix analogies; multiple-choice inductive reasoning, using objects/pictures.
Knowledge	Procedural knowledge at lower levels (child demonstrates named activity); child identifies or explains picture absurdities at higher levels.
Quantitative Reasoning	Variety of quantitative reasoning tasks, including block counting, manipulatives, multiple-choice visual quantitative series, and visual equations; spatial visualization or visual memory, in addition to reasoning ability, required on several items.
Visual–Spatial Processing	Formboard at lower level; form patterns (tangram-like activity) at higher level; task requires spatial visualization and visual–motor skills.
Working Memory	Object constancy, then block-tapping span, then a working memory version of block tapping; visual–sequential memory task, with working memory component at higher levels.
Verbal	
Fluid Reasoning	Lower levels require giving verbal descriptions of complex pictures, categorizing picture chips in different ways, and categorical labeling; higher levels involve verbal absurdities and analogies; reasoning ability and expressive language required.
Knowledge	Lower levels include body part naming and expressive labeling of nouns, then verbs; higher levels require defining words presented visually and aurally.
Quantitative Reasoning	Lower levels include oral counting and naming numerals; higher levels require solving word problems; pencil and paper are permitted, to minimize the impact of working memory.
Visual–Spatial Processing	Lower levels include use of spatial terms; higher levels include oral directions for map-like drawing and answering directional questions.
Working Memory	Lower levels require repetition of sentences; higher levels require answering a series of aurally presented questions, then repeating the last word, in order, of each question.

Note. Actual SB5 tasks differ according to which levels are administered.

vs. nonverbal, and the five-factor model) is supported. Extensive studies of special groups are also presented in the comprehensive technical manual. The floor of most of the subtests is not adequate for low-functioning examinees until about age 4-6, although Rasch-based "change-sensitive scores" are provided for the factor scores below the 2-0 age equivalent level. The ceiling appears adequate at all age levels. Full Scale scores can range from 40 to 160, and the change-sensitive scores provide for interpretation below and above those levels, making the SB5 especially useful for low- and high-functioning individuals.

The expansion of the factors assessed by the SB5 is welcome, and it is more closely aligned than the SB-IV was with current cognitive and neuropsychological theory. As is true with all of these screening measures, a number of important cognitive skills are not adequately assessed on the SB5, necessitating supplemental testing within our CHT model. The SB5 yields factorially complex tasks, with interpretation complicated by the extended age range (2–85+). The actual process demands of a subtest vary depending on the level administered, which in turn depends on the student's age and performance on the verbal or nonverbal routing task; all this makes interpretation somewhat inconsistent from child to child. Much practice with many different types of children will be needed before you can acquire good "head norms" about this test. As a result, it is essential to task-analyze a particular subtest, and this task analysis may change for different children of different chronological age. As the SB5 is a fairly recent addition to the test market, there has been little empirical examination of it thus far. It will be important to see how the SB5 is used for both clinical and research purposes in the years to come.

Wechsler Intelligence Scale for Children—Fourth Edition

The WISC-IV (Wechsler, 2003) is the most recent revision of the cognitive assessment instrument most commonly used in the schools. Moving beyond the Verbal–Performance dichotomy, this revision takes into account recent theoretical advances and research findings on cognitive functions and processes to provide a four-factor model. It also provides subtest and supplemental process scores (such as separate scores for Digits Forward and Digits Backward—a change that was warranted, given our [Hale, Hoeppner, & Fiorello, 2002] findings) to aid in the interpretation of strengths and weaknesses. The WISC-III (Wechsler, 1991) four-factor model has been revised and strengthened to make interpretation at the Index score level even more useful. There are fewer, but psychometrically stronger, subtests for the Verbal Comprehension, Perceptual Reasoning (formerly Perceptual Organization), Working Memory (formerly Freedom from Distractibility), and Processing Speed Indices. In addition, several supplemental tests can be used for hypothesis testing, including a new supplemental Verbal Word Reasoning subtest, which is useful in assessing verbal reasoning and abstraction. There has been an increase in the fluid reasoning aspect of the Perceptual Reasoning Index with the addition of Matrix Reasoning and Picture Concepts, and a deemphasis on speed and time bonuses. Table 1.3 provides information about the individual WISC-IV subtests and their interpretation.

The WISC-IV was standardized on 2,200 children from ages 6 to 16, stratified on age, sex, race, parental education level, and region of the United States. The standardization sample appears to match the 2000 U.S. census information quite well. Reliability studies indicate high reliability, with the FSIQ score reliability averaging .97 across the age levels. Individual subtests have average reliabilities ranging from .70 to .90, and the four Index scores have reliabilities ranging from .88 to .94. The WISC-IV provides considerable evidence of validity, including a concurrent validity index of .89 with the WISC-III. Studies relating the WISC-IV to measures of achievement, memory, adaptive behavior, and emotional intelligence have also been completed. Factor analyses confirm the structure of the test across the age groups, with some secondary loadings of subtests indicating the continued factorial complexity of this measure. We expect that the new WISC-IV will continue to be a popular measure of cognitive functioning, widely accepted by schools; it also moves closer to the neuropsychological model of cognitive functioning, and away from the oversimplified verbal–nonverbal split.

The WISC-IV thus appears to be a much better instrument than its predecessors, and it remains a psychometrically sound instrument consistent with the Wechsler tradition. Stimuli have been improved and directions simplified to reduce the impact linguistic deficits could have on understanding tasks, especially for the Processing Speed subtests. While this is a much improved measure, there are still a number of important cognitive functions that are indirectly assessed or not measured at all by the WISC-IV. For instance, there is no good measure of auditory processing/phonemic awareness, although the Working Memory and Verbal Comprehension subtests assess this indirectly. Most WISC-IV subtests remain factorially complex, making them rich clinically, but difficult to interpret at times. We recommend the continued use of the Information

TABLE 1.3. Wechsler Intelligence Scale for Children—Fourth Edition (WISC-IV)

Subtest	Constructs purportedly tapped
Verbal Comprehension	
Similarities	Expressive language needed to identify how two words or concepts are alike; task requires vocabulary/semantic knowledge, categorical thinking, and verbal reasoning ability.
Vocabulary	Early items require picture naming; later items require defining words presented aurally; requires vocabulary knowledge, crystallized abilities, and expressive language.
Comprehension	Child explains reasons for common social rules; task requires expressive language, implicit knowledge, and reasoning about social situations and conventions.
(Information)	Child answers factual questions from science, social studies, and the humanities; test of long-term memory retrieval and crystallized knowledge.
(Word Reasoning)	Child determines most probable response based on a sequence of verbal clues; task requires verbal comprehension, abstract verbal reasoning ability, and generation of alternative concepts.
Perceptual Reasoning	
Block Design	Child views a model or picture and reproduces it with red and white blocks; task includes time limits and time bonuses (untimed score available); measure of visual orientation, spatial processing, analysis and synthesis, and processing speed.
Picture Concepts	Child chooses a picture from each of two or three rows to form a group with a common characteristic; measure of fluid reasoning and abstract categorical reasoning ability.
Matrix Reasoning	Pictorial analogies, including pattern completion, classification, analogical reasoning, and serial reasoning; multiple-choice responses; measure of fluid reasoning and nonverbal concept formation.
(Picture Completion)	Child views a picture and identifies the important missing part; task requires visual scanning, long-term memory, spatial perception of meaningful stimuli, and part–whole relationships.
Working Memory	
Digit Span	Consists of two tasks—repeating a series of digits presented aurally in forward and then later in backward sequence; total score is combined, but process scores are available for forward (rote auditory–sequential memory) and backward (attention, working memory, and executive function).
Letter–Number Sequencing	Aurally presented letter and number sequences, repetition of numbers in ascending order and letters in alphabetical order; test requires attention, auditory working memory, mental manipulation, sequencing, and simple verbal expression.
(Arithmetic)	Child solves orally presented arithmetic problems within a time limit; task requires increased working memory load and decreased mathematical ability, as compared to WISC-III Arithmetic.
Processing Speed	
Coding	Child copies marks into symbols (younger) or symbols matched to numbers (older), according to a visually presented code; similar to Symbol Search, with more graphomotor and visual memory demands.
Symbol Search	Child visually scans and marks whether target symbols are in an array of abstract symbols; measure of visual perception of abstract symbols, scanning, processing speed, and graphomotor abilities (low).

(continued)

TABLE 1.3. (*continued*)

1. (Coding Incidental Learning Recall) and 2. (Coding–Symbol Copy)	1. Measure of paired-associate symbol recall, free recall, and paired-associate digit recall (task requires visual memory and graphomotor reproduction of symbols/numbers, as well as retrieval of numbers, symbols, and number–symbol associations). 2. Visual–motor/graphomotor/processing speed task.
(Cancellation)	Child scans pictures and marks target pictures; measure of processing speed, visual attention, vigilance, and visual neglect; process scores available for structured and unstructured presentation items.

Note. Subtests in parentheses are optional.

subtest, even though this is now an optional subtest. This subtest has a long history of sensitivity (but not specificity) for diagnosing learning problems, and it is probably one of the best measures of crystallized abilities available. It is also sensitive to memory retrieval problems. Similarly, we have always found the comparison of Arithmetic with achievement subtests measuring math computation useful, so we would suggest including it in some CHT evaluations. Because there has not been much research conducted with the WISC-IV, given its brief history, additional comment is difficult at this time. However, as was the case with the Wechsler Adult Intelligence Scale—Third Edition and now the WISC-IV, these tools are becoming increasingly useful in clinical practice and more closely aligned with current cognitive and neuropsychological theory.

Woodcock–Johnson III Tests of Cognitive Abilities and Tests of Achievement

The WJ-III series of tests (Woodcock et al., 2001) differs in two ways from the other cognitive assessment tools presented here: It was designed specifically to assess the full range of cognitive abilities according to the CHC theory, and it attempts to minimize factorial complexity by assessing specific, narrow abilities. In addition, CHC theory is in many ways compatible with current neuropsychological theories about cognitive functioning, and the test interpretation materials include clinical interpretations based on information-processing theory. This means that the WJ-III is an excellent source of individual subtests for CHT, despite the fact that it was not designed primarily as a neuropsychological assessment instrument. The scoring software provides clinical clusters measuring executive function, attention, and working memory. Table 1.4 presents information about a variety of useful tests from the WJ-III battery.

The WJ-III Cognitive was standardized on 8,818 people aged from 2 to over 80 years, stratified on age, sex, race, ethnicity (Hispanic or non-Hispanic), U.S. region, community size, type of school (public, private, or home), and parental educational and occupational level. The standardization sample appears to be an excellent reflection of the U.S. population, with the weighting procedure minimizing the effects of sampling differences. Reliability studies indicate high reliability, with the General Intellectual Ability (GIA) score having a median reliability of .97 (Standard) and .98 (Extended) across all ages, and the CHC clusters having median reliabilities ranging from .81 to .95. Individual tests have median reliabilities ranging from .74 to .97, with a few tests dropping below the .75 level at some ages. The WJ-III Cognitive has extensive evidence of validity, with content coverage of all of the major cognitive functions identified in CHC theory, which makes it an excellent source of supplemental tests for CHT. Factor-analytic evidence supports the cluster structure. Validity evidence includes concurrent validity indices of .71 to .76 with the WISC-III and .76 with the DAS. Predictive validity indices range from .58 to .72 for the GIA—

TABLE 1.4. Woodcock–Johnson III Tests of Cognitive Abilities (WJ-III Cognitive) and Selected Tests of Achievement (WJ-III Achievement)

Test	Constructs purportedly tapped
Comprehension–Knowledge (Gc)	
Verbal Comprehension	Task measures knowledge of spoken vocabulary—naming, synonyms, antonyms, analogies; sensitive to word-finding problems, not complex language.
General Information	Task assesses knowledge of general information/vocabulary; child answers function questions about objects.
Picture Vocabulary (Achievement)	Task measures semantic knowledge of picture–word associations; sensitive to word-finding problems.
Bilingual Verbal Comprehension*	Task taps lexical knowledge and language development in bilingual Spanish–English individuals.
Long-Term Memory and Retrieval (Glr)	
Visual–Auditory Learning	Test of word–symbol analogy learning and associative memory; "reading" visual rebus sentences; ability to benefit from feedback.
Visual–Auditory Learning—Delayed	Child recalls previously learned associations; measure of long-term memory retrieval.
Retrieval Fluency	Child names items within category, given time limit; measure of ideational fluency and retrieval.
Story Recall (Achievement) and Story Recall—Delayed (Achievement)	Narrative memory task; immediate recall of story elements presented aurally, and recall after delay.
Memory for Names* and Memory for Names—Delayed*	Associative memory task, using selective reminding format to associate nonsense names with pictures of aliens; long-term memory retrieval and fluid reasoning necessary.
Visual–Spatial Thinking (Gv)	
Spatial Relations	Child identifies part drawings that combine to make whole geometric figure; later items require mental rotation; multiple-choice format.
Picture Recognition	Task assesses visual working memory; pictures are presented briefly, and child recognizes stimulus from distractor array; verbal mediation and labeling minimized.
Planning	Child traces a series of geometric line drawings without duplicating a line or lifting the pencil; task requires spatial visualization and executive functions of planning and inhibition.
Visual Closure*	Child names common drawing represented by disconnected lines; measure of holistic perception, closure, prior knowledge, and verbal retrieval.
Block Rotation*	Child identifies two rotated drawings of a target drawing from group of distractors; test of visualization; spatial relationships, mental rotation.
Auditory Processing (Ga)	
Sound Blending	Child combines phonemes presented aurally to form English words; test of auditory attention, phonetic coding, auditory sequencing, and assembly.
Incomplete Words	Child identifies English words presented aurally with one or more phonemes deleted; test of phonetic coding, analysis, and closure.
Auditory Attention	After training of simple words presented aurally, child distinguishes words against increasing background noise; measure of auditory attention, speech sound discrimination, resistance to auditory distortion.

(continued)

TABLE 1.4. *(continued)*

Auditory Processing (*Ga*) *(continued)*

Sound Patterns—Voice*	Child indicates sound patterns differing in pitch, rhythm, or sound as same or different; test of sound discrimination without language component.
Sound Patterns—Music*	Child indicates whether sound patterns are the same or different (may differ in pitch, rhythm, or sound); test of sound discrimination with no meaningful language component.

Fluid Reasoning

Concept Formation	Child identifies rules underlying set formation, using simple geometrical figures; early items involve teaching and feedback; later items require use of "and" and "or" rules; inductive reasoning task with grammatical component.
Analysis–Synthesis	Child uses presented pictorial rules to solve color-combining problems; early items involve teaching and feedback; deductive/sequential reasoning task.
Number Series*	Child uses the mathematical principle underlying a number sequence to identify a missing number; quantitative reasoning task with no significant working memory load.
Number Matrices*	Child uses the mathematical principle underlying a matrix of numbers to identify a missing number; quantitative reasoning task with no significant working memory load.

Processing Speed

Visual Matching 1 and 2	Child finds matching figures (1) or numerals (2) in an array and circles them; measure of visual scanning and perceptual speed.
Decision Speed	Child chooses the two items from an array that go together conceptually and marks them; measure of attention and semantic processing speed.
Pair Cancellation	Child identifies pairs of objects matching a target pair in a full-page array and circles them; measure of attention, concentration, and processing speed.
Rapid Picture Naming	Confrontational naming of pictures under a time limit; test of rapid automatic naming skill.
Cross Out*	Child finds matching figures in a row of distractors and marks them with a pencil.

Short-Term Memory

Numbers Reversed	Auditory working memory task; child repeats an aurally presented list of digits in reverse sequence; measure of attention, working memory, and executive function.
Auditory Working Memory	Child encodes and retrieves a list of mixed items and digits presented aurally, repeating items in order, then digits in order; increasing role of strategic planning; good measure of working memory and executive function.
Memory for Words	Child remembers a list of unrelated words presented aurally; measure of auditory–semantic memory without significant working memory component.
Understanding Directions (Achievement)	Child points to elements in a complex picture in sequential order, corresponding to an aurally presented direction; test of attention, working memory, language comprehension, and praxis.
Memory for Sentences*	Child repeats sentences of increasing length; test of auditory–semantic memory and crystallized knowledge of syntax.

Note. Asterisks (*) indicate tests available in the WJ-III Diagnostic Supplement.

Standard and the WJ-III Achievement clusters for school-age children, generally exceeding prediction of those same clusters with the WISC-III FSIQ score. Special-group studies and bias analyses are also presented in the extensive technical manual. One of the most useful aspects of the examiner's manual is the section on adapting testing for students with disabilities.

A unique aspect of the WJ-III is the weighting of the GIA according to the g loading of each test at the individual age levels, making it a robust measure of overall cognitive ability if one should be needed. However, this can also affect the GIA if a child with a disability performs poorly on one of the highly weighted tests. The test authors have made significant attempts to limit the factorial complexity of the measures, which is both a positive and a negative aspect of the WJ-III. Limiting the factorial complexity gives you better diagnostic direction and a means to link assessment to intervention data. However, there is a drawback to such specific subtest construction. For instance, the WJ-III may not measure complex language as well as other measures. This is obviously good if you want to differentiate language from crystallized abilities, but not if you want to examine the integrity of the left hemisphere, as we will discuss in later chapters. Another similar pro-and-con decision involves the Spatial Relations subtest. In an attempt to avoid having motor skills and speed contaminate spatial processing, a multiple-choice response format is used, which makes this subtest very different from a perceptual organization/production task. Therefore, a child with poor spatial skills can deduce the correct answer (or at least get partial credit) by using a trial-and-error approach. Finally, although the WJ-III authors would probably not condone this, there is a tendency for practitioners to interpret these subtests with a "one construct, one subtest" mentality, which does not accurately reflect the cognitive skills required for the subtest (Hale & Fiorello, 2002). As we have suggested, you need to consider the input, processing, and output demands of all measures you administer. With all that being said, the WJ-III provides numerous subtests covering a wide variety of cognitive skills; it is thus a very useful CHT screening tool and source for supplemental tests for CHT evaluations.

A Practitioner's Guide to Intelligent Cognitive Assessment

Before we leave our blueprint for the practice of psychological assessment in the schools, we think it is important to take a minute to review the major points presented in the preceding sections. This blueprint serves as a foundation for much of the material presented in later chapters. Table 1.5 provides a number of suggestions we originally presented in a journal article a few years ago (Hale & Fiorello, 2001). You may have other points you would add to this synthesis, and this is a good idea. However, probably the most important thing you can realize from this discussion is that intellectual/cognitive assessment is a part of what we do, but it is by no means the only thing we should do as psychologists. These measures are only tools for use in a more comprehensive service delivery model. In the chapters that follow, we will demonstrate the utility of CHT evaluations in helping children with their learning and behavior problems. This is the true test of any psychological measure or approach.

Now that we have reviewed the basic issues related to intelligence/cognitive assessment, the factors involved in administration and interpretation of intelligence tests, and the commonly used measures of intellectual/cognitive functioning, let us turn our attention to several critical issues related to the practice of psychological assessment in the schools. These issues include identification of children with disabilities, complying with clinical and legal mandates, trends in service delivery, and linking assessment results to intervention.

TABLE 1.5. A Practitioner's Guide to Intelligence Testing.

- Intervene to assess. Reducing the number of referrals will result in better evaluations and ecological validity.
- Read recent theoretical, empirical, and practice-oriented literature on intelligence and its assessment.
- Explore neuropsychological literature for cognitive, achievement, and behavioral applications.
- Supplement core intellectual assessment tool with additional measures to ensure that all cognitive domains are assessed.
- Assess attention, memory, and executive functions as critical constructs related to school success.
- Interpret crystallized abilities in light of cultural, linguistic, and experiential background.
- Administer new measures of learning and memory to assess potential, rather than inferring it from crystallized measures.
- Interpret both level and/or pattern of performance based on individual child's profile.
- Interpret global intellectual scores only when there is no significant factor or subtest variability.
- Use demands analysis to examine input, processing, and output demands, but avoid "cookbooking," and test hypotheses to ensure ecological validity.
- Test assessment and intervention hypotheses over time, using single-subject experimental designs.
- Avoid confirmation bias; consider alternative hypotheses and interventions to meet child's unique needs.

Note. From Hale and Fiorello (2001). Copyright 2001 by the American Psychological Association. Adapted by permission.

CRITICAL ISSUES IN ASSESSMENT SERVICE DELIVERY

Identifying Children with Disabilities

Unlike private practitioners, psychologists in the schools (or any other individual team members, for that matter) cannot diagnose a child with a disability. The multidisciplinary team determines eligibility, placement, and services under special education law. Therefore, you are not individually responsible for identifying the child's problem or proposing a solution. How does this affect your diagnostic practice? First, differential diagnosis is determined by examining whether a child meets diagnostic criteria specified by professional consensus. A neurologist has criteria for diagnosing epilepsy, a psychiatrist has criteria for diagnosing Tourette syndrome, and a speech–language pathologist has criteria for diagnosing developmental aphasia. A particular professional does an evaluation and diagnoses the child as having a particular disorder. What are the advantages and disadvantages of such diagnoses? Are they relevant for identification, eligibility, placement, or treatment?

Does having a disorder automatically make a child eligible for special education services? The short answer is *no*; the school's multidisciplinary team must review and gather additional information to decide whether the child is eligible. You don't have to be intimidated into providing special education for a child just because a physician wrote "Dyslexia—provide special education" on a prescription pad! In fact, the word "dyslexia" has little utility in and of itself, other than to suggest that the child has a reading disorder. Several times, I (Fiorello) have been asked by interns whether they can "diagnose" a child. I tell them that as licensed psychologists, they may be professionally qualified to diagnose a child as having a specific disorder. But does the diagnosis make the child automatically eligible for special education services? The answer is no. Even though you are a school professional and a member of the multidisciplinary team, you cannot unilaterally decide that a child is eligible. This can be frustrating when you know a child has a disorder and meets requirements for clinical diagnosis, but does not meet the necessary IDEA criteria for services. It is important to remember that every referral must go through the team process to decide whether it meets all three eligibility questions:

- Does the child meet criteria for one or more of the existing disability categories?
- Does the child's disorder have an adverse impact on educational performance?
- Does the child need special instruction to ensure a free, appropriate public education (FAPE)?

You probably have appropriate concerns about diagnosing and labeling children, but it is important to consider that many children suffer negative effects when their school problems are obvious to teachers and peers, even without the label (e.g., see Riddick, 2000). A potentially more serious problem is the risk that a child's parents and teachers—and even the child—might have lower expectations because of the label (Rosenthal & Jacobson, 1968), although this tendency appears to decrease over time (Harris, 1991). Labels serve multiple purposes, but it is important to realize that they are only useful if they allow for accurate identification of child needs and help to identify appropriate services for the child. A label can tie together disparate problems, making them more understandable and manageable for all involved in the child's care. Is a child's attention problem due to ADHD, depression, learning disability, or a host of other possibilities? You cannot just have parents complete a checklist or respond to DSM-IV criteria and say, "Joey has ADHD, predominantly inattentive type." You must make every attempt to find out the exact nature of the attention problem, so that appropriate interventions can be attempted. We recommend the following principles for identifying or labeling children in order to maximize the benefits and minimize the costs:

- Never avoid clinical labels just because determining educational disability does not require them.
- Never use a label to "admire the problem"—ensure that it leads to appropriate interventions.
- Never label a child unless you professionally believe that the label is accurate.
- Never use a label as an excuse for a child's continued difficulty or failures.

Complying with Legal Mandates

As you are well aware, the IDEA and Section 504 of the Rehabilitation Act (1973a, 1973b), and the Americans with Disabilities Act (ADA, 1990) are the major pieces of legislation governing the practice of psychology in the schools. Intended to serve the educational needs of children with disabilities, the IDEA provides for identification of all district students with disabilities (i.e., "Child Find"); comprehensive evaluations of children's educational needs; and specially designed instruction and related services to ensure that each child receives an FAPE. Section 504 of the Rehabilitation Act and ADA are both civil rights laws that protect children and adults with disabilities from discrimination. Schools are required to provide reasonable modifications and accommodations to ensure that students have access to educational programs, but they are not required to develop an IDEA-specified IEP to serve the child. Instead, they should develop a 504/ADA plan that specifies the modifications and accommodations the student will receive. Qualifying for protection under 504/ADA is different from that under the IDEA. The student must have a "physical or mental impairment that substantially limits at least one major life activity"

(ADA, 1990), but there is little further definition of such terms as "substantial" or "limits." As a result, qualifying as disabled under 504/ADA is typically less stringent than qualifying under the IDEA. As a result, team members may see 504/ADA qualification as a backup plan for any student who doesn't qualify for IDEA services.

Sometimes the issue is not just serving children's needs; it also involves funding those services. Schools do not receive any federal money for providing 504/ADA accommodations, so from a strictly behavioral perspective, there is less incentive for serving children under these laws. This can be a real tragedy for some children, as needed services may be withheld until a struggling child falls far enough behind to qualify under the IDEA. Meeting children's needs should not be based on whether they fit categories or labels, but this is often the case. This is especially true in cases that are less clear-cut, when you may be pressured to identify a child as having a disability so that the child can receive services. In this case, legal and ethical expectations may come into conflict, leading you to a less than desirable outcome. As you are a child advocate, you must decide how to resolve this situation. You must remember that if children meet IDEA or 504/ADA criteria, they must be provided with services. However, it is important to remember that whether children are served under the IDEA or 504/ADA, they should be served in the least restrictive environment (LRE) to meet their needs. The fact that children are identified as having a disability doesn't mean that they cannot be fully served in a regular education or inclusive classroom. Being labeled with a disability doesn't automatically mean a need for segregation.

Trends in Service Delivery

Since the original passage of Public Law 94-142, special education law has called for students to receive a FAPE in the LRE, while still receiving a continuum of services. The law requires that each child's needs must be individually assessed, eligibility must be determined, and *then* the team must decide where the instruction should take place. You should never decide to label a child because you have room in this classroom, or a team member has time to work with him. It is presumed that the primary placement should be in general education with supplementary aids and services, but if that is not possible, more restrictive placement options must be available. Three factors need to be taken into account when deciding what the LRE is: the academic benefits versus costs of each setting for the student; the socioemotional benefits versus costs of the settings; and the degree of class disruption that makes satisfactory education impossible. These are somewhat vague factors, but considerations worthy of examination nonetheless.

Does this mean that the IDEA mandates inclusion? The answer is no. "Inclusion," and its predecessor, "the regular education initiative," are not part of the law; definitions in the research literature and schools vary, but inclusion is not synonymous with LRE. Inclusion is commonly defined as serving a student with a disability in the same class with necessary supports and services (e.g., Lipsky & Gartner, 1995). The major difference is that the IDEA requires a continuum of placements to be available if education in the inclusive setting is *not* working. A child with an auditory processing disorder will struggle in a lecture class without a note taker, written notes/instructions, tape recording, or some other accommodation to meet his or her needs. In addition, the IDEA considers resource room support to be part of the supplementary supports and services provided in the LRE (Heumann & Hehir, 1994), whereas many inclusion advocates consider resource room placement as noninclusive. However, full inclusion of a youth with mental retardation in an English literature class that studies Shakespeare is a clear example of a case when the LRE is not the regular classroom. It is important to remember that the LRE is really the LRE *that meets the child's needs*. What does the research tell us about inclusion? When appropriate services and supports are provided, the outcomes of inclusion are generally positive both for the student with a disability and for his or her classmates (McGregor & Vogelsberg, 1998). But if a student with a disability is placed in a general education classroom without appropriate services, continued academic and peer difficulties can be expected (Fiorello, Liebman, & Levine-Dawson, 1999). If regular education teachers are provided with training and staff resources, most are willing to serve children with disabilities in their classrooms. However, the team members must ensure that the child's IEP services are provided in the LRE, and must keep in mind that the LRE is not always the regular education classroom.

We have now examined your involvement in assessment and placement of children with disabilities, which have been the traditional concerns of psychologists practicing in the schools. However, these are not the only roles of school psychologists. Before we end this introductory chapter, it is important to consider one more area that has been largely neglected until relatively recently in the literature and in training programs. This role—one that is essential to serving the needs of children—may be the one that you feel least comfortable with: linking assessment results to intervention.

Linking Assessment Results to Intervention

Too many times, psychologists tend to see themselves solely as diagnosticians. As a psychologist conducting individual evaluations in the schools, you have *two* major objectives: identifying child strengths and difficulties (i.e., problem identification and analysis), and providing interventions to ameliorate the problems (i.e., instructional design, implementation, and evaluation). Linking assessment information to intervention is one of the main tasks of school assessment teams. Researchers examining aptitude–treatment interactions (ATIs) or the diagnostic–prescriptive model have attempted to identify links between specific assessment results and interventions. Early ATI researchers focused on identifying modality or perceptual weaknesses in children (e.g., auditory or visual); implementing group interventions to strengthen children who apparently had the weak modality; and, finally, assessing whether the targeted ability or related achievement improved as a result of the intervention. Reviews of that early research have consistently found limited support for either the modality or perceptual training model of instruction (e.g., Kavale & Forness, 1999; Ysseldyke & Sabatino, 1973), or for matching academic instruction to students' strongest learning modality (auditory, visual, or kinesthetic) (Braden & Kratochwill, 1997; Kavale & Forness, 1999).

Because most ATI research occurred when investigators had poor assessment instruments and a limited understanding of brain functions, early ATI research failures have been attributed to a variety of reasons. Many cognitive constructs were poorly defined or poorly measured (Ysseldyke & Salvia, 1974). Often, heterogeneous groups were simply divided at the median to define "high" and "low" groups. Treatments were also poorly defined or implemented without integrity checks (Reynolds, 1988). Because of the failure to find ATIs, Ysseldyke and Sabatino (1973) recommended assessing and remediating academic skill deficits instead of searching for "aptitudes." It is interesting to note that the seeds of Ysseldyke's fervent "paradigm shift" position advocating elimination of intelligence testing were probably sown after his own early ATI study was unsuccessful. As Braden and Kratochwill (1997) have noted, however, the fact that ATIs weren't established in the past doesn't mean that they can't be established in the future, especially at the single-subject level of analysis. Changing the focus from the *content* of test items (e.g., auditory, visual) to the underlying psychological *processes* (Reynolds, Kamphaus, Rosenthal, & Hiemenz, 1997) may be the key to understanding the true nature of brain–behavior relationships for individual children.

Since these early studies, research on ATIs has continued to be inconsistent. Psycholinguistic training, which identifies students' weaknesses and provides individualized, prescriptive instruction, has led to significant improvement in students' language skills (Kavale & Forness, 1999). In fact, speech–language pathologists, occupational therapists, and physical therapists frequently use single-subject designs to conduct ATIs. Another ATI study found that a mediated learning program was best for preschool special education students with language impairments, but that a direct instruction model was best for those with higher language skills (K. N. Cole, Dale, Mills, & Jenkins, 1993). More recently, performance on the CAS (Naglieri & Das, 1997) Planning, Attention, and Simultaneous and Successive Processing scales has been linked to intervention with the PASS Remedial Program (PREP). ATI studies using the PREP have shown improvement not only in Simultaneous and Successive Processing scores, but also in reading and mathematics scores (Das et al., 1994). Other ATI studies by Naglieri and his colleagues (Naglieri & Gottling, 1995, 1997; Naglieri & Johnson, 2000) found that children with low Planning scores improved their math scores more after planning- and strategy-based instruction than did children who initially scored higher on Planning. Other studies have used the Kaufman Assessment Battery for Children (Kaufman & Kaufman, 1983) simultaneous or sequential processing strengths to develop instructional interventions, but with limited success (Ayres & Cooley, 1986; Fisher, Jenkins, Bancroft, & Kraft, 1988; Good, Vollmer, Creek, Katz, & Chowdhri, 1993). However, as we will see in Chapter 3, this may be in part due to the assumption that the left hemisphere processes information sequentially and the right hemisphere processes simultaneous information—an assumption that does not adequately reflect current beliefs about hemispheric functioning (Bryan & Hale, 2001).

There have been numerous calls for ATI research that examines the multivariate nature of cognitive constructs, and that addresses the technical issues associated with treatment development and integrity (e.g., Braden & Kratochwill, 1997; Deno, 1990; Reynolds, 1988; Speece, 1990). In addition to improvements in the "aptitude" portion of the equation, the "treatment" portion needs attention. Two models, a deficit remediation model and a strength-based instructional model, are possible. When deficit remediation instruction is explicitly linked to academics, either during initial training or through a training transfer process, improvement in academic performance has been demonstrated. The strength-based model has theoretical support, but has been inadequately assessed (Reynolds, 1988). Because group models of ATI may obscure individual differences, single-case research using within-subject experimental methodology has been recommended as the preferred way to study ATIs (Braden & Kratochwill, 1997). In later chapters, we will argue that our CHT model—which is composed of neuropsychological interpretation of test data, verification of initial hypotheses, methods for ensuring ecological validity, and continual monitoring of intervention effectiveness—meets ATI standards, providing a method for individualized service delivery to children.

APPENDIX 1.1. Further Readings in the Intelligence Debate

Carroll, J. B. (1993). *Human cognitive abilities: A survey of factor-analytic studies.* New York: Cambridge University Press.

Das, J. P., Naglieri, J. A., & Kirby, J. R. (1994). *Assessment of cognitive processes: The PASS theory of intelligence.* Needham Heights, MA: Allyn & Bacon.

Elliott, C. D. (1990). *Differential Ability Scales: Introductory and technical manuals.* San Antonio, TX: Psychological Corporation.

Flanagan, D. P., & Ortiz, S. (2001). *Essentials of cross-battery assessment.* New York: Wiley.

Gardner, H. (1983). *Frames of mind: The theory of multiple intelligences.* New York: Basic Books.

Gottfredson, L. S. (1997). Why g matters: The complexity of everyday life. *Intelligence, 24,* 79–132.

Gresham, F. M., & Witt, J. C. (1997). Utility of intelligence tests for treatment planning, classification, and placement decisions: Recent empirical findings and future directions. *School Psychology Quarterly, 12,* 249–267.

Horn, J. L., & Noll, J. (1997). Human cognitive capabilities: Gf-Gc theory. In D. P. Flanagan, J. L. Genshaft, & P. L. Harrison (Eds.), *Contemporary intellectual assessment: Theories, tests, and issues* (pp. 53–91). New York: Guilford Press.

Jensen, A. R. (1998). *The g factor: The science of mental ability.* Westport, CT: Praeger.

Kamphaus, R. W. (2001). *Clinical assessment of child and adolescent intelligence* (2nd ed.). Needham Heights, MA: Allyn & Bacon.

Kaufman, A. S. (1994). *Intelligent testing with the WISC-III.* New York: Wiley.

Macmann, G. M., & Barnett, D. W. (1997). Myth of the master detective: Reliability of interpretations for Kaufman's "intelligent testing" approach to the WISC-III. *School Psychology Quarterly, 12,* 197–234.

McDermott, P. A., Fantuzzo, J. W., & Glutting, J. J. (1990). Just say no to subtest analysis: A critique on Wechsler theory and practice. *Journal of Psychoeducational Assessment, 8,* 290–302.

McGrew, K. S., & Flanagan, D. P. (1998). *The intelligence test desk reference (ITDR): Gf-Gc cross-battery approach to intelligence test interpretation.* Boston: Allyn & Bacon.

Reschly, D. J., & Ysseldyke, J. E. (2002). Paradigm shift: The past is not the future. In A. Thomas & J. Grimes (Eds.), *Best practices in school psychology IV* (Vol. I, pp. 3–20). Bethesda, MD: National Association of School Psychologists.

Sattler, J. M. (2001). *Assessment of children: Cognitive applications.* La Mesa, CA: Author.

Sternberg, R. J. (1997). The triarchic theory of intelligence. In D. P. Flanagan, J. L. Genshaft, & P. L. Harrison (Eds.), *Contemporary intellectual assessment: Theories, tests, and issues* (pp. 92–104). New York: Guilford Press.

Woodcock, R. W. (1993). An information processing view of Gf-Gc theory. *Journal of Psychoeducational Assessment (WJ-R Monograph),* 80–102.

CHAPTER 2

|_|_|_|_|_|_|_|_|_|_|_|_|_|

A Model of Brain Functioning

Science, like life, feeds on its own decay. New facts burst
old rules; then newly divined conceptions bind old and
new together into a reconciling law.

—WILLIAM JAMES

A DEVELOPMENTAL PERSPECTIVE

Child Neuropsychology, or Neuropsychology Applied to Children?

From the outset of our discussion on brain–behavior relationships, it is important to recognize
that there are important brain differences between children and adults. Every child neuropsychology text will make this proclamation with great conviction, and then report literature on adult
patients. Before you conclude that this is a condemnation of such texts, it is not. There is much
more literature on adults' brain functioning than there is on children's, so this limitation affects almost all neuropsychological texts, including ours. Our book is somewhat different, however, in
that we focus on developmental issues and primarily report literature relevant to clinical practice
with children. Although there is much less brain research on children than on adults, this situation is changing at a phenomenal rate. With the advent of noninvasive neuroimaging techniques,
there are more and more data both on typical children and on those with disabilities. The broad
conclusion that there are significant brain–behavior differences between adults and children is
true, but recent findings continue to dispel early beliefs that children with genetic or traumatic
causes for their learning problems do not suffer the same deleterious effects as adults with these
conditions. In fact, quite the contrary may be true: Some studies have suggested more adverse
outcomes for children, depending on the developmental level at which a disorder is first recognized and treated. In addition, it is important to realize that we are talking not just about developmental issues applied to genetics and trauma, but about the many types of learning disorders that
have been linked to abnormal brain development (Kolb & Fantie, 1997).

Development must be taken into account in any consideration of brain function and dysfunction. We always find it interesting when clinicians say that they can diagnose attention deficits in

43

3-year-olds. I usually say, "If children don't have attention deficits when they are 3 years old, I think something is wrong." The areas of the brain that control attention and executive function at this age are quite immature. Surely, given its deleterious effects on cognition and behavior, early identification of attention-deficit/hyperactivity disorder (ADHD) is a good thing; as we will see, however, the brain areas that help control attention are not well developed in preschoolers, and maturation of these areas is not complete until adolescence or early adulthood. We need to recognize that developmental changes occur in children, and at different rates for different children. Are the differences we are seeing during an assessment due to these developmental differences, to a genetic condition, to abnormal neural organization, to a "typical fall" head trauma, or to the psychometric characteristics of the test we're using? Only seasoned clinicians—as investigators with a wealth of clinical acumen—can answer these questions. However, let's begin our understanding with what we know about typical and atypical developmental changes and the brain.

Typical and Atypical Brain Development

Developmentally, many changes occur in the central nervous system even before birth, and they continue throughout life. There are four distinct phases of early brain development: the birth of neurons, cell migration, cell differentiation/maturation, and cell death/synaptic pruning (Kolb & Fantie, 1997). Once the neural tube develops, the process of cellular migration and neuronal differentiation can take place in earnest. As the brain is developing, neurons are differentiating and connecting with other neurons. The bumps (*gyri*) and crevices (*sulci*) are poorly defined during gestation, leaving the fetal brain looking somewhat like undifferentiated Jell-O until the last trimester. At birth, the brain has the differentiated neurons in the correct place (for typical children), but the brain weighs only about one-quarter of its final weight. What continue to take place after birth, and at extraordinary rates, are the branching and connections of dendritic "trees" and the myelination of axons, which account for the majority of hemispheric growth after birth (Majovski, 1997). *Myelin* is the substance that helps speed transmission of the nerve impulse, which is what "white matter" is all about. At the same time, a pruning of neurons and connections takes place, and this process also continues throughout the lifespan. The brain builds and destroys neuronal connections in an attempt to reach an equilibrium that optimizes beneficial pathways and minimizes dysfunctional ones. This is the genesis of complex cognitive processes through cortical maturation—a process that takes place primarily during the first 5 years of life (Whitaker, Bub, & Leventer, 1981). Cortical maturation begins with the primary sensory zones; it then progresses to the cortical areas that integrate information (association areas); and finally the frontal lobe, the last and most important cortical area, fully develops (Davies & Rose, 1999). The discontinuous nature of frontal lobe development is of particular importance, because changes in learning and behavior are associated with these changes (Thatcher, 1992). Interestingly, dramatic changes in cortical growth appear to coincide with Piaget's stages of cognitive development (Epstein, 2001).

There has been much debate about the critical periods for brain growth and recovery of function following brain injury, or the brain's "plasticity" (Johnson, 1999). Certainly there is evidence that the young child's brain is malleable or plastic, and that sparing of a cognitive function that should be lost can occur following brain damage (Hecaen, 1976); however, this may result in limitations for both the function that is spared *and* the other functions as well (Fletcher, Levin, & Landry, 1984). In the case of language recovery following left-hemisphere damage, the presumption is that the right hemisphere takes over for language functions. Unfortunately, some language functions, as well as some right-hemisphere functions such as spatial skills, may be lost. This is known as the "crowding hypothesis" (Teuber & Rudel, 1962), because language is said to "crowd" out the spatial skills. Interestingly, language may be more likely to crowd out nonverbal skills than vice versa (Teuber, 1975). Though it is now generally accepted that some behavioral dysfunction will occur following brain injury or insult to a child, the developmental stage clearly affects the manifestation of the cognitive and behavioral deficits observed (Kolb & Fantie, 1997). The brain-environment interaction is by definition bidirectional, affecting how brain structures develop propensities for information processing, and placing constraints on brain plasticity (Johnson, 1999). Although we are only now beginning to sort through the relationship between genotype and phenotype, it is clear that many psychological disorders have a genetic basis (see Goldstein & Reynolds, 1999). As we develop a greater understanding of the genetic basis of childhood disorders, such as learning disorders and ADHD, we can begin to evaluate their unique developmental pathways, and possibly to determine different developmentally appropriate assessment techniques and intervention strategies for each condition.

A REVIEW OF MAJOR BRAIN STRUCTURES

A Semantic Road Map

In addition to the terms and definitions found in Appendix 2.1, the following terminology review will help you navigate the following discussion of major brain structures. If this information is new to you, take a few minutes to study these terms and then quiz yourself. Recall that the central nervous system is primarily composed of *gray matter* (the nerve cells) and *white matter* (myelinated axons that speed transformation of information). We like to think of the gray matter as the houses and neighborhoods, and the white matter pathways as streets and highways. (Remember this metaphor later in the chapter, when we speak of the left hemisphere as having more houses and the right hemisphere as having more highways.) There are lots of bumps, each called a *gyrus* (plural: *gyri*), and each fissure or valley that separates the gyri is called a *sulcus* (plural: *sulci*). Clusters of axons, or *tracts*, often connect different brain areas and some are called *commissures.* The largest commissure is the *corpus callosum*, which serves to connect a majority of the left hemisphere with a majority of the right. In an intact brain, almost any information sent to one hemisphere is easily transmitted across this large commissure. A similar structure is the *cingulate*, which allows the front parts of the brain to communicate with the back parts. *Afferent* is related to input, or projections entering into a structure; *efferent* is related to output, or projections leaving a structure. *Ipsilateral* means the same side of the body, and *contralateral* means the opposite side. Basically everything above the lower brainstem crosses over, or *decussates*, from one side of the brain to the other half of the body. However, the increasingly important cerebellum subserves the ipsilateral side of the body. Structures are said to be *superior* or *dorsal* if they are on the top or in front, whereas *inferior* or *ventral* typically reflects bottom or posterior. Finally, *lateral* often refers to the side, away from the midline, and *medial* suggests the middle. There are many structures (especially subcortical ones) that are given different names or identified as belonging to different systems, depending on the resource. The important thing for you to remember is the general location of the structures and how they interact with each other. For further information and detail, please refer to Appendix 2.2.

Unless otherwise noted, the following five excellent sources have served as the basis for much of the following neuroanatomical and neuropsychological material. These resources include a classic neuropsychology text (Kolb & Whishaw, 1996), a neuroanatomy and neuropathology text (Reitan & Wolfson, 1985), a clinical child neuropsychology handbook (Reynolds & Fletcher-Janzen, 1997), a prominent neuroscience text (Gazzaniga, Ivry, & Mangun, 1998), and a renowned text on the left and right hemispheres (Springer & Deutsch, 1998). All are highly recommended for further reading.

The Supporting Cast: Subcortical Structures Serving the Neocortex

Although the majority of this chapter focuses on neocortical brain structure and function (i.e., the occipital, temporal, parietal, and frontal lobes), it is important to review the major forebrain and brainstem structures involved in neuropsychological and cognitive processes. Table 2.1 presents the major forebrain structures (which also include the neocortex) and their purported functions. This overview is a necessary oversimplification, but resources with greater detail are provided in Appendix 2.2. The basal ganglia have rich interconnections between cortical and subcortical structures, including the cerebellum. These ganglia were originally relegated to only a motor role, but our appreciation of their importance has grown in recent years; they are now known to be involved in executive, motor, and sensory functions (Middleton & Strick, 2000). In addition, dysfunction of the basal ganglia structures and their frontal cortical–subcortical loops has been linked to several childhood disorders, including ADHD, obsessive–compulsive disorder, and the disorder that has symptoms of both, Tourette syndrome. The amygdala is sometimes included as part of the limbic system, because it is involved in recognition and recall of emotional stimuli (Adolphs, Tranel, Damasio, & Damasio, 1995). The limbic system has been considered the "emotional brain" for many years, but the roles of the hippocampus in memory encoding, consolidation, and possibly retrieval, and of the cingulate gyrus in attention and executive control (Casey et al., 1997; J. D. Cohen, Botvinick, & Carter, 2000; Gehring & Knight, 2000), suggest that this conceptualization may not fully reflect the complexity of this system. Although significant research efforts continue to provide understanding into the functions of these structures, findings often reinforce their complex rather than simplistic nature.

We now move to the brainstem (see Table 2.2). The diencephalon consists of four structures that regulate body functions. The thalamus is of particular importance because almost all sensory and motor systems are influenced, making it the "Grand Central Station" of the brain. With its close partners, the frontal lobes and the basal ganglia, the thalamus is now being implicated in several childhood disorders. The hypothalamus, with its involvement in the endocrine system and maintaining homeostasis, is considered the autonomic center of the brain. It affects drives related to eating, drinking, sexuality, and rest. It is near the optic chiasm, where the vision "crosses over"

TABLE 2.1. Overview of Forebrain Structures

Brain area	Associated structures	Function	Associated activities
Basal ganglia/striatum	Caudate, putamen, globus pallidus	Motor	Posture, tone, motor activity, response coordination, sequencing, attention, working memory, executive functions
Limbic	Hippocampus	Memory	Encoding/consolidation
	Amygdala	Emotion	Approach–avoidance, emotional valence
	Cingulate	Executive	Orientation, inhibition, monitoring

TABLE 2.2. Important Subcortical Structures

Brain area	Associated structures	Function	Associated activities
	Diencephalon		
Epithalamus	Pineal body	Body rhythms	Sleep–waking and other activity cycles
Thalamus	Lateral geniculate body	Relay station	Visual
	Medial geniculate body	Relay station	Auditory
	Pulvinar	Attention	Sensory filter
Hypothalamus	Pituitary gland	Homeostasis	Regulation of hunger–thirst, temperature, sleep, and hormones
	Other subcortical structures		
Tectum	Superior colliculi	Vision	Visual modulation
	Inferior colliculi	Hearing	Auditory modulation
Tegmentum	Red nucleus	Motor	Voluntary movement
	Substantia nigra	—	(related to basal ganglia)
Cerebellum	Vestibulocerebellum	Body position	Balance, posture, eye movement
	Spinocerebellum	Gross motor	Sensory–motor integration for locomotion
	Neocerebellum	Fine motor	Movement initiation, maintenance, sequencing
Pons/medulla	Sensorimotor	Ascending–descending tracts, cranial nerves	
Reticular formation		Arousal	Level of consciousness

(see our discussion of the occipital lobe, below). Because it secretes melatonin, the pineal body of the epithalamus has been associated with circadian rhythms (e.g., sleep–waking cycles). Pineal tumors can occur during puberty, so dramatic changes in sleep patterns (outside the normal teenage experience!) should be evaluated further. The red nucleus and substantia nigra have rich interconnections with the basal ganglia structures, and, along with the cerebellum, are involved with regulation of motor functioning and learning. Among the other brainstem structures, the cerebellum has gained a great deal of attention in recent years. In fact, its involvement in many cognitive processes and its association with several psychological disorders suggest that it is almost a minibrain unto itself. It is interesting that the cerebellum affects the ipsilateral side of the body, suggesting that it is possibly serves the function of a cortical check-and-balance system, because the cortical areas all affect contralateral regions. Consistent with this hypothesis, the cerebellum seems to be intimately involved in timing, learning, memory, and coordinating cognitive functions (Ivry, 1993; Rapoport, van Reekum, & Mayberg, 2000). Finally, the net-like reticular formation, with its involvement in cortical tone, serves as an important mediator of attention as Luria's (1973) first functional unit—the unit for regulating tone, waking, and mental states. As we will see, many of Luria's principles and much of his theory still dominate the field of neuropsychology today. Although much has been discovered since his writings, and advances in the field have allowed us to reconceptualize Luria's (1973) *The Working Brain*, his seminal works still serve an important foundation purpose.

We have come to learn much more about these subcortical structures in recent years, and to appreciate the contributions they make during cognition. In fact, although humans can survive without the cortex, their daily lives would be quite limited, as they would be entirely dependent on others for survival. These subcortical structures are also implicated in many learning and other psychological disorders. However, subcortical dysfunctions are more likely to be recognized by physicians and neurologists, because their symptoms are often readily apparent and somewhat easier to assess than cortical dysfunctions. As a result, we place greater emphasis on the cortical brain areas in the following sections. Cortical deficits are likely to be identified by physicians as "soft signs" that require further neuropsychological investigation. They are also more likely to present as learning and behavior problems in the classroom. However, we believe that school practitioners should learn to identify the signs and symptoms of subcortical as well as cortical dysfunctions, as the processes subserved by both types of functions are intimately related and often clinically inseparable.

THE TWO-AXIS MODEL OF BRAIN FUNCTIONING

Laws of Cortical Functioning

To begin to understand how these cortical and subcortical structures interact with each other to produce cognition and behavior, we must identify two important dimensions or axes to aid in interpreting cognitive processes from a neuropsychological perspective: the "posterior-to-anterior axis" and the "left-hemisphere-to-right-hemisphere axis." First we describe each of the four lobes—the occipital, temporal, parietal, and frontal lobes. This section can serve as a guide for interpreting brain–behavior relationships on the posterior-to-anterior (input-to-output) axis. Following this section, we discuss lateralization of function—the second important distinction necessary to explore the differential processing capabilities of the left-hemisphere-to-right-hemisphere axis. Before we explore the nature of these axes, it is critical to note what we term the two fundamental "laws of cortical functioning" in our exploration of brain–behavior relationships:

1. No complex human behavior can be linked to one specific brain area; most brain–behavior relationships require an examination of interrelated brain networks.
2. There is much individual variability in cortical organization and function; differences within individuals can be greater than differences between individuals.

The Posterior–Anterior Axis and Cerebral Cortex

Table 2.3 provides an overview of the four lobes of the cerebral cortex. The four lobes, as well as the limbic system and basal ganglia (described earlier), constitute the telencephalon. An oversimplified, but useful, distinction among the functions of the four lobes is as follows: The occipital lobe processes visual information; the temporal lobe receives auditory information; the parietal lobe is responsible for the touch or somatic senses; and the frontal lobe governs motor output (and all behavior, for that matter). Therefore, the three posterior lobes are grossly associated with receiving afferent or input information, and the frontal lobe is responsible for efferent projections or output. However, all cortical structures have "superhighway" tracts or commissures that allow information to be sent to or received from other brain areas.

Before we begin to explore the function of each lobe in detail, it is important to review some important physical landmarks that will be referred to later. Figure 2.1 highlights some important gyri from a lateral (side) view. The two hemispheres are separated by the longitudinal sulcus or

TABLE 2.3. Overview of Cortical Structures and Major Functions

Brain area	Associated structures	Function	Activities
Cortex	Frontal lobe	Motor	Praxis—drawing/writing
	Parietal lobe	Somatosensory	Gnosis—feeling/texture/pressure
	Temporal lobe	Auditory	Hearing—understanding/memory
	Occipital lobe	Vision	Seeing—objects/words/faces/color

fissure, but commissures (connections) allow the hemispheres to communicate. The central sulcus separates the frontal motor area from the parietal somatosensory area. Simply put, anything posterior from the central sulcus is responsible for receiving afferent or sensory input; anything anterior is involved in efferent or motor output. However, as we will discuss later, the anterior and posterior areas interact with each other, so that they are involved in almost every aspect of cognition. The lateral sulcus (often called the sylvian fissure) separates the frontal (motor output) from temporal (auditory input) lobes, and one can see the central sulcus extends laterally to separate the frontal from parietal (somatosensory input) lobes. For the other demarcations, the boundaries are less clear. This is not without reason: The occipital, parietal, and temporal lobes have intricate interconnections that are necessary for processing complex visual, somatosensory, and auditory information. So the parietal–occipital–temporal "junction" is not typically demarcated clearly, as this region processes all types of information, not just one sense. Given this caveat, the boundary between the parietal and occipital lobe is conveniently named the parietal–occipital sulcus, and the preoccipital notch is sometimes identified as separating the occipital lobe from the temporal lobe.

Luria's Working Brain and the Two Axes

Over three decades ago, the noted Russian neuropsychologist A. R. Luria provided us with a conceptual understanding of how the posterior–anterior and left–right axes work together to produce

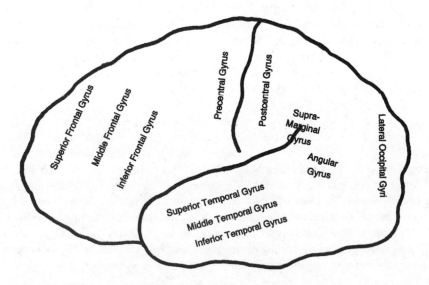

FIGURE 2.1. Lateral view of major gyri.

complex behavior. Although parts of his theory have been questioned, and many of his initial findings about patients with brain damage have been elaborated and expanded upon, Luria's *The Working Brain* (1973) still serves as a seminal work in neuropsychology. His ideas provide a conceptual understanding of the basics of brain–behavior relationships, which will serve you well as you begin to explore the posterior–anterior axis represented by the four lobes of the neocortex. There are three basic tenets of Luria's model: (1) The brain is hierarchically organized (from basic zones to complex zones); (2) the cortical areas diminish in specificity (from simple processing of stimuli to complex integration demands); and (3) they increase in lateralization of function (from undifferentiated cells to unique hemispheric systems). In-Depth 2.1 elaborates on these basic tenets of Luria's theory, the "laws of functional organization."

IN-DEPTH 2.1. Luria's Working Brain

Luria's first law of functional organization is his principle of *hierarchical organization* of individual cortical zones. This has to do with how information is processed and/or behaviors are produced. According to this model, the body sends afferent information to the subcortical structures and then to the *primary* cortical zones. There are three primary zones for the different senses—one each in the occipital (vision), temporal (auditory), and parietal (somatosensory) lobes. This information is then elaborated on in *secondary* zones or *association cortex*. Finally, there is the *tertiary cortex* or the "zone of overlapping," where all information is eventually processed, regardless of origin and type. It is in the tertiary cortex that the highest levels of comprehension and understanding take place. According to Luria's model, input proceeds in a hierarchical fashion from primary to secondary zones and then to the zone of overlapping, the tertiary cortex. For motor functions, the opposite occurs: The tertiary cortex provides the idea and plan; next, the secondary motor cortex provides a motor program; and then the primary motor cortex dutifully carries out the act. Luria's notion *is* largely accurate in representing how the brain processes information and produces behavior, but current research suggests that there are multiple parallel pathways and processes, some of which bypass different zones. However, Luria (1973) correctly noted that these zones form an interdependent system, and that disruption in one zone is likely to affect another. It is well known that a focal brain lesion can cause initial loss, and then subsequent loss of function in the interconnected areas in the system—a process called *diaschisis*.

Luria's second law of functional organization suggests that there is *diminishing* specificity as one ascends the hierarchical zones (or *increasing* specificity as one descends the frontal motor route from tertiary to primary cortex). That is, the primary cortex is very specific in addressing only one sensory modality, whereas the tertiary cortex can address all of them. At the occipital–parietal–temporal "crossroads" described later, structural boundaries become blurred, and multiple complex cognitive processes take place within this "zone of overlapping."

Luria's third law of functional organization is related to the progressive *lateralization* of function. As information ascends the sensory hierarchy, and is processed by association cortex that is less modality-specific, it is more likely that subsequent processing will take place in one hemisphere or the other. Although some have interpreted Luria (1973a, 1980b) as suggesting that successive processes occur in the left hemisphere, and that the right hemisphere processes simultaneous information, this is an oversimplification of his theoretical and clinical presentation. According to Luria's model, it is not the type of information that distinguishes between the hemispheres; it is the manner in which they organize and represent information (Majovski, 1997). It is this third law—the one addressing lateralization of function—that has evolved dramatically since Luria's time. These changes are discussed in the section of this chapter on the left–right axis.

It is also important to note that Luria (1973) described three "principal functional units" in the brain. As noted earlier, the reticular system and related structures are primarily responsible for Luria's first functional unit, which is the unit for regulating tone or waking. Luria noted that without the first functional unit, higher levels of cognition are unlikely. Quoting his colleague Pavlov, Luria noted that optimal cortical tone is critical for organized goal-directed activity. You can easily envision this construct of "cortical tone," especially when your morning coffee is wearing off! The posterior occipital, parietal, and temporal areas represent Luria's second functional unit—the unit for receiving, analyzing, and storing information. The anterior (output) cortex is responsible for Luria's third functional unit—the unit for programming, regulating, and verifying mental activity. As the cortical area responsible for the third functional unit, Luria described the frontal lobes as the "superstructure" responsible for governing the entire brain. Through this claim about the frontal lobes may seem somewhat overzealous, current evidence suggests that Luria's contention is largely correct, especially for higher-level mental activities. The frontal lobes are the "brain manager" (Hale & Fiorello, 2001), basically governing almost every aspect of cortical functioning.

Concerning the development of function, Luria (1973) argued that there is a gradual development of cognitive skills from anterior to posterior: New skill acquisition requires more of the (anterior) third functional unit, but once a skill becomes mastered or routinized, the (posterior) second functional unit becomes more important in performing the learned task (Goldberg, Harner, Lovell, Podell, & Riggio, 1994). More importantly, as we describe later in the chapter, there appear to be hemispheric differences in processing novel and routine information. We now begin our discussion of the four lobes of the brain, but keep in mind that there is support for Luria's notion that the four lobes work concertedly to perform most cognitive tasks, in a type of gradiential fashion (Goldberg, 2001). As you will see, disruption or damage to one area is likely to affect the others. Is this patttern of performance due to primary dysfunction to a particular area, or is it due to another area that affects the performance you see? You will learn to ask yourself this question repeatedly in clinical practice. For instance, neglect of self and environment may look like frontal ADHD, but it is caused by dysfunction of the parietal lobes. Why is this important for us to know? The frontal type of ADHD is more likely to respond to medication treatment. This is why differential diagnosis requires a thorough understanding of the complexity of neuropsychological processes before these processes can be related to achievement and behavior domains.

AN AXIS DIVIDED: I. VISUAL PROCESSES AND THE OCCIPITAL LOBE

Visual Pathways: From Eye to Occipital Lobe

Before visual information can be processed by the occipital lobe, the information must be processed by the eye and sent to it. Afferent information from the retina of the eye is sent to the occipital lobe mainly via the optic nerve, thalamus, and superior colliculus. The left visual field projects to the right hemisphere, and the right visual field goes to the left hemisphere. Damage to the pathways can lead to loss of vision in one eye—or, if the damage 'is after the optic chiasm (where crossover occurs), then it is likely to cause loss of vision in half of each eye contralateral to the injury. Several cranial nerves control horizontal or vertical eye movement, iris (pupil) size, and eyelid movement. When you are concerned about a child's visual functioning, it is important to check each of the visual fields (each eye has four quadrants) and look for differences in pupil size or reaction to light, as well as eyelid function. After entering the lateral thalamus, two main types of pathways emerge from the lateral thalamus to the occipital lobe: the *M-pathway*, which will eventually lead to processing of motion and contrast; and the *P-pathway*, for eventual processing of contrast, color, location, and orientation. This visual division of labor continues and becomes more detailed in the occipital lobe, where the P pathway divides in two (one P pathway leads to perception of color and contrast, and the other to perception of location and orientation). Working in concert with the pulvinar, the superior colliculus affects these processes in the occipital lobe. It is responsible for detection and orientation to visual stimuli, and has been associated with visual attention (Gazzaniga et al., 1998). However, as we will see later, the concept of attention is multifaceted and requires several interconnected brain regions.

Occipital Lobe Structure and Function

The occipital lobe has several distinct areas that process different aspects of visual stimuli and are depicted in Figure 2.2. These regions are identified as the *striate*, or *primary visual cortex*, and the *extrastriate*, or *association visual cortex*. Simply put, the primary visual cortex receives the information from the visual pathways described above, and then sends this information to the association cortex, where "interpretation" begins. Sometimes you will read descriptions of brain areas in terms of Brodmann's (1909) areas (e.g., 17, 18, 19), and sometimes you will read descriptions using a contemporary V nomenclature (V1, V2, dV3, VP, V4, V5). For the purposes of clinical assessment, it is important to note that different areas exist and do different things. Afferent information from the M and P pathways is received by the primary cortex. In Figure 2.2, the lower visual field is represented *above* the calcarine sulcus, and the upper visual field is represented *below* this landmark. If a stimulus is located in the peripheral visual fields, it will be processed medially. If it is in the center of the visual field, it will be processed by the most posterior cortex. This suggests that damage to the most posterior part of the occipital lobe could lead to loss or partial loss of vision in the center of the visual field, but that such an injury is less likely to affect peripheral vision. The different aspects of processing are discussed in In-Depth 2.2, but for the remainder of this

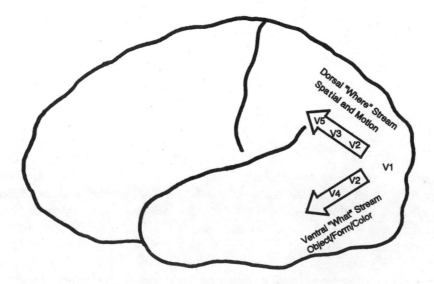

FIGURE 2.2. Structure and function of the occipital lobe.

IN-DEPTH 2.2. The M and P Pathways

For the primary visual cortex, Gazzaniga and colleagues (1998) provide a nice summary of the three distinct processing areas related to the M and P pathways. As can be seen in the table below, the structures related to the two P pathways include some for color and contrast perception (called *blobs*) and some for form, location, and orientation (called *interblobs*). The M pathway is important for processing contrast and motion, and has been associated with reading disorders. This pattern is continued in the secondary association cortex, but here the structure of the cortex has led to a different distinction—one of "stripes" (thin, thick, and pale). As can be seen, the M pathway cells lead to perception of motion and contrast, whereas the two P pathways lead to perception of color, contrast, location, and orientation.

	M pathway	P pathway	
		Occipital lobe structures	
V1	Layer 4b	Blobs	Interblobs
V2	Thick stripes	Thin stripes	Interstripes
		Cell stimulus response	
Contrast	High	High	Low
Location	Low	Low	High
Motion	High	Low	Middle
Color	Low	High	Middle
Orientation	Middle	Low	High

It is important to note that the pathways are responsive to other stimuli as well. This differential response is important, because damage to one occipital region but not another can lead to "blind spots" (scotomas) in the visual cortex, and to misperception of form, color, motion, or location. Individuals with these blind spots are usually not aware of them, because rapid eye movements (nystagmus) help compensate or "fill in" the missing information. Although this compensation is important, task performance may be impaired or slowed as a result.

section, we refer to these areas as *primary cortex* and *association cortex*. Those interested in further discrimination of association areas can also refer to the sources mentioned earlier, or to other sources in Appendix 2.2.

From the primary cortex to the secondary and other association areas, the pathways become quite complex and interrelated, but their distinction becomes important in our study of visual-perceptual brain–behavior relationships. These pathways extend *beyond* the occipital lobe to the parietal and temporal lobes, so differential diagnosis requires an independent understanding not only of the occipital, temporal, and parietal lobes, but of how they interact with each other. As stated earlier, the differentiation of the M and P pathways continues in the primary cortex and becomes elaborated in the association cortex. From there, the beginning of the *dorsal stream* (occipital lobe to parietal lobe) and *ventral stream* (occipital lobe to temporal lobe) becomes apparent in the association areas. The dorsal stream receives input that originated in the M pathway system, but the ventral stream receives input coming from both the M and the two P pathways. To make the connection between the occipital and respective lobes, the dorsal stream requires the superior longitudinal fasciculus, and the ventral stream uses the inferior longitudinal fasciculus. Although an oversimplification, you may read literature that talks about the dorsal stream as the "where" pathway and the ventral stream as the "what" pathway (Ungerleider & Mishkin, 1982). Recognize that these two streams form the basis of many learning and possibly psychological disorders discussed later. In-Depth 2.3 provides you with a greater understanding of these important visual processes.

In our example of the baseball player diving for the ball in the introduction to this book, he needed his dorsal stream—not only to track the trajectory of the ball, but also to be aware of his own body and glove position in relation to the ground and the other fielder's movements. Whereas egocentric (self) space is likely to be related to dorsal stream functions, allocentric (other) space is likely also to require the ventral stream. Because object perception and recognition are related to visual memory, the center fielder needed his ventral stream to recognize objects, people, faces, uniforms, the grass, the ball, and so on. This is consistent with evidence that visual association areas and the ventral stream are associated with long-term visual memories for faces and objects (Kosslyn et al., 1993). In addition, the ventral stream helped the center fielder realize that the left fielder's changing image suggested he was moving vigorously toward the center fielder and then stopping. The ventral stream doesn't detect movement per se; it allows a viewer to recognize that regardless of his or her position, and the position of the object, it is still the same object. To attempt to catch the ball, the center fielder needed an understanding of his body in relation to other objects and their relative movement and shape, necessitating the interaction of the dorsal and ventral streams. His dorsal stream helped the center fielder recognize the motion of the left fielder and his own actions in space, but this ventral stream helped him to recognize the different perspectives of the left fielder. The fielder's actions, as well as such activities as driving or reaching for a door, require coordination of the two visual streams. However, be-

IN-DEPTH 2.3. Further Examination of the "Where" and "What" Pathways

Milner and Goodale (1995) provide a more detailed examination of the "where" and "what" pathways that reflects their complexity. For the dorsal stream, V3A and VP are involved in recognition of spatial forms, and V5 is important for motion perception. As a result, the "where" stream may more accurately be considered the "how" stream. For the ventral stream, V3 is responsible for dynamic form recognition or object constancy, and V4 is important for color/form recognition. As discussed later, the dorsal stream is important for recognizing spatial relationships and motion, and the ventral stream is critical for perception and recognition of a variety of objects. They serve very different functions, but seldom work independently of each other in the real world. Differentiating the relative adequacy of the functions mediated by the dorsal and ventral streams can have implications for academic and behavioral intervention. For instance, a child with a writing problem may have difficulty with fine or gross motor skills (probably a frontal lobe problem), but if the difficulty is related to spatial processing, and visual feedback to the motor system, the areas associated with the dorsal stream may be implicated, particularly in the right parietal lobe. If integration of the dorsal and motor systems is in question, the corpus callosum may be implicated, because spatial–holistic skills tend to require right parietal functions, and handwriting skills tend to require left frontal functions in right-handed people.

cause these streams project to different lobes, it is important to recognize their differential impairment and/or dysfunction. Further evidence for the relevance of the dorsal and ventral streams in psychological practice can be found in Application 2.1.

Occipital Lobe Summary

To summarize the functions of the occipital lobe, it is the primary processor of visual information. It is thought to have the following attributes:

1. Visual processes are both hierarchical and parallel. There is a check-and-balance system that allows some sparing of visual perception, even though there may be damage to small regions of the visual cortex. If this is the case, you will see a child display *nystagmus* (rapid eye movements) to compensate for the damage.

2. The separate M and P pathways that project to the occipital lobe process different types of information. The M pathway is most closely related to contrast and motion. The P pathway divides into two P pathways in the occipital lobe—one more related to contrast and color, and the other more related to location and orientation.

3. After initial processing of information in the primary cortex, different pathways emerge in the association cortex: a dorsal stream that projects to the parietal association areas, and a ventral stream that projects to the temporal association areas.

4. The ventral stream is important for recognizing objects and for integrating form and color, regardless of object orientation ("dynamic form").

5. The dorsal stream is important for detecting motion and spatial relationships, providing perceptual feedback to the motor system so that a person can respond to the environment.

6. Both streams are needed for complex interactions between the individual and the environment; however, recognizing these functions can help you tease apart visual processes and determine whether they are differentially affected in learning and behavior disorders.

APPLICATION 2.1. Streams in the Classroom?

Take a minute to think about how the dorsal and ventral streams are relevant in the classroom. When are the dorsal and ventral streams needed in the classroom during a particular task? This task would require children to recognize objects, and then to guide their movements in response. Although there are many possibilities, one that comes to mind is copying notes from the board during a lecture—a common occurrence in the classroom, and one that gives children with some disorders considerable difficulty.

In this case, the ventral stream is specifically needed for recognizing the drawings and words on the board, and the teacher's shape and relative position (i.e., stretching an arm above the head and facing the board mean that the teacher is writing). The letters are symbols that represent words; they are objects, just as the teacher is an object. Children need the dorsal stream to guide their hands in forming and spacing the letters as they write. Of course, they must integrate this visual information with auditory information as well. All of this sensory information must be coordinated with the motor system, and managed by the "brain boss," the frontal lobe. When you think of all the complex systems that must be coordinated, it is no wonder that children with certain disorders have such a difficult time taking lecture notes in class.

AN AXIS DIVIDED: II. AUDITORY PROCESSES AND THE TEMPORAL LOBE

Auditory Pathways: From Ear to Temporal Lobe

The outer, middle, and inner ears have complex functions that translate sound information to electrical information in the auditory nerve via the cochlea. Because many children with reading problems have had frequent ear infections (otitis media), it is critical for referred children to be given audiological examinations to ensure adequate auditory acuity. However, as explained later, frequent ear infections can cause reading disorders even in the absence of frank hearing loss. The auditory nerve transmits information via the cochlear nucleus to the inferior colliculus, and two separate pathways emerge, with one going to the dorsal medial thalamus and the other to the ventral medial thalamus. The ventral pathway directly influences the primary auditory cortex, whereas the dorsal pathway influences the auditory association cortex. Unlike the visual system, where complete crossover takes place, auditory information is represented bilaterally. For instance, a sound made in the left ear is primarily sent to the contralateral auditory cortex of the right hemisphere (crossover), but it is also represented in the ipsilateral auditory left-hemisphere cortex.

Temporal Lobe Structure and Function

The lateral or sylvian fissure serves as an important landmark for separating the frontal lobe from the temporal lobe, and for locating the primary auditory cortex in Heschl's gyrus (see Figure 2.3). This superior temporal area, and the surrounding auditory association areas, are especially important for processing of language (Newman & Tweig, 2001). The tissue surrounding and within the superior temporal sulcus (STS), which separates the primary auditory cortex from the association and ventral stream areas, contains complex multimodal (i.e., pertaining to different senses) association cortex. The visual areas described earlier are below this region, in the lateral–ventral temporal cortex. There are several important areas in the medial temporal lobe. This medial temporal cortex includes the perforant pathway, which connects to the hippocampus (needed for forming new long-term memories) and limbic structures such as the amygdala (needed for affective tone

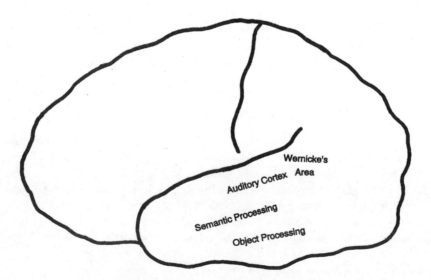

FIGURE 2.3. Structure and function of the temporal lobe.

or valence). However, as noted earlier, this is an oversimplified explanation of the medial areas, because they are part of an exceedingly complex interconnected circuit affecting attention, memory, and emotion. There are multiple connections between the temporal lobe and other lobes—including two interhemispheric commissures, the anterior commissure and the corpus callosum, and the uncinate fasciculus (an important emotional–memory link between the frontal–temporal areas). As can be seen, the temporal lobe has several different important roles in cognitive processes. It participates in auditory processing and comprehension, memory consolidation and storage, emotional processing, and visual object recognition.

We now have an oversimplified understanding of the complexities of the temporal lobe. The superior and dorsal medial temporal areas are involved in processing sounds; the ventral–lateral area serves as the ventral visual stream; and the medial surface is involved in memory encoding and emotional valence. Let's look at each of these independently. First, the processing of sounds and language is of primary importance in the study of reading disorders. Even when they are detected as early as infancy (Molfese, 2000), auditory processing weaknesses can lead to poor phonemic awareness and reading disorders (Vellutino, Scanlon, & Tanzman, 1994). In addition to genetic studies, the Molfese infant study suggests that some causes of reading disorders are genetic or occur at some time prior to birth (see Chapter 5); however, others may be caused by auditory pathway or temporal lobe dysfunction/disruption, which can be caused by recurrent ear infections, so an audiological examination should be undertaken whenever there is concern about reading. Even when hearing is intact, a history of ear infections can result in reading impairment, but this may be related to the time when the ear infections occurred during development of the auditory association cortex.

As is the case with the visual cortex, auditory processing begins in the primary auditory area within Heschl's gyrus. High-frequency sounds are processed in the posterior–medial part of this area, and low-frequency sounds are processed in the anterior–lateral section. The sounds are elaborated and integrated in the association areas, where comprehension probably occurs in Wernicke's area, the multimodal STS region, and the medial region (the insula). The primary cortex is involved in auditory attention and sensory memory, which are short-lived. It "registers" the auditory input for further analysis. Information is then integrated, organized, and categorized in the association cortex, allowing comprehension of auditory information to occur. As noted in In-Depth 2.1, the tertiary areas of the planum temporale—including Wernicke's area—are involved in comprehension of language, regardless of the input modality (Michael, Keller, Carpenter, & Just, 2001). As discussed later, this area has been found to be important in developing an association between sounds and symbols, and with the closely associated supramarginal and angular gyri of the left parietal lobe, has been implicated in phonemic awareness, sound–symbol association, and reading skills. It is the temporal lobe boundary of the occipital–parietal–temporal multimodal "crossroads" area. However, linking reading disorders to one region is difficult, and as we will see later, there appear to be significant hemispheric differences in auditory and language processing.

The ventral visual stream, as discussed earlier, is important for object identification and object constancy, and this is obviously linked with long-term memory. Long-term memory for objects has been linked to these lateral ventral temporal lobe areas. However, the medial temporal lobe areas are also associated with long-term semantic memory (Daselaar, Veltman, Rombouts, Raaijmakers, & Jeroen, 2002). The distinction is related to the cognitive processes of long-term memory *encoding* and *consolidation* for the medial area, and long-term memory *storage* for the lateral–ventral area. Medial temporal lobe and hippocampal damage can lead to anterograde amnesia (loss of memory for events after an accident), but not to retrograde amnesia (loss of memory for events prior to an accident). When combined with evidence showing that lateral temporal lobe damage can lead to retrograde amnesia, this conclusion seems warranted. However, there is evidence that the hippocampus also becomes active during long-term retrieval, especially for contextual memories, so this distinction may not be entirely accurate. Interestingly, if the medial damage affects the amygdala, emotional memories may also be impaired. The search for *where* long-term memories are stored is further examined in In-Depth 2.4.

Temporal Lobe Summary

To summarize the functions of the temporal lobe, it is the primary processor of auditory information. It is thought to have the following attributes:

1. The superior–posterior temporal lobe is where auditory information is received from the ear and auditory nerve, with the main projections contralateral; however, there are also ipsilateral projections as well, which is unlike the other sensory systems.

2. Comprehension of auditory information takes place in the auditory association areas, which include the insula, areas within the STS, and Wernicke's area (located within the planum temporale, an area often implicated in language comprehension and reading disorders).

3. The ventral–lateral temporal lobe is where the ventral visual stream is received from the occipital lobe. It is important in object recognition and probably long-term memory storage for objects, but long-term memory is widely distributed, primarily to the areas that process or perform the information originally (i.e., visual memory in the occipital lobe, auditory memory in the temporal lobe).

IN-DEPTH 2.4. The Search for Memory

Although it is clear that memories and emotions are affected by medial temporal lobe damage, it is unlikely that long-term memories are "stored" in these structures. Instead, a growing body of evidence suggests that semantic long-term memory is stored in the left temporal lobe. For instance, whereas facial processing tends to be a right temporal lobe task, memories for familiar or famous faces is found in the left temporal lobe (Damasio, Grabowski, Tranel, Hichwa, & Damasio, 1996). In fact, memories for living things (people, animals) tends to be associated with the left anterior temporal lobe, and memories for objects tends to be located in the left temporal–occipital region (Damasio et al., 1996). This is also supported by positron emission tomography (PET) studies that demonstrate temporal and frontal lobe activity during retrieval of past memories (Tulving & Markowitsch, 1997). Additional support comes from studies showing noun deficits following temporal lobe injury, but verb deficits following frontal injury (Daniele et al., 1994). These findings appear to show a lateralized effect, with long-term memories for semantic information likely to be found in the left temporal lobe (Gourovitch et al., 2000; Strauss et al., 2000; Wiggs, Weisberg, & Martin, 1999). Left temporal lobe activation is common throughout learning trials, as part of the consolidation process for forming long-term memories (Kopelman, Stevens, Foli, & Grasby, 1998).

These findings suggest that whereas long-term memory for learned information is likely to be associated with left temporal lobe functions, memories for hearing, vision, somatosensory, and motor functions are probably related to the same areas that perform those functions (Goldberg, 2001). *The implications are significant for both assessment and intervention.* If someone has a particular sensory or motor deficit, then the memories of those functions may also be impaired. This could account for the well-known finding that damage to the left-hemisphere motor regions can lead to apraxia.

4. The medial temporal lobe serves as an important component of the cortical link with the limbic structures associated with attention, learning, memory, and emotion.

5. Connections between the temporal lobes and other cortical areas probably serve different functions. The connections between the temporal lobes are likely to be important for linking object recognition processes, and for linking temporal lobe functions with limbic functions. The temporal–parietal lobe connections are important for linking the dorsal and ventral streams. The connections with the frontal lobes may have to do with the medial temporal lobe functions and long-term memory storage and/or retrieval. The temporal lobe connections with the occipital lobes are important for the ventral stream.

AN AXIS DIVIDED: III. SOMATOSENSORY PROCESSES AND THE PARIETAL LOBE

Somatosensory Pathways: From Skin to Parietal Lobe

The major pathways for the somatosensory cortex project from the brainstem to the parietal lobe via the thalamus. As is the case with vision and hearing, two pathways emerge. The dorsal pathway leaves the dorsal column of the spinal cord and projects to the thalamus, where it then goes to the primary somatosensory area. Consistent with this organization, the dorsal pathway is important for perception of touch, pressure, and proprioceptive movement (kinesthesis). The other pathway leaves the lateral spinal column and projects to the lateral posterior thalamus and pulvinar, and then on to the somatosensory cortex. This lateral pathway is important for perception of pain and temperature. Consistent with what we have seen for the other sensory systems, the lateral pathway affects the secondary somatosensory areas, not the primary cortex.

Parietal Lobe Structure and Function

Figure 2.4 presents several pertinent parietal areas discussed in this section. As noted earlier, the primary somatosensory cortex processes touch, pressure, and movement for the body. Important

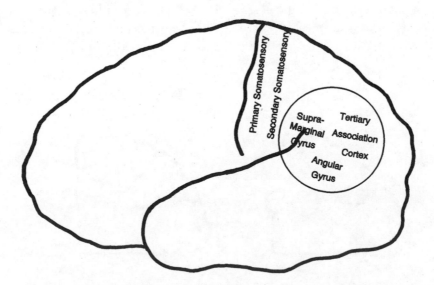

FIGURE 2.4. Structure and function of the parietal lobe.

distinctions can be made in regard to what parts of the body are represented in what parts of this primary cortex. Figure 2.5 presents the body area representations in the primary motor cortex (left side of figure) and somatosensory cortex (right side), called a *homunculus* ("little man" in Latin). As can be seen on the right, there are large amounts of somatosensory cortex for the hands and face, with smaller amounts for the limbs and torso. The disproportionate representation allows for more sensitivity in important sensory areas (e.g., lips, fingertips), and less sensitivity in other areas. The organization of the cortex is important, because damage to the lateral somatosensory cortex can result in problems with facial feeling, whereas damage to the medial portion can result in loss of feeling in the feet. After medial area damage, a child is more likely to lose feeling in both feet, because of the close proximity of the medial somatosensory cortex in the left and right hemispheres. Can you guess what might happen if damage occurs in the lateral section? Not only might the child have problems with speaking and eating (because the tongue and jaw are represented there), but he or she could also have problems with auditory processing (as this area is close to the auditory cortex). From the primary area, the sensory information is integrated in the somatosensory association cortex. This area is responsible for somatosensory integration and interpretation, and it has important connections or commissures with motor cortex in the frontal lobe. These connections are important for providing sensory feedback to the motor system, and this feedback is reciprocal. These areas are also responsible for tactile recognition of shapes and textures, and deficits can lead to agnosia (loss of perception); this in turn can lead to constructional apraxia (loss of motor program), which is discussed in the next chapter.

The remainder of the parietal cortex is multimodal association cortex, including the dorsal visual stream discussed earlier. The supramarginal gyrus and angular gyrus and associated temporal lobe areas, as noted earlier, serve to integrate visual, auditory, and somatosensory information. This is the parietal boundary of the occipital–parietal–temporal "crossroads," where the most complex forms of multimodal comprehension take place—Luria's tertiary area (see In-Depth 2.1). These cells are more likely to respond to many types of stimuli—not just auditory, visual, or somatosensory. This is also where the dorsal stream projects, and thus where important visual–spatial and motion information can be integrated with the other senses. Given the complexity of this region, it is not surprising that it has connections or commissures with the prefrontal cortex and frontal eye fields, discussed in the next section. It is also crucial to recognize that this multimodal association cortex is the most lateralized tissue of any receptive cortical area, and that these

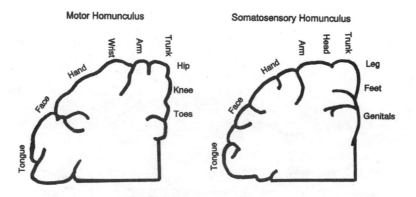

FIGURE 2.5. Motor homunculus and somatosensory homunculus.

differences have important ramifications for understanding complex cognitive processes, including reading, math, and writing. Consistent with Gerstmann syndrome, damage to the left parietal area can lead to finger agnosia, left–right confusion, acalculia, and dysgraphia. Interestingly, angular gyrus dysfunction has been associated with reading disorders, and supramarginal gyrus dysfunction has been associated with math disorders. We will return to these findings in Chapters 5 and 6, respectively.

Dysfunction or damage in these regions can cause problems with sensory integration, self-awareness, environmental neglect, right–left orientation, and academic performance. Since self-awareness and environmental awareness are related to parietal lobe functioning, it is not surprising that damage to these regions can cause attention problems and poor self-awareness (Rushworth, Paus, & Sipila, 2001). As noted earlier, these symptoms are quite similar to the symptoms seen in children with ADHD. However, a child who has attention problems due to parietal lobe dysfunction will probably not respond to stimulant medication or will respond only minimally (most of us would benefit from having a little stimulant—e.g., a cup of coffee!), so differential diagnosis becomes crucial. A child with this type of attention problem cannot be detected by behavioral criteria alone, as highlighted in Case Study 2.1. In a case like this, only neuropsychological testing will reveal the true nature of the child's deficits, and thus the appropriate course for treatment.

Parietal Lobe Summary

To summarize the functions of the parietal lobe, it is the primary processor of somatosensory information. It is thought to have the following attributes:

CASE STUDY 2.1. The Untreatable Boy with ADHD

Bill had been diagnosed with ADHD, depression, and social skills deficits several years before coming to our clinic. Originally diagnosed via *Diagnostic and Statistical Manual of Mental Disorders*, fourth edition (DSM-IV) criteria and behavior rating scales, Bill had been unsuccessfully treated with several types of stimulants and antidepressants for several years. In fact, his social and academic skills were reportedly deteriorating, despite years of special education support. His writing was also quite messy, and he was seeing an occupational therapist. Bill's parents, teacher, and physician were quite concerned at his poor treatment response.

After the physician referred Bill to us, we met with the parents, who presented a clinical picture that just didn't quite fit with ADHD. Sure enough, Bill qualified as having ADHD according to DSM-IV criteria, but when he underwent our double-blind placebo medication trial of methylphenidate (Ritalin), he showed few neuropsychological signs of ADHD. We could see why others thought he had ADHD, as his behavior ratings confirmed problems with attention, self-awareness, and interpersonal relationships. However, further neuropsychological testing suggested that he had the classic signs of right parietal dysfunction, affecting the dorsal stream. His "motor" problems, originally thought to be consistent with his ADHD diagnosis, were actually related to poor visual feedback to the motor system. Both Bill and children with "true" ADHD have behavioral signs of ADHD, but the interventions we use will have very different effects on these two types of children. We ended up using social skills instruction to help Bill identify facial affect and prosody, and metacognitive ("thinking about thinking") strategies to help him monitor his performance and behavior—strategies that would be difficult for most unmedicated children with "true" ADHD.

1. The primary somatosensory cortex has different pathways. One projects to the primary cortex and processes touch, pressure, and kinesthesis, while the other projects to the secondary cortex and processes pain and temperature.

2. The primary somatosensory cortex is arranged like a homunculus ("little man"). Large portions of cortex are needed for sensitive areas, such as the fingertips and lips; less sensitive areas, like the limbs, have less somatosensory cortex. The lateral surface is more likely to be involved in facial areas, and the medial areas are related to the lower extremities.

3. The secondary somatosensory association cortex has rich connections with both the primary areas and frontal lobes to control movements, and, with the dorsal stream, is responsible for spatial perception and guiding actions in response to the environment.

4. The posterior–ventral parietal lobe, and associated temporal regions, are where the highest form of understanding takes place. The occipital–parietal–temporal "crossroads" serves as the important non-modality-specific comprehension zone. It has numerous interconnected and bidirectional connections with the frontal lobe, discussed in the next section.

5. Parietal lobe dysfunction, especially on the left side, can result in difficulty with sound–symbol association for reading, perceptual–motor difficulties for writing, and arithmetic computation skills. Damage to the left parietal lobe is most often associated with Gerstmann syndrome, characterized by finger agnosia, left–right confusion, acalculia, and dysgraphia.

6. Parietal lobe dysfunction, especially on the right side, can cause neglect of oneself and the environment, leading to symptoms (poor attention and self-awareness) that appear to be ADHD. However, the differential diagnosis is critical, as this type of attention problem is unlikely to benefit from stimulant treatment.

AN AXIS INTEGRATED: HIGHER-LEVEL PROCESSES AND THE FRONTAL LOBE

Motor Pathways: From Frontal Lobe to Muscles

So far, we have examined the afferent system, with the occipital, temporal, and parietal lobes all related to afferent information, or sensory input. Whereas the posterior brain regions are important for understanding, the frontal lobe is responsible for *action*. Notice that the heading for this section starts with the brain (frontal lobe) and then extends to the periphery. Instead of the association cortex being the end of the path, as it is for the sensory systems, the motor system starts with association cortex, where motives and plans for motor activity are developed. These areas are discussed in the next paragraph. After receiving the motor directions from the association areas, the primary motor cortex is charged with carrying out the action. The primary motor cortex has a similar body representation (homunculus) described in the parietal lobe section (see the left side of Figure 2.5). From this area, two separate pathways emerge: the ventral–medial and lateral motor systems. Simply put, the ventral–medial system is responsible for whole-body, or gross motor, movement; the lateral system is responsible for skilled, or fine motor, movements. A description of these systems, and of their interaction with subcortical and posterior cortical sensory structures, would be exceedingly complex and is beyond the scope of this text. However, recall that the basal ganglia, tegmentum, cerebellum, and cranial nerves all play important roles in motor as well as other cortical functions. As suggested earlier, the variety of sensory and motor connections with subcortical regions not only allows for complex behavior to emerge, but also serves a regulatory check-and-balance function. Think of it as a judicial system that keeps the congressional posterior lobes and the presidential frontal lobe in check.

Frontal Lobe Structure and Function

Depicted in Figure 2.6, the primary motor cortex is the cortical endpoint of motor programs, not the beginning, as is the case with the primary visual, auditory, and somatosensory cortices. Anterior to the primary motor area are the secondary motor areas—one related to body motor skills (e.g., writing) and one related to eye motor skills (e.g., visual tracking). The secondary motor area is divided into the lateral or *premotor* area, and the medial or *supplementary motor* area. The premotor area affects motor functions indirectly through the primary motor cortex, and directly through cortical–spinal connections. Although there is some debate over the issue, the supplementary motor and premotor areas provide for different motor functions, depending on the type of activity and the amount of experience the individual has with a task. The supplementary motor area is thought to regulate internally guided motor programs (e.g., getting dressed for the day); it is critical for developing and programming self-directed motor sequences. The supplementary motor area is also important for bimanual coordination (using both hands together). Alternatively, the premotor area provides for movement in response to external stimuli (e.g., the center fielder's reaching out to catch that baseball). Consistent with these propositions, the premotor cortex is active in learning novel motor sequences, but the supplementary motor cortex is more active during previously learned or routinized motor patterns (Jenkins, Brooks, Nixon, Frackowiak, & Passingham, 1994). Interestingly, the left motor association and prefrontal areas have been found to be related to memories for verbs (representing action) and imagined tool use (a motor skill) (Daniele, Giustolisi, Silveri, Colosimo, & Gainotti, 1994; Moll et al., 2000). The other secondary motor area is the frontal eye field. It has numerous connections with cortical and subcortical structures to guide eye movements, which are important for visual search, scanning, and tracking (O'Driscoll et al., 2000). Consistent with the other secondary areas, one area is for self-directed movement, and the other is for responding to external stimuli. You will not be surprised to find that these areas have connections with the dorsal and ventral visual streams discussed earlier, as well as subcortical areas involved in movement (see In-Depth 2.5).

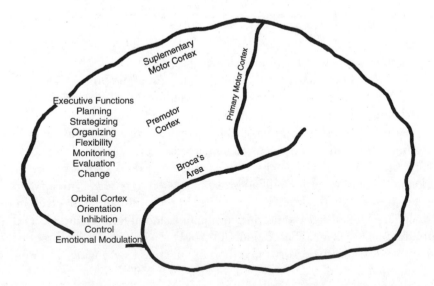

FIGURE 2.6. Structure and function of the frontal lobes.

IN-DEPTH 2.5. The Big Five Loops

There are at least five reciprocal frontal–subcortical circuits that are involved in the highest levels of self-management and emotion regulation. They are sometimes referred to as "loops," because information exchange is reciprocal. Lichter and Cummings (2001) provide us with the following understanding of how these interrelated circuits, born out of distinct physiological and functional systems, give rise to the complexity of human goal-directed behavior. All five circuits are related to the frontal lobe, basal ganglia, and thalamus. The dorsal system is responsible for executive control, and the ventral system is responsible for emotional tone, with both systems represented in dorsal and ventral areas of their related structures. The five circuits are as follows:

- Motor circuit—related to premotor, supplementary motor, and primary motor functions (ecological validity check: handwriting).
- Oculomotor circuit—related to frontal eye field, prefrontal, and parietal cortex functions (ecological validity check: reading words).
- Dorsolateral prefrontal circuit—related to anterior-lateral prefrontal executive functions (ecological validity check: turning words into equations during math word problems).
- Orbital prefrontal circuit—related to inferior-medial prefrontal functions (ecological validity check: raising hand and waiting turn during class discussion).
- Anterior cingulate circuit—related to anterior cingulate (ecological validity check: finishing work in a timely manner).

Deficits in the motor or oculomotor circuits can lead to problems with motor control and activity, or with visual attention and scanning, respectively. Dorsolateral prefrontal circuit dysfunction leads to the classic signs of attention deficits and executive dysfunction, such as problems with planning, strategizing, organizing, monitoring, evaluating, shifting, and changing behavior (Hale & Fiorello, 2001). Orbital prefrontal circuit dysfunction is often related to emotional lability and disinhibition or poor impulse control. Finally, anterior cingulate dysfunction can lead to problems with motivation, persistence, and on-line monitoring of performance. Hale, Bertin, and Brown (2004) argue that children with ADHD probably experience dysfunction in one or more of these loops, especially the dorsolateral (inattentive type) and orbital (hyperactive–impulsive type) circuits.

To gain an understanding of the remainder of the frontal cortex, the prefrontal cortex, it is best to think of it as the "brain manager" or "boss" of the rest of the brain (Hale & Fiorello, 2001). It is Luria's (1973) "superstructure"—the seat of all volitional goal-directed activity. The dorsolateral prefrontal cortex serves as the highest cortical area responsible for motor planning, organization, and regulation. This area is often associated with executive functions. Before you continue reading, try to brainstorm all of the things a company executive or your boss does, and you will know the definition of *executive functions*. The boss does not do the work per se; he or she manages the workers, the work environment, and relations with the public. Similarly, the dorsolateral prefrontal cortex does not do the brain's work per se, but it is intimately involved in planning, organizing, strategizing, initiating, monitoring, evaluating, modifying, changing, and shifting (requiring flexibility) our behavior (Hale & Fiorello, 2001). These activities all require Luria's "superstructure" frontal lobes to govern all other brain areas, serving as a gating or filtering mechanism for mental control of information (Shimamura, 2000).

To ensure that the "big picture" isn't lost, the brain executive also needs *working memory* to carry out the various activities described above. Working memory is required for temporary storage, manipulation, and monitoring of information processing (Owen, Lee, & Williams, 2000).

Thought to be an appropriate substitute for the cognitive construct of short-term memory, working memory represents volitional mental action on information acquired through sensory memory. Sensory memory, as you will recall, is thought to be passive and represented in the associated sensory cortical areas (e.g., primary visual, auditory, and temporal cortices); however, some have noted that this passivity perspective may underestimate the interrelationship between posterior attention/sensory memory and anterior working memory functions (Collette et al., 1999). Related to working memory is the notion of temporal information processing, or processing sequences of information over time, which is the responsibility of the prefrontal and related basal ganglia areas (Rammsayer, Hennig, Haag, & Lange, 2001; Sirigu et al., 1998). As noted by Luria (1973), this area is also important for both verbal fluency and nonverbal fluency (Baldo, Shimamura, Delis, Kramer, & Kaplan, 2001), which are related to locating and retrieving information from memory storage.

Damage to this prefrontal region leads to problems with organizing and segregating events in memory (Milner, 1995). Not only is working memory necessary for encoding of information into long-term memory storage, which is apparently the role of the left frontal areas; it is also needed for retrieval of semantic information from long-term memory storage, which seems to be the responsibility of the right frontal lobe (Cardebat et al., 1996; Dalla Barba, Pariato, Jobert, Samson, & Pappata, 1998; Fletcher, Shallice, & Dolan, 1998; Fletcher, Shallice, Frith, Frackowiak, & Dolan, 1998; Kopelman, Stevens, Foli, & Grasby, 1998; Wiggs, Weisberg, & Martin, 1999). Although lateralization of encoding (new learning) and retrieval (accessing old memories) processes is currently a source of debate, there is convincing evidence that the frontal lobes provide the executive skills necessary for these functions (Demb et al., 1995; Gershberg & Shimamura, 1995; Wheeler, Stuss, & Tulving, 1995). It is more likely that as retrieval demands increase, bilateral prefrontal cooperation is required (Ranganath & Paller, 1999).

It is important to recognize that the dorsolateral prefrontal cortex is not the seat of all executive functions, since additional cortical and subcortical circuits are needed to ensure efficient executive control. These cortical–cortical and cortical–subcortical circuits are required for all complex mental activity. Executive functions are also likely to require the functions of the orbital frontal cortex, part of the ventral prefrontal cortex. The orbital frontal cortex has intricate subcortical connections to help initiate and maintain performance, inhibit irrelevant responses or actions, and modulate emotional responsiveness. In concert with the dorsolateral region, it mediates initiative and decision-making behavior, especially during complex probabilistic situations (Elliott, Rees, & Dolan, 1999). A medial frontal cortex area including the anterior cingulate is often identified, but this area is sometimes considered part of the limbic system. The anterior cingulate probably serves a crucial executive-attention function, ensuring efficient interactions between the multiple posterior and prefrontal areas (Posner & Raichle, 1994). It is involved in responding to novelty, self-monitoring performance, inhibiting automatic responses, shifting cognitive set, and complex decision making (Posner, 1994). Combined, these anterior areas serve as the executive attentional system, responsible for guiding and directing all other aspects of consciousness (Posner & Petersen, 1990). (See In-Depth 2.5 for further discussion.)

A discussion of the frontal lobes also has to include another motor area of interest to school psychologists and speech–language pathologists: the well-known Broca's area. Broca's area is an important site for expressive language, but it is also involved in syntax (the rules of language) and possibly other motor functions (Sirigu et al., 1998). It is connected to Wernicke's area by the arcuate fasciculus—an important commissure that will be discussed further in Chapters 5 and 7. As noted earlier, the prefrontal cortex has many other important direct or indirect connections with almost every other area of the brain, especially the posterior association cortex. Important additional frontal–posterior connections for sensory processes include the superior longitudinal fasciculus and inferior occipital–frontal fasciculus. In contrast with some intellectual researchers, it is important to recognize that the frontal lobes, not the left hemisphere, are responsible for sequential or successive processes (see Lichter & Cummings, 2001). As discussed later, there is a left-hemisphere advantage for processing stimuli related in time, and it is intimately related to processing of details, but temporal processing is a bilateral phenomenon (Corballis, 1996).

As we can see, Luria's (1973) description of the frontal lobes as the "superstructure" above all other brain areas seems appropriate. It is interesting to note that few early researchers focused on the structure and function of the "silent" frontal lobe (for a discussion, see Goldberg, 2001), because several studies had shown that frontal damage did not result in decrements in "intelligence" as measured by IQ tests. Like many of the findings reported in this book and in the field, this may have more to do with the measures and methods used to study brain–behavior relationships. If you assume that intelligence tests measure intelligence, and that intelligence is not harmed by frontal lobe damage, then you might conclude that studying frontal lobe functioning is not very important. On the contrary, as we have seen, the frontal lobes are the source of higher-level cognition; they serve as manager of the anterior–posterior axis, as well as of the left–right axis. Unfortunately, few intelligence tests tap these higher executive processes well, and even neuropsychological measures may not fully tap the true nature of these functions. We will return to this issue in the next chapter.

Frontal Lobe Summary

To summarize the functions of the frontal lobe, it is primarily involved in motor activity. It is thought to have the following attributes:

1. The primary motor cortex has a "little man" structure similar, but not identical, to that of the primary somatosensory cortex. The head's motor activities are associated with the lateral portions, and those of the lower body are linked with more medial sections.

2. The primary motor cortex is linked to two separate areas of association cortex: the premotor and supplementary motor cortices. The premotor cortex is more responsible for directing movements in response to the environment and is involved during learning of motor scripts. The supplementary motor area is more involved with self-directed movement, and is active during previously learned or routinized motor skills. Motor skill learning has also been linked to the frontal-basal ganglia–cerebellum circuit, which is bidirectional.

3. The prefrontal area consists of the dorsolateral prefrontal cortex, the orbital frontal cortex, and the medial section (including the anterior cingulate). These regions have rich interconnections with almost every area in the cortex, and either directly or indirectly with almost every subcortical area, especially the basal ganglia and limbic system.

4. The dorsolateral and orbital cortices can be differentiated from each other. The dorsolateral region is considered the "brain boss" or "brain manager," in charge of executive function and working memory activities, whereas the orbital frontal region is responsible for behavioral and emotional regulation.

5. The anterior cingulate also plays an important role in this executive "superstructure," including responding to novelty, self-monitoring of performance, inhibiting automatic responses, shifting cognitive set, and complex decision making.

6. Part of the lateral frontal association cortex includes Broca's area, long identified as the source of expressive aphasia. It is located between the executive area and the facial motor areas; it

is involved in symbolic expression, including language, and has been associated with language rules and other motor activities. It is connected to the posterior speech zones via the arcuate fasciculus.

THE LEFT–RIGHT AXIS AND THE CEREBRAL HEMISPHERES

Early Findings: The Dominant and Nondominant Hemispheres

Before the late 20th century, there were basically two brain–behavior camps: the "localizationists," who argued that separate brain areas are responsible for unique mental processes, and the "antilocalizationists," who argued that the brain is an "equal-opportunity" organ and that all parts are involved during all cognitive processes. Gall's phrenology was an early and unsuccessful attempt at supporting the localizationist position, whereas Lashley argued in favor of a mass action and equipotentiality for all cognitive processes (Das & Varnhagen, 1986). The seminal works by Paul Broca and Carl Wernicke in the late 1800s furthered the localizationist cause, as they identified damage to the left-hemisphere association areas in several patients with expressive and receptive aphasia. Since language was thought to be a left-hemisphere process, researchers concluded that visual–spatial skills must be a right-hemisphere process—a finding they then confirmed in numerous studies. These verbal–nonverbal results, often based on studies of patients and animals with brain damage, predominated during most of the 20th century.

The relationship between left-hemisphere language functioning and right-hand preference (handedness) provided further evidence for the localizationists. The localizationist camp gained greater recognition as this concept of "cerebral dominance" permeated the early neuropsychological research efforts. Studies demonstrating anatomical hemispheric differences confirmed the left hemisphere's propensity to control language and handedness (Galaburda, LeMay, Kemper, & Geschwind, 1978). These arguments, especially when combined with findings suggesting that language problems (aphasia) and many types of motor problems (apraxia) are more likely to occur following left-hemisphere damage (Liepmann, 1908), led to the reification of the left hemisphere's role as the "dominant" hemisphere and the right hemisphere's role as the "minor" hemisphere (Goldberg, 2001). Because children with learning disorders were found to have a greater incidence of left-handedness, several concluded that incomplete hemispheric dominance can result in learning disorders (Geschwind, 1983); this led some to try to "correct" left-handedness in chil-

TABLE 2.4. Theories of Differences in Left- and Right-Hemisphere Processing

Left hemisphere	Right hemisphere	Source
Leading	Automatic	Jackson (1868)
Verbal	Nonverbal	Weisenberg & McBride (1935)
Analytic	Holistic	Levy (1974)
Routinized	Novel	Goldberg & Costa (1981)
Sequential	Simultaneous	Kaufman & Kaufman (1983)
Local	Global	Delis, Robertson, & Efron (1986)
Microstructural	Macrostructural	Glosser (1993)
Fine	Coarse	Beeman (1993)
Successive	Simultaneous	Das, Naglieri, & Kirby (1994)
Concordant/convergent	Discordant/divergent	Bryan & Hale (2001)

dren. What followed was a plethora of "dichotomania"—theories and measures that claimed to reflect processing differences between the hemispheres (see Table 2.4).

Despite the overwhelming belief in the dominant-verbal and nondominant-nonverbal dichotomy, there were opponents to these localizationist views. Noting the ability of young children to acquire language following left-hemisphere damage, Lenneberg (1967) took up the antilocalizationist cause by arguing that the hemispheres are equally capable of developing language, but equivocated by arguing that lateralization is gradually realized through adolescence. Supported by the finding that brain damage occurring early in life is less debilitating than damage occurring in adults—a concept known as the "Kennard principle" (Kennard, 1938)—many suggested that the brain may be equally capable of performing all tasks. This also led to the popular belief that humans only use a small portion of their brains, and that much "brain power" is untapped, left in reserve should something go awry. These findings and beliefs led many to view localization of function as a worthless endeavor and to regard functionalist views as more pragmatic, especially in work with children. This gave clinicians treating brain damage in children a sense of optimism that the children could recover, regardless of the insult; however, subsequent research suggests that such optimism may not be warranted (Pirozzolo & Papanicolaou, 1986), as noted in Application 2.2.

As is the case for many debates in psychology, the "truth" about damage and recovery lies somewhere between the localizationist and antilocalizationist perspectives. When it comes to lateralization, controversy over whether the hemispheres act independently, interactively, or in domain-specific ways (Teeter & Semrud-Clikeman, 1995) is likely to continue, as arguments can be made for both invariant and progressive lateralization (Kinsbourne, 1997). As we have seen,

---

APPLICATION 2.2. The "Benign" Head Injury

It seems as if we are hearing a good deal from parents or teachers about kids' hitting their heads and suffering no long-term consequences. About half of the children we see in clinic have scars on their heads—evidence of past injuries (especially now that shaved or very short hair is back in vogue). Discussing the incidents with the parents during an interview, we usually get similar responses: "She fell from the high chair and hit her head on the table," or "They were throwing rocks, and one of the other boys mistakenly hit him," or "He fell off his bike and hit his head, but he only got a headache." The next sentence is usually "You know, these things happen to children; they fall and hit their heads all the time." True, children fall and children hit their heads, and many children apparently suffer no long-term effects. However, the children we see are often said to have learning and attention problems of unknown origin, but a careful examination often reveals a possible genetic, physical, or environmental determinant in a majority of these cases.

I (Hale) remember one child who was in a car accident and hit his head. When I asked the parent about possible indications of brain trauma (headache, nausea, vomiting, dizziness, etc.), she replied, "Oh, no, he was fine, but he did get the flu that night." She never returned to the hospital to get this "flu" evaluated, and the boy could have died. We are especially bothered by emergency/rescue television dramas that discuss children who "miraculously" survive brain trauma. Yes, a child's brain is remarkable in its ability to recover function after even a serious cerebral insult, but such a child is likely to experience considerable attention and learning problems, with the length of coma directly related to the degree of impairment. This is not to say that we should automatically assume that every little bump and scrape leads to significant head injury, but we should be ever vigilant for the possibility that a reportedly "minor" incident has indeed affected a child's brain and his or her current functioning.

brain areas have many different structures and functions, but the brain also has an amazing ability to recover following an insult, and the same insult does not always produce the same behavioral outcome in all children. That is why we need to be on our clinical toes! We must recognize that each child is unique and malleable, and that intervention has much to do with the success of a child's outcome, regardless of the nature or cause of the deficits or strengths. Similar to early conceptualizations of posterior–anterior brain functions, much of the initial work in hemispheric differences was based on measures and methods that limited accurate interpretation of left–right differences. Early conceptualizations were often based on adults with brain lesions or animal models. Just as many researchers and practitioners neglected the frontal lobes in early research, since frontal damage did not apparently affect "intelligence," early lateralization researchers were overly focused on measures of language and prior learning, which are more likely to be impaired following left-hemisphere damage. In other words, the methods and measures shaped the questions, and the results easily confirmed those early predictions.

Contemporary Interpretation of the Left–Right Axis

As much of our discussion has indicated, it is not surprising that these early beliefs have been modified or dismissed as we gain a greater understanding of hemispheric function. Although it is not completely inaccurate, the suggestion that the left hemisphere is "verbal" and the right is "nonverbal" is an oversimplification of hemispheric differences. Do you ever wonder why the Wechsler Intelligence Scale for Children—Fourth Edition (WISC-IV) auditory–verbal and visual–spatial subtests do not always hold together, even though you've been taught that they reflect left- and right-hemisphere processes, respectively? What about the Cognitive Assessment System successive and simultaneous model, or the Kaufman Assessment Battery for Children sequential and simultaneous model? Though subtest scatter can certainly be related to the differential cognitive processes described in the previous sections, it is also related to left–right differences. However, as noted earlier, the original conceptualization of the left- and right-hemisphere processes was often based on the performance of adults with brain damage on verbal and nonverbal tasks. The findings of these early lateralization studies probably told us more about the tasks used than about true differences in hemispheric functioning (Gazzaniga et al., 1998). It is now clear that hemispheric asymmetries are *process-specific*, not stimulus-specific (Reynolds, Kamphaus, Rosenthal, & Hiemenz, 1997).

The advent of functional neuroimaging techniques helped to dispel early misconceptions about hemisphere differences. We now can study typical adults and children engaged in mental activities. Results from these and other studies confirm that verbal *and* nonverbal cognitive processes occur in *both* hemispheres. As we will discover, *the hemispheric division of labor is determined by the neuropsychological processes required, not the stimulus (input) or response (output)*. This is an important distinction—one that will advance psychological assessment and intervention practices in the years to come. When we could not correlate brain activity with mental processes, we were left with interpreting input and output, much as a behaviorist must rely on observation of overt antecedents, behaviors, and consequences. Although stimulus input and motor output remain important, we must now examine neuropsychological processes as well.

As one would expect, given this premise, current neuroimaging research suggests that *both* hemispheres are likely to be engaged during most tasks. It is the hemispheric division of labor that differs from one task to another, depending on the processes required. This baffled many researchers, as they found right-hemisphere involvement during language processing, and left-hemisphere involvement during visual–spatial processing. However, within the neuropsychological paradigm shift we will discuss, this makes perfect sense. After reviewing the literature on hemispheric differences in In-Depth 2.6, we will provide you with a greater understanding of why the old conceptualizations must give way to a new understanding of hemispheric processing differences. This synthesis evolved from the seminal work of Goldberg and Costa (1981), recently updated in Goldberg's (2001) highly readable and highly recommended treatise on frontal lobe functioning, *The Executive Brain*. Their work, in combination with the other findings presented below, provides us with the impetus to pursue this neuropsychological paradigm shift—a dramatic shift from focusing solely on input and output demands, to interpreting them in relation to neuropsychological processing demands.

A Monumental Step in the Right–Left Direction

Based on physiological differences and other clinical evidence, Goldberg and Costa (1981) concluded that the right hemisphere has a greater capacity to deal with informational complexity and multimodal representations, while the left hemisphere is specialized for tasks requiring single-modal representations that are well known and automatic. Therefore, the right hemisphere specializes in processing disparate information, whereas the left hemisphere is specialized for processing routinized codes. This is not to suggest that that the hemispheres work independently. It is not surprising that Goldberg, as a student of Luria, sees the hemispheres as interconnected and mutually dependent. The hemispheres necessarily work concertedly on most tasks, with the major difference being related to how much they are involved in any given activity. According to Goldberg's (2001) gradiental theory, the interconnected nature of brain systems makes it difficult to determine whether symptoms are related to one structure or another, and damage to one system will necessarily affect another.

One research group has shown bilateral hemisphere activation during many different types of cognitive tasks, but their conclusions are somewhat different from ours. Belger and Banich (1998) conclude that information complexity determines the amount of hemisphere involvement, which is somewhat consistent with the position stated above. However, they conclude that as in-

IN-DEPTH 2.6. The Asymmetrical Brain Divided

Although at one level the left and right hemispheres are symmetrical, there are numerous structural differences between them—not only in terms of their general anatomy, but at the cellular level as well. Of the physiological differences, several are related to auditory and other temporal lobe processes. The left planum temporale and insula are often larger than their right-side counterparts, and this asymmetry has important implications for language representation. The sylvian fissure is longer and the occipital lobe is wider on the left side. The postcentral gyrus and other secondary somatosensory areas have been reported to be larger on the left; this is similar to the pattern found in the frontal motor areas, including Broca's area. Interestingly, Broca's area is buried deeper on the left and has more surface area on the right. Asymmetries favoring the right side include a larger Heschl's gyrus, because there are two of them in the right hemisphere; a larger occipital–parietal–temporal association area; and a wider frontal lobe, especially the prefrontal cortex. Most importantly, the right hemisphere is heavier and contains more white matter than the left, but gray matter is disproportionately represented on the left. As a result, the left hemisphere has more primary cortex and does more within-region processing, whereas the right hemisphere has more association cortex and does more between-region processing.

formation complexity increases, an individual is likely to "recruit" the right hemisphere to help out the left hemisphere. This fits well with earlier notions about the "dominant" left hemisphere, but it also fits nicely with our model. If an activity requires novel (or more complex) processing, then the right hemisphere will predominate. If a routinized, automatic code exists to aid in processing the incoming information, the left hemisphere will predominate. Language is a well-routinized code. It is symbolic (letters, words, and concepts) and highly structured (syntax and grammar), so it is not surprising that conventional language use is better represented by left-hemisphere processes. This model does not supplant the left/verbal–right/nonverbal dichotomy per se; instead, it recognizes that the hemispheres are specialized for different processes, not different stimuli. Most verbal processes, especially those tapped by standardized measures that require a "correct" answer, require the left hemisphere's specialization for routinized codes. Conversely, the right hemisphere is specialized for global, holistic, novel processes. As a result, it is responsible for solving complex nonverbal performance tasks—tasks that require integration of multiple sensory, motor, and executive skills. The "hemisphere load" argument does not truly encompass this apparent difference between the two hemispheres, as suggested by the evidence presented in the following sections.

Empirical Examination of Left–Right Processes

Let us explore the empirical evidence supporting this new model of hemispheric interaction. As noted earlier, previous studies that had adults with brain damage perform dichotic listening or visual field tasks predominated during the early study of hemispheric differences. Given these early methods, which focused on stimulus inputs and motor (either speech or fine motor) outputs, clear and convincing evidence for the left hemisphere as "verbal" and the right hemisphere as "nonverbal" emerged (Springer & Deutsch, 1998). The concept of cerebral dominance was probably invoked to explain how a nonverbal behavior (carrying out motor acts or praxis) could also be carried out by the left hemisphere. However, with the advent of neuroimaging techniques and other technologies, researchers and clinicians have had to revise their thinking about hemispheric processes. The convergence of these findings within the theoretical framework described earlier is both enlightening and exhilarating. These technologies have allowed us to move beyond this stimulus–response mentality to one of understanding neuropsychological processes—a perspective that is congruent with Goldberg and Costa's (1981) propositions about novel/right–routine/left processes more than two decades ago.

If you ask many people, they will tell you that music is a right-hemisphere process. One area of research supporting these novel–automatic distinctions has to do with the processing and playing of music. With its distinctively nonverbal quality but auditory demands, the early findings that music was processed in the right hemisphere seemed to confirm that this hemisphere is specialized for nonverbal processes. Early research confirmed that deficits in processing of melody and other nonverbal sounds were associated with damage to the right, but not left, hemisphere—a finding confirmed during anesthetization of the right hemisphere (Gordon & Bogen, 1974). Left-hemisphere damage is likely to cause disruptions in temporal or rhythmic musical interpretation, but right-hemisphere damage limits understanding of pitch and melodic contour (Peretz, 1990). However, while studies suggest that processing of music for novices reveals a right-hemisphere advantage, concert musicians use the left hemisphere for music skills (Bever & Chiarello, 1974), and left-hemisphere damage can lead to aphasia for words and music in musicians, especially for familiar musical pieces (Zatorre, 1984). This is consistent with a PET study of concert musicians that showed bilateral activity during listening, reading, and playing of classical music, but the activity was greater in the left hemisphere, especially in occipital–parietal and frontal association areas (Sergent, Zuck, Terriah, & MacDonald, 1992).

Therefore, auditory processing of music is consistent with a right/novel–left/routine perspective. Could this theory also apply to language? One line of research has focused on the acquisition of linguistic processing skills in children. Using an electrophysiological technique called *event-related potentials*, Dennis Molfese and his colleagues have measured the brain activity of children in response to auditory-phonemic stimuli for over 20 years. They have even followed these children longitudinally, and found that *bilateral* auditory processing skills 36 hours after birth predicted whether children would have reading disorders (Molfese, 2000). Interestingly, Molfese and his colleagues have consistently demonstrated this bilateral activity during phonemic processing in young infants, but as language skills develop, the left hemisphere is responsible for most auditory–verbal skills. Could it be that early language acquisition requires right-hemisphere processes? The findings by this research group certainly confirm that bilateral processes are important, and that auditory processing undergoes a significant reorganization in the first years of life (Simos & Molfese, 1997). These right–left differences seem to be related to the amount of familiarity or experience infants have with stimuli, regardless of the modality (e.g., verbal–nonverbal), and to initial versus later processing demands (Molfese, Morse, & Peters, 1990). These findings are consistent with cerebral blood flow studies showing that the right hemisphere is dominant for cognitive processing during the first 3 years (Chiron et al., 1997), and with findings that right-hemisphere damage early in life leads to later language deficits (Eisele, Lust, & Aram, 1998).

For many years, people thought that deaf people use their right hemispheres to process American Sign Language (ASL) (Poizner, Klima, & Bellugi, 1987). After all, ASL does not require auditory–verbal skills; it requires visual recognition of hand movements to understand language, and motor skills to express oneself. If it is visual–motor, it must be a right-hemisphere task, right? However, studies have consistently shown that the left-hemisphere is used for processing ASL (Bavelier et al., 1998), and that left-hemisphere damage leads to aphasia-like symptoms in deaf signers (Hickok, Bellugi, & Klima, 1996). This may be because the left hemisphere preferentially processes grammatical structures (Weber-Fox & Neville, 1996), or it could be due to the fact that language is an automatized skill, as we have suggested here. Finally, while praxis is a visual–tactile–motor phenomenon, it is well known that apraxia and aphasia are more likely to occur following damage to the left, not right, hemisphere (Springer & Deutsch, 1998). This could explain why apparently "visual–motor" tasks are deficient in children with language-based reading disorders (Ramus, Pidgeon, & Frith, 2003). Children with apparently very different symptoms (language and motor problems) have these deficits because praxis—like language—requires recall of well-known routinized knowledge and action.

Though there is overwhelming clinical evidence that language deficits (for both verbal language and ASL) occur following left-hemisphere damage, they also occur following damage to the "nonverbal" right hemisphere. When cases of "crossed aphasia" following right-hemisphere damage were discussed in the clinical literature, it was generally concluded that these individuals must have had language lateralized to the right hemisphere. Clinicians and researchers originally accounted for these differences by suggesting that language is not always lateralized to the left hemisphere. However, studies in the late 20th century began to shed light on this apparent paradox. Indeed, language processes are represented bilaterally in all individuals; the different *neuropsychological processes* are what determine the participation of each hemisphere. Our traditional aphasia instruments readily tapped typical language processes, and adequately assessed individuals who were afflicted with traditional left-hemisphere aphasias. The left hemisphere appears to be specialized for closely related words, single interpretations, and semantic integration, but the right hemisphere is important for exploring multiple word meanings and distant semantic relationships (Chiarello, 1998). The findings that people with right-hemisphere damage are more likely to have difficulty with comprehending voice intonation or prosody, drawing inferences, understanding metaphors, recognizing humor, analyzing multiple word connotations, and interpreting implicit or figurative speech (for reviews, see Bryan & Hale, 2001; Van Lancker, 1997) suggest that they miss the "gist" of social discourse (Hough, 1990). Although they are not typically deficient in understanding grammar, because it is largely rule-governed, they have difficulty with complex syntactic structures (Caplan, Hildebrandt, & Makris, 1996). Because they are overly focused on routinized literal interpretations and expressions during discourse, children with right-hemisphere dysfunction fail to adapt to the subtleties of social exchange.

Individuals with right-hemisphere dysfunction have no difficulty with typical language tasks, but they may have difficulty retrieving verbal information from long-term memory. Recall that activation in the left frontal areas occurs during encoding, and that retrieval requires right frontal activation (Fletcher, Shallise, & Dolan, 1998; Fletcher, Shallise, Frith, et al., 1998), but that both frontal areas are involved in more complex memory tasks. At first glance, this seems to run counter to our right/novel–left/routinized distinction. But if we consider that encoding requires convergent processes to categorize and place information in long-term memory, and that retrieval requires a divergent search for information, this makes perfect sense. The left frontal processes during retrieval are involved in prototypic semantic connections (e.g., "cool" = low temperature), whereas the right hemisphere represents diversity beyond immediate associations, examining indirect or implicit associations (e.g., "cool" = good) (Schwartz & Baldo, 2001).

In addition to the linguistic and memory-related aspects of right-hemisphere deficits, children with such deficits are likely to have difficulty adapting their language and behavior during social exchange, largely because they can't recognize subtle differences in behavior and flexibly explore multiple word/phrase connotations during discourse. For instance, imagine saying, "Don't put all your eggs in one basket," to Mary, a person with right-hemisphere dysfunction. She might respond, "Well, I put my eggs in the refrigerator," or "I don't have any eggs, and I don't even have a basket to put them in." Her literal interpretation is that you were giving advice about what she should do with her eggs, and that she should put some of them in the basket, but keep some of them outside the basket. As discussed further in Chapter 8, right-hemisphere disorders result in both verbal and nonverbal deficits. We may not readily recognize these problems, or may not detect them with standardized intellectual and achievement measures. However, these are some of the "strange" children we see—those who show good routinized skills, and get decent IQ and achievement scores (at least during the early school years), but appear to have significant psychosocial problems and behavior disorders. Preferring to use left-hemisphere *convergent* processes that are *concordant* with their existing thoughts, children with right-hemisphere dysfunction are unlikely to integrate new *discordant* social information flexibly as the conversation proceeds, or to engage in the *divergent* thinking necessary to adapt reliably to the social situation (Bryan & Hale, 2001).

The left hemisphere detail-fine and right hemisphere global-coarse distinction has been validated as well. In visual field studies, the right hemisphere appears to be specialized for global perceptions, such as gender, and the left hemisphere can identify known persons (Sergent, 1995). This may be because the left hemisphere is specialized for high spatial frequencies, whereas low spatial frequencies are processed by the right hemisphere. In an ingenious experiment, Delis, Robertson, and Efron (1986) asked patients with left- and right-hemisphere damage to draw the figures they saw. Figure 2.7 depicts the stimulus and the types of responses given by typical patients with left- or right-hemisphere damage. As one can see, the typical left-hemisphere patient

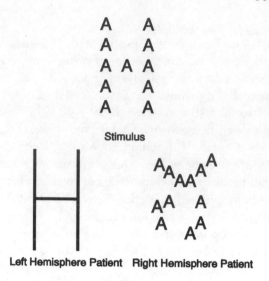

FIGURE 2.7. Global–local responses in patients with left- or right-hemisphere brain damage. Data from Delis et al. (1986).

drew the global shape, and the typical right-hemisphere patient drew a disorganized mess of letters. These left/local–right/global processes are consistently found in empirical studies, but their relation to spatial frequency is currently being debated (Blanca, Zalabardo, Garcia-Criado, & Siles, 1994; Evans, Shedden, Hevenor, & Hahn, 2000; Fink, Marshall, Halligan, & Dolan, 1999). This is why the left parietal lobe is sensitive to local stimulus characteristics like direction, orientation, and patterns of stimuli, whereas the right parietal lobe is sensitive to global, holistic, spatial configurations (Suchan et al., 2002)—a distinction that is useful in understanding performance differences on traditionally "nonverbal" tasks, such as WISC-IV Block Design. This global–local distinction fits nicely with our novel–routine perspective, as the right hemisphere looks for multiple pieces of information to obtain the "big picture," and the left hemisphere is focused on specific details and predictable stimuli.

   Finally, the right/novel–left/routinized distinction is accumulating supportive evidence on a regular basis, mostly from patient and neuroimaging studies. These studies are perplexing for those with a verbal–nonverbal orientation, but are quite consistent with the novel–learned position we present. For instance, there has been some debate over convincing evidence that visual imagery (e.g., visualizing your favorite lake in the woods) is a left temporal–occipital (ventral stream) phenomenon (for a review, see Farah, 1995). This doesn't make much sense from a verbal–nonverbal perspective, because it's visual. However, because visual imagery requires memory, it is likely to be related to previous learning, so it is a left-hemisphere task. (It is interesting to note that recommendations for children with left-hemisphere dysfunction often include use of visual imagery, because it has been presumed to be a right-hemisphere function!) Henson, Shallice, and Dolan (2000) found that right occipital activation was common during initial exposure to visual stimuli, in keeping with the traditional role of the right hemisphere; once the participants were familiar with the stimuli, however, the homologous left-hemisphere region was active. In another learning experiment, which used both verbal and visual stimuli, bilateral activity was found during acquisition of the information, but right-hemisphere activity diminished with learning (Martin, Wiggs, & Weisberg, 1997). Bilateral frontal activity, especially on the right side, has been found during initial learning of motor sequences, but this activity declines with learning (Muller, Kleinhans, Pierce, Kemmotsu, & Courchesne, 2002; Staines, Padilla, & Knight, 2002). Because of its role in working memory, frontal lobe activation is highest during initial learning stages, and there is a gradual shift from right to left frontal lobe activation when learning takes place (Gold, Berman, Randolph, Goldberg, & Weinberger, 1996; Raichle et al., 1994). This activation does not appear to be due to the verbal–spatial dichotomy; rather, the type and complexity of processing are what determine prefrontal activation for working memory tasks (D'Esposito et al., 1998; Postle & D'Esposito, 2000). D'Esposito and colleagues (1998) found the ventral region to be responsible for active maintenance of information in working memory, and the dorsal region to be responsible for manipulation and monitoring of ventral processes, with right-sided activation greater during the complex working memory task.

Implications of the New Left–Right Axis

If the verbal–nonverbal dichotomy no longer accurately represents the left and right hemispheres, we must understand how verbal and nonverbal information differs in terms of the neuropsychological processes of each hemisphere. The right hemisphere gets the "big picture"; it processes novel, holistic, global, and discordant information. The left hemisphere is more concerned with rote, detailed, local, and concordant information. We can't just look at children's WISC-IV Verbal Comprehension and Perceptual Reasoning scores and determine left–right differences. We must look at patterns of performance. Moreover, we must recognize that some verbal tests require novel problem solving (e.g., Arithmetic), and that some nonverbal tests require prior knowledge and memory retrieval (e.g., Picture Completion). Although it is interesting to note that the novel–learned perspective fits nicely with data supporting the *Gf-Gc* approach to understanding intelligence (Pallier, Roberts, & Stankov, 2000), even these tests require veridical decision making, so the involvement of both hemispheres is required on virtually all measures requiring "correct" answers. Obviously, response format makes a difference: A multiple-choice format taps the left hemisphere to a greater extent, and a free-recall format taps the right. The right hemisphere processes information in a coarse fashion to explore multiple associations; the left hemisphere is specialized for making finely detailed distinctions (Beeman, 1993). The following two sentences highlight these differences:

> "He stopped at the bank because he had to make a deposit."
> "He stopped at the bank because he had to stay dry."

You probably needed less time to comprehend the first sentence than the second sentence, because "bank–deposit" is a common association and was easily processed by your left hemisphere, whereas the less common "bank–dry" association required additional processing time. To make this second association, you needed more right-hemisphere activity to explore multiple meanings of "bank" in reference to "dry." The association between "bank" and "money" is such a strong one that you may have thought, "Is he going to buy a raincoat or an umbrella?", but then you probably thought to yourself, "OK, 'bank' refers to 'river bank.'" Had we included the word "river" in the second sentence, both sentences would have required familiar associations, which are primarily the responsibility of the left hemisphere.

It is no wonder that traditional aphasia tests, as well as most academic skills, tap left-hemisphere cognitive processes, because these tests and skills require correct answers. How are right-hemisphere processes important for learning? The answer is that right-hemisphere processes are *essential* for learning, but we typically don't assess these processes well with our standardized measures. Without the right hemisphere, learning new information becomes difficult if not impossible—a finding consistent with neuropsychological studies of children with "nonverbal" learning disorders, who often acquire language later than other children (Rourke, 1994). Not only do these children have difficulty acquiring new skills; they are unlikely to generalize known skills beyond highly structured tasks and situations. They may perform reasonably well on veridical tasks that require correct answers, but they can't provide adaptive responses, which is the real key to success in society (Goldberg, 2001). All the facts and details in the world can't help a person overcome considerable problem-solving deficits and an inability to adapt to novel situations.

Learning is about acquiring new information, and children with right-hemisphere dysfunction are likely to prefer relying on previously learned information rather than adjusting to the novel demands of a new learning situation. This may not be a problem during early learning experiences, as these children use their good rote learning skills to acquire basic academic skills. They enjoy rote drill and instruction, so in many ways they are perfectly adapted for early educational experiences. However, as the demands of learning become more self-directed, and as information becomes more complex, implicit, and ambiguous, these children are likely to have significant difficulty. This pattern has implications for psychosocial functioning as well. If children cannot adapt to new learning and social situations, they are likely to be perceived as unmotivated, oppositional, or preoccupied. Combined with limited self-awareness and difficulty recognizing the feelings and situations of others (i.e., poor "theory of the mind"), these children are at considerable risk for interpersonal problems (Surian & Siegal, 2001). The resulting alienation, as Rourke (1994) has noted, can have devastating effects on psychosocial adjustment. However, because these children typically have positive academic experiences, we are often left to wonder: Do these children end up in classrooms for behaviorally disordered or seriously emotionally disturbed students because no one recognizes their neuropsychological deficits? To close this chapter, let's look at some examples that highlight how the left and right hemispheres work together when presented with a problem (see Applications 2.3 and 2.4).

APPLICATION 2.3. The Civil War: Whose Side Are You On?

When you are asked a factual question, such as "Was Illinois part of the Confederacy or the Union during the Civil War?", you must use language comprehension, long-term memory to access facts about geography and the U.S. Civil War, and expressive language to give the answer. But there are three types of people out there. There is a group who will know where Illinois is, and will know enough about the Civil War to know that it was in the Union. All of these people will probably require left-hemisphere, routinized processes. However, if you don't know where the Mason–Dixon line was located, or much about geography in the United States, right-hemisphere processes will have to come into play. You'll need to think about what you know about Illinois, and to make some associations: "Illinois—Chicago, it's cold in the winter, it's the Windy City, it was a cattle town and industrial town at the time of the Civil War," and so on. Also, you'll have to try to think of the Mason–Dixon line separating the Confederacy from the Union during the Civil War, and try to recall where major battles took place. You may try to visualize the various regions of the country, and to locate the Midwest.

All of these processes require left-hemisphere functioning, but the right hemisphere is active as well, because it has to help you explore and connect the proverbial dots. But the right hemisphere is also involved in the people who know *too much* about Illinois during the Civil War. How can that be? Certainly industrial Chicago and northern Illinois wanted to stay in the Union, but many in southern Illinois supported their Confederate neighbors in the struggle to secede from the Union. The right hemisphere is required to give this answer: "Illinois was in the Union, officially, but the issues were hotly contested by Illinois politicians." This example also highlights how individual differences in prior knowledge, or crystallized abilities, can influence cognitive and academic performance. (By the way, the nickname "Windy City" came from the talkative politicians in City Hall, not the weather!)

Is every oral or written comprehension question the same? Let's explore how the brain copes with answering typical and atypical comprehension questions. Read the story carefully, and then answer the teacher questions that follow.

> Jack and Jill went up the hill on their way to the candy store. Jill opened the door for Jack and then followed him inside. Both said "Hi" to Ms. Smith, the store manager. They went to the candy counter, and each child picked out two pieces of 5-cent candy. They went to the register, where they gave Ms. Smith the money for the candy and waved goodbye to her. Ms. Smith said, "Have a nice day," and the children left.

Teacher questions:

1. What were the names of the boy and girl?
2. Did they go up or down the hill to get to the store?
3. Who held the door open for the other child?
4. What did Ms. Smith say when the children left the store?
5. What was the cost of the candy?
6. What will they do next?
7. What are all the things they could do after they leave the store?

The first four questions are explicit comprehension questions—those typically asked of most school-age children. Teachers typically assume that children have adequate reading comprehension if they can answer such questions. These questions are difficult for children with reading disorders and left-hemisphere dysfunction. You may have answered the fifth question quickly, but then said, "Well, it depends on what you meant by the question." Some of you probably thought 20 cents total, others may have thought 5 cents for each piece of candy, and a third group of readers may have thought 10 cents for each child. This question is purposely written to be ambiguous. It requires right-hemisphere activation to explore multiple possibilities, and left-hemisphere processes to impose a "structure" on the question. It also requires greater executive or frontal involvement to direct the right hemisphere to explore the various possibilities, mentally calculate a sum for the "total cost," and organize the response so it is accurately spoken. None of the three possible answers are wrong, but you have to add "total" or "each piece" or "per child" to make sure you are right. This is also true for the sixth question. Most of you may think that the children will eat the candy next. There are numerous possibilities, but this answer is "correct" in the sense that it is the most probable answer, given the other information in the passage. You need to rely on the story *context* to arrive at this conclusion (which necessitates right-hemisphere processes) and then decide on the "best" answer available (which requires left-hemisphere processes). Again, executive and working memory demands are higher for this question than for the first four questions. A teacher might ask the seventh question after a student answers the sixth one with "They are going to play at Jill's house." This question helps break down the task. It imposes a structure to help children with executive or right-hemisphere dysfunction realize they need to explore multiple possibilities before responding to the sixth question. This linking of assessment information to interventions for children with neuropsychological processing differences is the focus of the remaining chapters in this book.

APPENDIX 2.1. Glossary of Neuropsychological Terms

a-   Prefix that means "without," but often can reflect "difficulty with" as well (see **dys**).

Absence seizure   Disorder characterized by brief lapses of attention; may be mistaken for ADHD.

Acalculia/dyscalculia   Inability to perform/difficulty in performing mathematical operations.

Afferent   Signal that is going toward the central nervous system (CNS) and from lower to higher levels of processing.

Agenesis/dysgenesis of corpus callosum   No development or (more typically) partial development of the corpus callosum—a disorder that interferes with efficient transfer of information between hemispheres.

Agnosia   Complete or partial failure to recognize stimuli, even though senses are intact; associated with problems in sensory association cortex.

Agonist   A drug that facilitates the effects of a neurotransmitter.

Agraphia/dysgraphia   Inability to write/difficulty in writing.

Anarthria/dysarthria   Inability to speak/difficulty with speech, caused by motor cortex or cranial nerve damage.

Anomia/dysnomia   Total or partial inability to name things or find words, common in Broca's or nonfluent aphasia.

Anosodiaphoria   Indifference, typically caused by right parietal lobe dysfunction.

Anosognosia   Failure to recognize deficits, typically caused by right parietal lobe dysfunction.

Antagonist   A drug that inhibits the effects of a neurotransmitter.

Anterior   Toward the front.

Anterograde amnesia   Inability to recall events/learn new information after a brain insult.

Aphasia   Loss of or difficulty with receptive and/or expressive language.

Apperceptive agnosia   Difficulty in recognizing objects, though senses are intact.

Apraxia   Inability to understand/difficulty with voluntary movement, due to sensory and/or motor deficits.

Aprosodia   Inability to understand/difficulty with understanding speech prosody, primarily due to right temporal lobe damage.

Asomatognosia   Loss of or difficulty with body awareness, primarily due to right parietal lobe damage.

Association cortex   Higher-level cortex that integrates across sensory and/or motor functions.

Astereognosis   Inability to recognize/difficulty with recognizing objects by touch, typically due to parietal lobe dysfunction contralateral to the affected hand.

Ataxia   Muscle coordination problem leading to irregular motor performance.

Autotopagnosia   Inability to name/difficulty with naming body parts, such as finger agnosia.

Bilateral   Pertaining to both sides of the body.

Broca's aphasia   Nonfluent aphasia resulting in halting/absent speech, low verbal fluency, and word-finding problems.

Coarse processing   Right-hemisphere processing that explores multiple aspects of stimuli simultaneously.

Commissure   White matter that connects the two hemispheres.

Concordant/convergent thinking   Left-hemisphere process of looking for similarities among stimuli and arriving at a single answer; contrasted with **discordant/divergent thinking** (see below).

Concussion   Injury to the brain resulting in a temporary loss of consciousness; likely to lead to subtle impairments often undetected by standard assessments.

Conduction aphasia   Type of fluent aphasia characterized by poor word repetition but adequate comprehension of language.

(continued)

Constructional apraxia   Inability to perform/difficulty in performing complex graphomotor or visual–motor constructional movements, despite adequate elementary vision and motor functions. Problems with writing and puzzles/blocks could be due to this disorder.

Contralateral   Pertaining to the opposite side of the body.

Contralateral neglect   Tendency to ignore stimuli on the side of the body opposite the injury; probably due to parietal disorders, more often right parietal (affecting left side of the body).

Coup injury   An injury to the brain in which the head is hit by a moving object (e.g., a baseball).

Coup–contrecoup injury   Common deceleration injury in which the moving head hits an object (e.g., a wall), causing a contusion to the brain (coup), and then the brain moves back and forth, causing another contusion to the opposite side of the brain (contrecoup).

Crossed aphasia   Term invoked to explain language deficits after right-hemisphere damage, based on the assumption that the individual must have right-hemisphere language localization; now probably explained by known right-hemisphere language processes.

Cross-modal   Integrated across senses and/or motor systems; assumed to be related to the integrity of white matter transmission of information.

Crowding hypothesis   The belief that undamaged brain areas can "take over" for damaged brain areas, resulting in some **sparing of function** (see below), but that both the spared and original functions subserved by the undamaged brain area are subsequently depressed.

Declarative memory   Prior knowledge or crystallized abilities; probably related to the integrity of the medial and lateral temporal lobes.

Decussation   Crossed sensory and motor pathways, which allow the right brain to control the left side of the body and the left brain to control the right side of the body.

Deep dyslexia   Use of a sight word approach to compensate for poor phoneme–grapheme correspondence; thought to be right-hemisphere reading.

Developmental deficit hypothesis   The assumption that brain-based learning and behavioral problems are due to developmental deficits suggesting brain dysfunction; largely accepted as a result of research refuting the **maturational lag hypothesis** (see below).

Diplegia   Damage to the midline motor cortex, which causes muscle weakness/paralysis of the legs more than the upper body.

Diploplia   Double vision, or seeing multiple objects as one.

Discordant/divergent thinking   Right-hemisphere process of looking for multiple possibilities among stimuli and brainstorming multiple answers; contrasted with **concordant/convergent thinking** (see above).

Distal   Going away from the point of reference.

Dorsal   The anterior/superior part of the brain.

Dorsal stream   The "where" occipital–parietal stream, necessary for perceiving spatial relationships and self-perception in relation to the environment.

Double dissociation   Controversial method of establishing localization of function in patients with brain damage; involves demonstrating that damage to one area leads to a neuropsychological deficit, but damage to another area does not.

Dys-   Prefix that means "difficulty with."

Dysarthria   See **anarthria**.

Dyscalculia   See **acalculia**.

Dysdiadochokinesis   Shifting from one motor response to another; related to prefrontal and premotor functioning.

Dysgenesis of corpus callosum   See **agenesis of corpus callosum**.

Dysgraphia   See **agraphia**.

Dysnomia   See **anomia**.

(continued)

Efferent   Signal that is going from the CNS and from higher to lower levels of processing.

Executive functions   "Brain manager" functions for planning, organizing, strategizing, implementing, monitoring, evaluating, changing, and modifying behavior; thought to be functions of the prefrontal cortex and basal ganglia.

Explicit memory   See **declarative memory**.

Fine processing   Left-hemisphere processing that examines details and specificity of stimuli.

Finger agnosia   Inability to recognize or difficulty with recognizing fingers by touch.

Fluent aphasia   See **Wernicke's aphasia**.

Gerstmann syndrome   Finger agnosia, right–left confusion, acalculia, and agraphia resulting from left parietal damage.

Global processing   Right-hemisphere processing of multiple aspects of stimuli for a holistic "big picture" ("whole" of part–whole relationships).

Grapheme   Smallest group of letters that conveys meaning.

Gray matter   Neuron cell bodies, more common in the left hemisphere; contrasted with **white matter** (see below), which is more common in the right hemisphere.

Gyri   The "hills" or "bumps" that have valleys (**sulci**; see below) between them.

Hemianopia   Loss of vision in one visual field in both eyes, resulting from damage posterior to the optic chiasma in the hemisphere contralateral to the visual field loss.

Hemiparesis/hemiplegia   Muscular weakness or paralysis of one side of the body

Hierarchical organization   Principle suggesting that processing is least complex in primary areas and most complex in tertiary areas; works in concert with **parallel processing** (see below).

Homunculus   Literally, "little man" in Latin; the arrangement of known body area representations in the somatosensory and motor cortex. The legs are represented in the medial areas, and the face is represented in the lateral areas.

Hyperlexia   Well-above-average word reading without adequate comprehension, possibly related to **Wernicke's aphasia** (see below) or right-hemisphere dysfunction.

Ideational apraxia   Difficulty with the concept of a motor activity, even though the individual motor acts can be carried out; probably due to frontal–basal ganglia or temporal lobe damage.

Ideomotor apraxia   Difficulty with carrying out the individual motor acts, even though the individual maintains the concept of the motor activity; probably due to problems with supplementary motor cortex.

Implicit memory   Automatic performance of a routinized skill; likely to be related to cerebellar/basal ganglia and frontal circuits.

Inferior   Toward the bottom of the brain.

Ipsilateral   Same side of the body; the cerebellum affects motor functioning on the same or ipsilateral side of the body.

Kennard principle   The belief that early CNS damage is less likely to result in long-term deficits than later damage; unlikely to be uniformly true.

Kindling   Initially contested finding that repeated seizures result in further brain damage.

Kinesthesis   Movement perception or position of body parts, related to parietal lobe functioning; important for providing feedback to the motor system.

(continued)

Lateral   Toward the side of the brain or body.

Lesion   Any damage to the CNS.

Local processing   Left-hemisphere processing of single aspects or minutiae of stimuli, for a detailed "part" analysis.

Maturational lag hypothesis   The assumption that brain-based learning and behavioral deficits are due to developmental delays; largely replaced by research supporting the **developmental deficit hypothesis** (see above).

Medial   Toward the midline of the brain or body.

Morpheme   The smallest meaningful part of a word (e.g., "mean-ing-ful" has three morphemes).

Multimodal   Association cortex that processes more than one type of information; see **tertiary cortex**.

Nonfluent aphasia   See **Broca's aphasia**.

Nystagmus   Rapid eye movements that can result from cranial nerve damage or can serve as a compensatory mechanism to "fill in the gaps" when there is damage to the occipital lobe.

Object constancy   Identification of objects as the same objects, regardless of the viewpoint; a ventral stream function.

Papilledema   "Bulging eyes," signaling cerebral spinal fluid increase due to brain damage.

Paragraphia   Writing the wrong word; see **paraphasia**.

Parallel processing   Simultaneously processing information in multiple ways; works in concert with **hierarchical organization** principle (see above).

Paraphasia   Saying the wrong word (semantic paraphasia) or letter (phonemic paraphasia).

Pathognomonic signs   Symptoms that are clearly diagnostic of a known disorder; also known as "hard signs."

Perseveration   Saying or doing the same thing over and over again; suggestive of frontal–basal ganglia dysfunction.

Phoneme   Smallest unit of sound in words.

Plasticity   The ability of the brain to change structure and function to compensate for damage to other areas. See **crowding hypothesis** and **Kennard principle**.

Posterior   Toward the back.

Pragmatics   The functions of language in relation to the environment; probably governed by the right hemisphere.

Praxis   Movement governed by the premotor cortex (in response to the environment) or supplementary motor cortex (self-directed).

Primary cortex   The first cortical zones to process information (superior temporal, posterior occipital, anterior somatosensory), or the last cortical zone to carry out a motor activity (posterior frontal).

Procedural memory   See **implicit memory**.

Prosody   Rate, rhythm, and intensity of speech; related to right-hemisphere functioning.

Prosopagnosia   Inability or difficulty in recognizing faces; probably due to right (unfamiliar) or left (familiar) ventral stream, depending on familiarity with the face; also occurs with right parietal dysfunction.

Proximal   Close to the point of reference.

Ptosis   Drooping eyelid, indicating cranial nerve (oculomotor) damage.

(continued)

Retrograde amnesia Loss of preinjury memory following brain damage, suggesting more global cortical destruction. See **anterograde amnesia**.
Right–left confusion Poor orientation to self or other (including object); symptom of left parietal lobe dysfunction.

Scotoma Small blind spot due to occipital damage, compensated for by nystagmus.
Secondary cortex Intermediary cortex between **primary cortex** and **tertiary cortex** that perceives input (sensory) or prepares for output (motor).
Semantics Prior knowledge of the meaning of language; probably related to left temporal lobe functioning.
Short-term memory Short-lived rote memory for stimulus input; requires **working memory** (see below) for higher level processing.
Sleep apnea Difficulty with breathing; can cause sleep disruption and subsequent attention problems.
Sparing of function See **crowding hypothesis**.
Stereognosis Recognition of objects by touch; probably requires both parietal lobe somatosensory and temporal lobe long-term memory store.
Sulcus The "valleys" between one gyrus and another (see **gyri**).
Superior Toward the top of the brain.
Surface dyslexia Phonological letter-by-letter approach to reading, with extreme difficulty with sight words or morphemes; probably impairs reading fluency and comprehension.
Syntax Language rules for putting words together; likely to be a left frontal function.

Tertiary cortex Luria's sensory "zone of overlapping" (occipital–temporal–parietal junction) and motor "superstructure" (prefrontal cortex), which govern the highest levels of cognition.

Ventral The posterior/inferior part of the brain, contrasted with **dorsal** (see above).
Ventral stream The "what" visual stream between the occipital and temporal lobes, providing object recognition.
Visual agnosia Inability to recognize/difficulty in recognizing objects; likely to be a ventral stream problem.
Visual neglect Inattention to stimuli in the contralateral hemispace; probably due to parietal lobe damage, especially in the right hemisphere.

Wernicke's aphasia Fluent aphasia characterized by clear speaking without meaning ("word salad"); also difficulty with language comprehension; due to damage to Wernicke's area.
White matter "Superhighway" pathways allowing for intermodal connections and complex behavior; more prevalent in the right hemisphere, and contrasted with **gray matter** (see above), which is more prevalent in the left hemisphere.
Working memory Executive function memory that "works" on information in short- and long-term memory; important for encoding to and retrieval from long-term memory.

The following books and Web sites or pages are useful further readings in brain–behavior relationships. Our list provides relatively few sources; there are hundreds if not thousands available, many of which are cited in the chapter text and worth further examination.

Print Resources for Brain–Behavior Relationships and Neuropsychology

Gazzaniga, M. S., Ivry, R. B., & Mangun, G. R. (1998). *Cognitive neuroscience. The biology of the mind.* New York: Norton.

Goldberg, E. (2001). *The executive brain: Frontal lobes and the civilized mind.* New York: Oxford University Press.

Goldstein, S., & Reynolds, C. R. (Eds.). (1999). *Handbook of neurodevelopmental and genetic disorders in children.* New York: Guilford Press.

Kolb, B., & Whishaw, I. Q. (1990). *Fundamentals of human neuropsychology* (4th ed.). New York: Freeman.

Lichter, D. G., & Cummings, J. L. (Eds.). (2001). *Frontal–subcortical circuits in psychiatric and neurological disorders.* New York: Guilford Press.

Lyon, G. R., & Krasnegor, N. A. (Eds.). (1996). *Attention, memory, and executive function.* Baltimore: Brookes.

Reitan, R. M., & Wolfson, D. (1985). *Neuroanatomy and neuropathology: A clinical guide for neuropsychologists.* Tucson, AZ: Neuropsychology Press.

Reynolds, C. R., & Fletcher-Janzen, E. (Eds.). (1997). *Handbook of clinical child neuropsychology* (2nd ed.). New York: Plenum Press.

Spreen, O., Risser, A. H., & Edgell, D. (1995). *Developmental neuropsychology.* New York: Oxford University Press.

Springer, S., & Deutsch, G. (1998). *Left brain right brain: Perspectives from cognitive neuroscience* (5th ed.). New York: Freeman.

Yeates, K. O., Ris, M. D., & Taylor, H. G. (2000). *Pediatric neuropsychology: Research, theory, and practice.* New York: Guilford Press.

Web Sites or Pages for Brain Structures, Function, and Brain-Based Developmental Disorders

American Academy of Child and Adolescent Psychiatry. http://www.aacap.org

American Academy of Clinical Neuropsychology. http://www.theaacn.org

American Board of Clinical Neuropsychology. http://www.theabcn.org

American Board of Professional Neuropsychology. http://abpn.net

Atlases of the Brain. http://medlib.med.utah/kw/brain_at

Division 40 of the American Psychological Association. http://www.div40.org/

Kennedy Krieger Institute. http://www.kennedykrieger.org/accessible

Learning Guide for the Human Brain. http://www.marymt.edu/~psychol/brain.html

National Academy of Neuropsychology. http://nanonline.org

National Institute of Mental Health Laboratory of Neuropsychology. http://neuron.nimh.nih.gov

Neuropsychology Central. http://www.neuropsychologycentral.com

New York University Child Study Center. http://www.aboutourkids.org

Society for Neuroscience Brain Briefings. http://web.sfn.org/content/Publications/BrainBriefings

Virtual Hospital: The Human Brain. http://www.vh.org/adult/provider/anatomy/BrainAnatomy

The Whole Brain Atlas. http://www.med.harvard.edu/AANLIB

Yale Child Study Center Developmental Disabilities Clinic. http://info.med.yale.edu/chldstdy

CHAPTER 3

Ⅼ⏐⏐⏐⏐⏐⏐⏐⏐⏐⏐⏐Ⅼ

Neuropsychological Approaches
to Assessment Interpretation

DEVELOPMENTAL NEUROPSYCHOLOGICAL ASSESSMENT

Developmental Differences in Practice

The developmental differences among children can be significant and can have tremendous implications for neuropsychological interpretation of assessment data. Moreover, children are not merely small adults; their test performance is both quantitatively and qualitatively different from that of adults (Fletcher & Taylor, 1984). As a result, applying neuropsychological principles in school settings requires not only substantial training, skills, and clinical acumen, but an awareness of the broader developmental context. In working with each child, developmental criteria should shape the nature of the assessment, interpretation of results, and recommendations for intervention. Therefore, it is critical that different assessment practices should be used for different children, and that interpretation should vary depending on children's unique patterns of performance within the context of their current developmental level.

This is not to say that we should deviate from standardized test administration practices. Instead, it suggests our rapport building and maintenance activities will vary from child to child, and that summative scores (e.g., global IQ) provide little insight into the developmental nature of the child's performance. For instance, it would be inappropriate to conclude that a 7-year-old girl who gives only 1-point responses on the Wechsler Intelligence Scale for Children—Fourth Edition (WISC-IV) Similarities subtest has good "abstract verbal concept formation," just because her score is above average. This suggests that clinical observations and idiographic interpretation must be developmentally sensitive as well. This flexibility in observation and interpretation is important, but some people think that it is contrary to a neuropsychological approach to interpretation. Indeed (and unfortunately), many view a neuropsychological orientation as one that focuses on static, intractable brain problems (Rourke, 1994), and that views all strengths and weaknesses as alike, regardless of developmental level. This "medical model" orientation is seldom supported by those who practice pediatric neuropsychology. Most practitioners recognize the dynamic interplay between brain development and experience, which shapes and modifies a child's development course in a bidirectional manner (Johnson, 1999). As a result, most neuropsychologists today place greater emphasis on understanding children's deficits than on determining whether they have localized brain damage (Groth-Marnat, 2000a). Although children tend to obtain developmental milestones at certain ages, each child is unique in his or her acquisition and manifestation of skills. Assessment practices must examine both the vertical (i.e., nomothetic) and horizontal (i.e., idiographic) developmental variations at each level (Bernstein, 2000), because each child shows skill differences in progressing from one developmental level to the next.

Continuum of Typical and Atypical Development

Important to these developmental processes is how the brain develops under typical and atypical conditions (Tramontana & Hooper, 1997). What do "typical" and "atypical" mean, however? It is important for you to recognize that there is no clear dichotomy; the brain's various structures and pathways develop along a continuum of typical and atypical development *for each individual child*. A child's chronological age can serve as a starting point or marker for expected physical, cognitive, and brain development (Dennis, 2000), but developmental strengths and weaknesses must be examined in relation to each other. Some deviations are to be expected, but developmental benchmarks can be used to guide appropriate interpretation of test data, because what is appropriate at one developmental level may be problematic at another. Brain development is dramatic during infancy and childhood, and corresponding changes in performance can be expected at each developmental level (Reynolds & Mayfield, 1999). You must decide whether a child's presenting problem is due to the environment, a delay, or a deficit, or (as is likely) to some combination of the three. For instance, most children should master the calculation skills required for the WISC-IV Arithmetic subtest by the early school-age years. For very young children, poor mathematics achievement can account for poor Arithmetic performance; for older children, however, other plausible explanations for failure responding should be entertained (Kaufman, 1994), including limited auditory attention, working memory, and executive function. Uniformly interpreting Arithmetic as a measure of quantitative skills is both inaccurate and misleading (Hale, Fiorello, Kavanagh, Hoeppner, & Gaither, 2001). In addition, while summative test results can convey normative differences, the clinician must relate these findings to the developmental demands a child faces in their environment. For example, a child who is not expected to clean his or her room will be unlikely to meet this developmental criterion on an adaptive behavior inventory. You must determine how moderator (e.g., environmental) variables influence the child's basic neuropsychological processes (Fletcher & Taylor, 1984).

Conducting Developmentally Sensitive Evaluations

As young children are quite variable in their responses to assessment demands, you must try to be quite enthusiastic and engaging during an evaluation. Multiple sessions may be required for younger children. It does no good to test a child for 6 hours and then determine that the results are invalid because of fatigue or motivation problems. During testing, it is important to maintain rapport while moving quickly through the measures, keeping the child engaged and interested in the test materials. Supplemental instructions (if allowed) are frequently needed for young children and should be provided as necessary. This, of course, depends on the nature of the task. For instance, a memory test item cannot be practiced prior to administration. Young children also speak, read, and write differently from older children. Whereas errors of articulation, grammar, and letter sequencing (e.g., reversals) are common in young children, these are signs of pathology in older children. As young children explore their vocabularies, they commonly use words inappropriately, but this hardly suggests that they have a semantic paraphasia (an important linguistic problem to be discussed later).

Luria's (1973) model can provide us with insight into the developmental issues affecting neuropsychological performance in children. According to Luria, the developmental progression begins with the first functional unit and the primary sensory and motor areas; it then proceeds to the secondary areas; and it finally moves to the occipital–parietal–temporal "zone of overlapping" and frontal "superstructure," which are the last areas to reach full maturity, often late in adolescence (Anderson, 1998). The developmental timeline is both dynamic and relative. It would be inappropriate to conclude that children have no prefrontal activity before they reach school. In fact, different executive functions are likely to develop at different ages. For instance, sustained attention and freedom from distractibility are typically developed by school age; inhibition and problem-solving skills are developed by middle childhood; and planning and foresight are accomplished by adolescence (Welsh, Pennington, & Groisser, 1991).

Although there has been some variation in these findings, this general developmental perspective is worth noting. For instance, most infants are engaged in simple sensory and motor acts, and reflexive behavior predominates. As secondary cortical areas become functional, reflexive behavior diminishes, and symbolic behavior emerges. Finally, the development of tertiary areas allows for complex understanding and volitional behavior to predominate, but hemispheric differences continue to emerge throughout this time. It is important to recognize that young children engage in more effortful processing (Bjorklund & Green, 1992) and that they become increasingly automatic in the execution of complex behaviors with age (Hooper & Boyd, 1986), suggesting a gradual developmental shift from right- to left-hemisphere processes during task performance. What may be a novel task for one child may be routinized for another, even at the same chronological age. As can be deduced from Chapter 2, this novel–routine distinction may dramatically affect both a child's performance and the interpretation of the results (Hale & Fiorello, 2001).

Developmentally appropriate assessment techniques are meaningless unless we can link them to developmentally appropriate interventions. Linking assessment to intervention requires an understanding of developmental processes and of differences in pedagogy from one age level to the next. For instance, a child with right-hemisphere dysfunction may not need reading comprehension instruction in the early grades, but will need extensive help as he or she enters middle school (Rourke, 1994). This is because the child is likely to have difficulty with implicit and inferential questions—questions that are seldom asked in the early grades. In addition, whereas remediation may be important for young children, compensatory strategies become essential for older children, depending on the nature and severity of the deficits. At all levels, some compensation and some remediation should take place; it is the amount of each that varies according to developmental level. Developmentally sensitive interventions take into account the chronological age of the child, and the child's relative strengths and needs, as highlighted in Case Study 3.1.

Most schools have curriculum scope and sequence charts that can help you determine developmentally appropriate teaching sequences. Through task analysis of the goals, teaching successive steps, and shaping success, we can help these children make developmental gains. If we have unrealistic objectives or overwhelming tasks, our help will become a punisher to such children.

CASE STUDY 3.1. Terrance's Dislike of the Resource Room

I (Hale) once conducted a clinical interview with Terrance, a boy who had received special education resource room services for several years. I asked him what he thought about his teacher and the services he received. Terrance said that he liked the help and the teacher was nice, but that he didn't like being in the class and being a "sped." He hated being pulled out of his regular class, and he wished he was like the other boys in class—not "stupid" like the rest of the "speds."

What led Terrance to these feelings? Some of this could be related to the appropriateness of his placement, or to his segregation from peers. However, when I asked him about it, my early behavioral training became important in understanding his perspective. From Terrance's perspective, the resource room was a punisher, because the teacher always focused on the one subject he had a difficult time with and liked the least! He seldom experienced success in this class, and the focus was always on what he couldn't do.

Helping children like Terrance experience high rates of success by teaching at the instructional rather than the frustration level requires an understanding of developmentally appropriate curricula and teaching techniques. In addition, interspersing remedial activities (resolving weaknesses) with compensatory ones (teaching to strengths) allows you to use the Premack principle (use compensation to reinforce remediation) effectively to foster motivation and perseverance.

After years of experiencing failure, older children can begin to become disillusioned and oppositional toward those trying to help them. They may skip classes or become defiantly disruptive in the classroom in an attempt to avoid showing their weaknesses to their peers. Their social awareness tells them that it's better to look "bad" than to look "dumb." We don't do a very good job of helping older children and teens understand their disabilities, or normalize their experiences for them. Part of the problem is related to the labeling and self-fulfilling prophecy; they have become "disabled" youth. Helping children understand their disability does not convey a message that they must fit some label. It is no wonder that many of our children with differences dislike special education and school in general; it is an aversive experience for them, one that focuses on their weaknesses. Normalizing their experience by suggesting that all of us have developmental differences in cognition and behavior can help alleviate this problem. In addition, older or more impaired children may benefit from recognizing their strengths rather than focusing on their weaknesses (Reynolds & Mayfield, 1999). Operating from a developmental and historical perspective, you can truly understand the dynamic and ever-changing relationship between brain and behavior—a key to successful assessment practices and intervention strategies for children of all characteristics and needs.

THE SCIENTIFIC METHOD IN NEUROPSYCHOLOGICAL ASSESSMENT

Examining Prereferral Data and Referral Questions

As discussed in Chapter 1, the systematic prereferral interventions you attempt will provide you with a good starting place for formulating hypotheses about each child's strengths and needs, and for developing your assessment battery. After you examine the prereferral data, the referral question(s) can further define the nature of the child's difficulties and help shape the battery. Unfortunately, many referral questions are written from a global perspective, with summative rather than objective terminology. For example, a referral might read, "Johnny is out of control, he's mean, and he refuses to follow classroom expectations." You could conclude that Johnny has some problem with following teacher directions or completing work, and that he probably displays some negative behaviors (e.g., name calling, hitting, destroying property) toward his peers and/or the teacher. But these assumptions can get you in diagnostic hot water, so after you receive the teacher referral, it is critical to clarify any vague or ambiguous information. Even if the teacher or parent can pinpoint the overt symptom of the problem (e.g., inattention), it is still up to you to determine if the problem is due to developmental delay, a learning disorder, a psychiatric problem, or whether it is truly ADHD (Reynolds & Mayfield, 1999). Although we focus primarily on learning disorders and ADHD in this book, as they are the most common referral problems (Shaywitz, Fletcher, & Shaywitz, 1995), it is important to be aware of other disorders that involve learning and attention difficulties.

This referral information can provide an important link between the environment and subsequent assessment data, but it is important to realize that the teacher could be partially or completely wrong about the problem behavior. Because the referral question tends to represent the teacher's opinion and is influenced by the teacher's perceptions and interpretations (Sattler, 2001), you must keep an open mind. This common phenomenon, in our opinion, is one of the biggest problems associated with problem-solving consultation that relies on teacher impressions to define the problem and develop interventions: What if the teacher is *wrong*? When a teacher says that a child has an "attention problem," you should consider multiple possible reasons for the attention issues, only one of which could be ADHD. Teachers rarely say that their teaching techniques are at fault, even though we know that environmental determinants are the cause of some problematic classroom behaviors. You can help a teacher see that a poor "goodness of fit" between a child and the environment can lead to problem behaviors and achievement; these are rarely just child problems. Even if the teacher is found to be "wrong" in the end, it is critical to use your consultation skills to help the teacher reframe his or her impressions so that they are congruent with the objective data, as suggested in Case Study 3.2. Otherwise, you've eliminated an important opportunity to work collaboratively with the teacher.

Conducting a Screening Battery Assessment

Your choice of assessment tools should occur in stages, beginning with the screening battery evaluation. Choosing the screening instruments depends on the prereferral data previously collected and the initial teacher, parent, and/or child interviews regarding the referral question. At this initial assessment stage, you should address environmental/historical issues thoroughly, as factors such as educational, cultural, linguistic, medical, emotional, behavioral, psychosocial stressors, and expectations can all influence current functioning and test performance (Sbordone & Purisch, 1996). You should at least attempt to include behavior ratings and interviews (with a teacher, a parent, and [if applicable], the child); a systematic classroom observation; a measure of intellectual/cognitive functioning; and a multidimensional (e.g., reading, math, spelling) achievement measure. Even if a learning disabilities teacher or other teacher conducts the team achievement evaluation, we believe that you should still collect some achievement information, as this will help you formulate your diagnostic impressions and treatment recommendations. Although this basic "screening battery" should be administered to all children, there are circumstances in which you may wish to use additional measures (or eliminate others) during this screening stage.

The initial evaluation should take place during one session, if possible (with adequate breaks offered, depending on the child's developmental level). However, teachers can be reluctant to

CASE STUDY 3.2. **Reframing Billy's Referral Question**

I (Hale) once consulted with a kindergarten teacher who was frustrated with Billy's "disruptive" behavior, and complained that he was always in time out. She said he needed special education for his "outrageous and uncontrollable behavior," which is hardly behavioral terminology. A functional analysis revealed that he only called out, talked to his peers, and played with objects during teacher lectures to the whole class. The teacher never engaged Billy during these times; moreover, she always conducted the lectures from the front of the room, and Billy sat in the back row. Finally, the time-out chair was in a play area in the back of the room, with a walled partition separating the child from the rest of the class. Time out, which should last only the length of the child's age, was for over 20 minutes. Peering over the partition, I noticed Billy quietly playing with the boxes of toys during time out. Needless to say, I did not think that an evaluation was necessary.

In meeting with the teacher, I showed her the results of my observation, and we brainstormed possible things she could do to help Billy. We eventually agreed to change his seat to the front, to increase his participation by calling on him, improving teacher proximity, and to make time out less appealing by removing all interesting objects from the time-out area. These interventions resulted in a decrease in Billy's disruptive behavior. Had these strategies not worked, then a formal evaluation might be necessary, with our major concern being a problem with auditory attention, auditory processing, or language comprehension.

---

have children tested over an extended period. At one extreme, a teacher may tell you to test a child only during one class period, which is typically less than an hour. This should be avoided, as repeated test sessions disrupt rapport and violate standardized test administration requirements. Because your evaluation will follow this child throughout his or her academic career, you must make every attempt to get valid data. For administering and scoring the tests, excellent sources, such as Kamphaus (2001), Kaufman (1994), and Sattler (2001), are available to refresh your memory about collecting assessment observation data and administering tests. However, In-Depth 3.1 provides you with several additional issues related to using neuropsychological principles when conducting evaluations.

After completing this initial evaluation, most psychologists score and interpret their data and write their reports. They base their diagnostic and treatment recommendations on their observations, interviews, rating scales, assessment impressions, test results, and interpretation of data. This is certainly appropriate if the data obtained are all within normal limits. We should not continue to test children with numerous measures in an attempt to find a deficit (Lezak, 1995), because as the number of measures increases, the likelihood that one will be discrepant is likely. This is the Type I error that we are told to avoid in statistics—saying that there is a problem when there is indeed none. The null hypothesis is that there is "no problem," and we should reject the null hypothesis only when there is convincing evidence of deficient performance. However, if there is an apparent problem during the initial screening battery assessment, we cannot stop here; we must validate our apparent findings. Typical school psychology practice does not afford an opportunity to confirm our clinical impressions. We are instead asked to make diagnostic "leaps of faith" (Reschly & Gresham, 1989), which serve to limit our effectiveness in understanding children and helping them learn and behave in the classroom. But with fewer formal evaluations (due to the intervention assistance team's [IAT's] effectiveness!), this initial evaluation is designed to help us generate hypotheses about a child's strengths and needs, and to test hypotheses until we have incremental validity supporting our interpretation.

IN-DEPTH 3.1. Administration and Interpretation Issues

The following issues can affect the validity of your interpretation and the utility of your assessment results:

- *Maintaining rapport requires talking to the child at his or her developmental level, but not violating standardized administration and scoring of the measure.* Too often children's global test scores change because of administration differences—a source of error that can be avoided. The bottom line is that you must adhere to the manual's directions, and score the behavior you obtain from the child.
- *If you think that the results do not reflect the child's current functioning, you should test the limits (TTL) to obtain maximal performance.* When you are using TTL results, report a score according to standardized administration, then calculate another using the raw score obtained during TTL, and report both scores. Don't assume that a child can do something if he or she doesn't; objectivity in administration and scoring is paramount.
- *Rigid adherence to the test manual and directions is likely to interfere with rapport, so supplement standardized instructions with rapport-maintaining activities.* Maintaining rapport requires minimal "casual conversation" between subtests and "checking in" with children to ensure they are motivated and understanding what is expected of them. It does no good to report extremely low scores or numerous "spoiled" subtests, which render the overall evaluation invalid (this does happen from time to time).
- *If doing so is not contraindicated, you should supplement or paraphrase instructions or ask the child what he or she is supposed to do, to ensure that the child understands the task.* After using standardized instructions, you may need other techniques to ensure that the child understands the task demands, unless such techniques are explicitly contraindicated in the manual. As this is *not* possible for memory, fluid reasoning, and executive function tasks, you must administer such tests as specified, and then report any deviations that occurred during your TTL. You can't decide to change the wording of instructions because they are poorly written (even though some are!), because the children in the norming sample also had those poorly written instructions. However, you may have to modify your administration and interpretation after the child performs very poorly with the standardized procedure.
- *You must describe any deviations from standardized administration, indicating that the results are not valid and that interpretation should be made with caution.* Psychologists are often reluctant to say that their results are invalid, as if this suggests they did something wrong. Although reporting that the results are invalid limits your findings, this option is better than (for example) having a child fly through the Differential Ability Scales (DAS) Speed of Information Processing subtest and receive a scale score of 2 because he or she didn't attend to or understand the directions.
- *Because a child will have higher motivation for preferred tasks than for difficult ones, you must record all responses and behavior during testing.* We all have a tendency to like the things we are good at, and to dislike things that are difficult for us. During testing, it is important for you to be energized and motivated, so the child will work hard during the evaluation. In your observations, note whether motivation waxes and wanes, or whether affect changes, within or between subtests. A good dose of empathy can encourage and support children when they have difficulty on test items, as will be the case on any subtest where they miss multiple items on their way to a discontinue rule.

(continued)

IN-DEPTH 3.1. *(continued)*

• *Scribble observation notes all over your protocol, and write down all responses, regardless of whether they are correct or not.* Sometimes "seasoned" psychologists barely write anything on protocols, just the scores. This tells us little about a child's performance and behavior. Also, only noting error responses provides clues to the child about his or her performance.

• *Subtest demands and a child's neuropsychological profile can influence test-taking motivation and behavior.* What hemisphere is more likely to be involved during the beginning of a subtest? You may think of the right hemisphere, because the task is novel when it is first introduced. However, the correct answer depends on the type of task and the individual's proficiency on the measure. For instance, on most achievement measures, the earlier the item, the more the left hemisphere will be engaged because the answer is automatic; the right hemisphere will be more involved during later, more complex items. The beginning of novel cognitive tasks requires right-hemisphere processes until the child becomes accustomed to the task demands and chooses a problem-solving strategy. Input, processing, and output demands can even change during a subtest. For instance, initial Block Design performance can deteriorate when the block lines are removed from the stimulus design. This unexpected task change happens in the middle of the task, so the early–late principle varies according to the nature of the task demands.

Cognitive Hypothesis Testing and Successive Levels of Interpretation

Whether you are conducting problem-solving consultation with or without standardized cognitive and neuropsychological data, you should use the scientific method when conducting evaluations and/or interventions. A plausible theory calls for an empirical test of its validity. After you develop a testable hypothesis, and collect and interpret the data, you evaluate the validity of the theory. This is what our cognitive hypothesis-testing (CHT) model is all about. CHT is not unlike approaches that have been advocated by neuropsychologists for some time (see D'Amato, Rothlisberg, & Rhodes, 1997; Fennell & Bauer, 1997). However, unlike other empirical methods that focus on overt behavior, CHT calls for you to go one step further: examining the *input, processing,* and *output demands* of the tests you administer, and relating the findings to all other obtained data. Of course, the input and output demands are easy to see, but processing demands are more difficult to ascertain, as all we really have are observable and measurable behaviors from which to draw inferences about neuropsychological processes. As noted previously, just looking at observable input and output demands led to over a century of misconception about how the hemispheres process information, and many misguided attempts at establishing aptitude–treatment interactions (ATIs) as a result.

Each hypothesis derived during the initial evaluation should be subsequently evaluated for its validity. There are numerous measures available to test hypotheses, and most are easy to administer and score. It is important to critically examine these measures carefully before use—not only to ensure their technical quality, but also to examine their characteristics in relation to the child's functioning (Telzrow, 1989). Although your instrument choice will depend on the initial results, it is often important to use measures of attention/concentration, learning, and memory, as these are the most common symptoms of dysfunction (Reynolds & Mayfield, 1999). However, you must be selective in choosing measures, as excessive testing will lead to fatigue and poor test performance (Spreen & Strauss, 1998). Exactly which measures you administer will depend on the data previously acquired, their technical characteristics, and the number and types of hypotheses you have. However, you must be flexible in understanding the results of individual subtests, and not remain tied to one interpretation conclusion for each subtest, as highlighted in Case Study 3.3.

When you are choosing additional measures for hypothesis testing, it is important to make sure that they vary according to simple–complex, rote–novel, and single-modality–modality demands (Rourke, 1994), and to look for similarities and differences on the measures that tap similar constructs (Sattler, 2001). From the previous chapters, it should be clear that even the simplest of tasks requires cooperation among almost every brain area. Therefore, you need to examine the various instruments available to you, and choose several measures within the context of what you know about the child's history, the existing data, and brain–behavior relationships. You may have a good idea of why the child is failing math tests or arguing with peers, but further analysis is required. A critical component of the CHT model is trying to *refute* your hypotheses; that is, you must try to maintain the null hypothesis, or run the risk of confirmation bias. Reject the null hypothesis only when you have considerable evidence to support your conclusions. Don't fall into a pattern in which you look for confirming evidence and avoid other data that does not fit with your hypothesis. Instead, keep an open mind, and explore multiple possible explanations for the child's behavior. Table 3.1 highlights important questions to ask yourself when interpreting test results, especially when the subtest data don't fit well with your other findings.

Which measures should you use for CHT? In Chapter 1, we have described several intellectual assessment tools, and subtests from these measures can be used for hypothesis testing. In Chapter 4, we describe a number of neuropsychological assessment tools we find useful in CHT. We primarily report measures that have good psychometric characteristics, but we realize that

---

CASE STUDY 3.3. Joey's Auditory Processing Problem

Joey, aged 10-3, apparently had an auditory processing problem. He had difficulty following class directions and frequently asked for repetition. Examination of his permanent products, and of his Wechsler Individual Achievement Test—Second Edition subtest data, revealed he was well below average in reading and spelling—apparently due to sound–symbol association deficits (presumed dysfunction in the superior temporal gyrus, angular gyrus, or secondary visual areas). However, on the Woodcock–Johnson (WJ-III), Joey's *Ga* Sound Blending subtest score was significantly below average (supporting the hypothesis), but his Incomplete Words subtest score was in the average range (refuting the hypothesis). Interpreting the WJ-III *Ga* cluster was obviously inappropriate (a significant subtest difference), so an examination of the subtests was in order. Was this subtest difference due to motivation, subtest construction, or differences in test demands? Joey seemed to try hard on both tasks, but an examination of the subtest sample space revealed very little at the upper age ranges, so a couple of errors could account for a fairly large SS difference.

Although this could possibly explain the difference, an examination of the task demands revealed an important distinction between the subtests: The Incomplete Words subtest requires auditory closure, whereas Sound Blending requires sequencing and phonological assembly skills. Further analysis of phonemic processing (left hemisphere), global processing (right hemisphere), and sequential processing (frontal lobes) helped delineate the exact nature of the problem. Joey did have phonological processing problems due to difficulties related to the superior temporal lobe, but he compensated for these by using good auditory closure skills on the Incomplete Words subtest. Several children with this deficit do well on this subtest; they hear part of the word (even if they miss some phonemes), and are still able to provide a plausible response. Concluding that they have adequate auditory processing skills on the basis of the *Ga* cluster score would be inappropriate and misleading, which is a risk with interpreting global or factor scores when significant variability exists (Fiorello et al., 2001).

TABLE 3.1. Seven Questions for Effective Interpretation of Performance Variability

- Are subtest input, processing, and output demands reflective of the construct of interest?
- Could a particular input, processing, or output demand change the subtest score?
- Does the subtest measure something different for a child because a particular strategy was used?
- Is the subtest sensitive to and specific for the construct of interest?
- Does the subtest have adequate technical characteristics?
- Could the child's behavior before, during, or after the subtest help explain performance?
- Did a change in my interaction style or test administration affect the results?

many "clinical" tools have a long history of use in clinical neuropsychology and can be useful for establishing incremental validity. However, it is important to realize that CHT and the application of neuropsychological principles in daily practice are difficult enough that we do not want to support continued use of "clinical" tools that have not been standardized or received enough empirical support. Recall that your assessment tools and your administration, scoring, and interpretation should meet the criteria described in the *Standards for Educational and Psychological Testing* volume (American Educational Research Association, American Psychological Association, & National Council on Measurement in Education, 1999). You need to examine test coverage, content validity, and comprehensiveness (Rourke, 1994). Many tests may be sensitive to deficits or dysfunction (e.g., attention problems), but have little specificity (ADHD-only attention problems). As discussed in In-Depth 3.2, the use of clinical tools must be limited to supporting empirical judgments, not the other way around.

IN-DEPTH 3.2. The Value of Clinical Judgment

Is there a place for clinical judgment in CHT? In addition to examination of normative data, "clinical norms" (sometimes referred to as "head norms") may have to be used when you are interpreting neuropsychological data (Reynolds, 1997). Although a qualitative clinical approach provides you with tremendous insight, it is difficult to learn; it does not allow for verification of results; and it does not readily allow for determination of treatment efficacy (Rourke, 1994). However, we don't want you to assume that qualitative, clinical approaches are meaningless. Instead, we stress that diagnoses should not be made in the absence of adequate norm-referenced measures (Reynolds, 1997). Test scores are only useful insofar as they allow for clinical interpretation (Lezak, 1995), and understanding the processes a child displays during testing can have intervention implications (D'Amato et al., 1997). You should not get "stuck on psychometrics" (i.e., fixating on numbers that may or may not accurately represent the child's true level and pattern of performance).

Every child is a single-case study, in which you must decipher the relationships among overt behavior, psychological processes, and neuropsychological systems (Bernstein, 2000). Ultimately, while the numbers remain important, and their consistency helps determine the confidence you have in your conclusions, it is up to you to make appropriate clinical judgments. There is often an inherent tradeoff between sensitivity (detecting a problem) and specificity (discriminating among problems), so we must strive for a balance between the two (Reynolds, 1997). It is important to remember that the costs associated with diagnostic error are constant; a Type I error (identifying a problem when none exists) is as bad as a Type II error (identifying no problem when one exists). Good diagnostic decisions are based on both actuarial and clinical factors (Willis, 1986).

After you have carefully collected additional data from these measures during the hypothesis-testing stage, you should reexamine all of the data to determine whether your original theory was accurate. Some data will be consistent, while other data may not. Again, it is important to look at all data, not just supporting evidence that confirms your hypotheses (Hale & Fiorello, 2002). There are many reasons why the data may not fit, one of which is that your original theory was not quite right. If your theory appears to be accurate, then a crucial search for ecological validity can be undertaken. Only after ecological and treatment validities are established can you be entirely sure that your theory appeared to be a good one.

The Missing Link: Ecological and Treatment Validity

Ecological validity is one of our biggest concerns about practitioners' adopting and using CHT and demands analysis strategies. Many educators complain that neuropsychology has everything to do with diagnosis, but nothing to do with intervention. Although finding objective data to support inferences can be difficult, understanding how these inferences relate to the child's daily functioning is critical (Matarazzo, 1990). There is growing empirical interest in the ecological validity of neuropsychological assessment results, and a corresponding focus on enhancing practical everyday skills in intervention (Stringer & Nadolne, 2000). You must bridge the gap between neuropsychological knowledge and everyday practice. For each child, you will need to find evidence in the classroom, the home, or some other setting that relates your test findings to the natural environment. Without confirming evidence of ecological validity, no matter how convinced you are, your findings should at best be considered a "working hypothesis." Ecological validity data are acquired through examination of all existing data; follow-up direct observations; and consultation with parents, teachers, and/or the child. Finding ecological validity data is not as difficult as you think, as suggested by Application 3.1. Try to develop lists of ecological validity signs on your

---

APPLICATION 3.1. Auditory Processing Problems in the Classroom

Think of some things you might see during an observation that might suggest an auditory processing problem in a child. During interviews and observations, we have seen the following signs of ecological validity for auditory processing problems:

- Asks to have questions repeated.
- Does not understand oral directions or displays perplexed look during such directions.
- When repeating words or sentences, substitutes words that sound similar.
- Does not recall some or most of a phrase just heard.
- Does not pronounce words clearly.
- Fails to take notes, or looks at other children's notes, during lecture.
- Relies on context clues and discussion before answering questions.
- Performs better on written than on oral exercises.
- Uses sight word approach when reading, and avoids decoding unknown words.
- Has spelling errors that do not make phonemic sense.
- Reports being confused in classroom, especially when it is "too loud."
- Has limited verbal interactions during noisy, unstructured activities.
- Asks for frequent help during oral activities.
- Uses both hand and facial gestures or props to further communication efforts.
- Has receptive language problems, despite a normal audiological examination.

---

own—not only for auditory processing problems, but for problems with other types of cognitive processing as well. Some helpful ecological validity examples tied to various brain areas can be found in Appendix 3.1.

There are several sources that can provide you with the ecological validity you need. Parent and teacher reports should be analyzed for concurrent validity, and children should be encouraged to discuss their own perspective as well (Baron, Fennell, & Voeller, 1995). You should compare and contrast your results to other data sources, and determine what could account for any discrepancies. It is amazing to find how parent or teacher perspectives can shed light on clinical data. For instance, during an initial interview, a mother described her son as inattentive, unkempt, and socially inept. He showed classic signs of asomatognosia during testing, so I (Hale) asked her to tell me about his language understanding and prosody. She said that he had a hard time understanding jokes, and that he couldn't tell whether she was angry or happy when she talked to him. However, the teacher did not recognize this pattern at school; this is not an uncommon occurrence, given the difference in setting demands or differential tolerance of problem behaviors (McBride, 1988). Discrepancies may suggest different behavior in the home and school, but may suggest different expectations as well (Sattler, 2001). In addition to parent report, teacher report, and child self-report, it is important to establish ecological validity by determining how the assessment results affect classroom behaviors (through direct observation) and classroom performance (through examination of permanent products, such as classroom assignments and tests). Direct observation in different settings and time periods not only helps you establish ecological validity, but also lays the foundation for intervention development, implementation, and evaluation.

What about those pesky clinical hunches you have regarding a child? You may have clinical beliefs about your child's performance and underlying characteristics, but they should be considered tentative working hypotheses until you have established ecological validity. As stated earlier, quantitative and qualitative data are interrelated and essential to substantiate clinical conclusions (Lezak, 1995), and both types can be used during consultative sessions to establish ecological validity and develop intervention plans. However, you must remember that even qualitative clinical judgments need objective support. At the same time you search for support for your clinical judgments, work just as diligently at ruling out other possible causes for your findings (Bernstein, 2000). If these attempts are thorough and ecological validity is established, you will hear from parents and teachers what we have heard on numerous occasions—the rewarding phrase "How did you get to know him so well?"

Discussing Evaluation Results and Planning Interventions

Once you have established ecological validity, and your data support your conclusions, you now have a theory as to why the child is having a particular difficulty. This theory is then discussed with the parent and teacher as part of the problem-solving process, where you and the teacher agree about the nature of the problem and possible remedies. Your knowledge of neuropsychological principles puts you in a unique position of helping other team members recognize the underlying processes that contribute to what they have seen (Bernstein, 2000). However, avoid the temptation to "label" the problem during this discussion. We left-hemisphere types want a definitive answer—the "cause" of a problem—but it is never that clear cut, and the problems associated with labeling are too numerous to list here. It is best to talk about the child's current functioning, in order to avoid the expectancy effects that are more likely to result if the child is labeled (Sattler, 2001). This initial conversation should build upon previous discussions and should focus on understanding the nature of the child's strengths and needs, not on bringing finality to the process by assigning a label to the child. Your credibility with the teacher will be enhanced if you use examples of what you've seen in the classroom and during testing, as well as what the teacher reported during the interview. Allen and Graden (1995) provide us with several important problem-solving considerations to remember when we enter the problem-solving phase:

1. All children have the potential to learn.
2. Learning is an interaction between the child and the environment.
3. Assessment and intervention require multidimensional approaches.
4. Problem solving is about solutions, not "problem admiration."
5. Service delivery is about meeting children's needs, not solely determining eligibility.
6. Assessment and intervention is necessarily idiosyncratic to the child and situation.

Evaluation and intervention are two sides of the same coin (Holmes-Bernstein, 2000). What you did at the beginning of CHT, you continue during the intervention phase. The problem-solving model takes over within this paradigm. You and the teacher brainstorm possible intervention strategies, develop an intervention plan, and agree on the methodology for carrying out and evaluating the intervention. Data collection begins, and you modify/recycle your hypothesis as necessary. The fact that you have a good understanding of the problem doesn't mean that the intervention you choose will automatically work. As we noted earlier, the CHT model begins with the collection of prereferral and evaluation data; it does not end with it. Just as a hypothesis needs recycling after you refute it, the same is true when it comes to interventions. The CHT results only give you a better understanding of the problem and a greater likelihood of choosing an appropriate intervention. Intervention efficacy, or treatment validity, is still required. If your original theory does not appear to be entirely accurate, a new theory should be developed and tested. The hypothesis testing is repeated until you have convincing evidence regarding your theory's validity and the child shows documented gains in the problematic areas. As stated earlier, the comprehensive evaluation is not the endpoint; you need to monitor the child's learning and/or behavior over time. This is possible, given that a majority of referrals are now handled by the IAT.

Good interventions are adaptive, flexible, and ecologically valid. It does no good to have children learn to draw in the sand when they need to learn to write with a pencil on a piece of paper. One of the biggest drawbacks of specific interventions that are designed to improve brain functioning, but that do not include naturalistic task demands, is that they are seldom generalized to the classroom setting (Taylor, 1989). We believe it is important to use interventions that focus on the skills required in the classroom or other naturalistic setting. Listed in later chapters are a number of excellent sources to help you develop a good understanding of interventions in academic and behavioral areas; however, they must be realistic, adapted to the individual situation and the resources available (Rourke, 1994). The teacher is an excellent resource for developing interventions, but if your academic program didn't require a class in special education, you may wish to consider purchasing some of the texts listed in Chapters 5–7 to get a better understanding of teaching. We disagree with problem-solving advocates who suggest that the teacher should know all the strategies, and that your job as consultant is merely to facilitate the teacher's decision making. True, that is one of your objectives. However, if you can demonstrate a knowledge of and interest in the teaching process, this will give you much more credibility. The field has not done a good job of individualizing interventions in the past (Reynolds, 1988), so it is up to you to establish individual ATIs at the single-subject level (Braden & Kratochwill, 1997). In your efforts to help individual children, you should build a "theory of pedagogy" to truly link neuropsychological assessment findings to effective interventions (Bernstein, 2000).

INTERPRETING TEST RESULTS FROM A NEUROPSYCHOLOGICAL PERSPECTIVE

Specifying the Interpretive Sequence

One of the most common ways to interpret neuropsychological test data is to follow the procedure for interpreting the Halstead–Reitan Neuropsychological Test Battery outlined by Reitan (1974). Reitan specified four steps in the interpretive process:

1. Levels of performance.
2. Patterns of performance.
3. Left–right (and posterior–anterior) differences.
4. Pathognomonic signs.

The levels-of-performance interpretation compares the individual's performance to that of the normative group for the measure in question. By its very nature, it is a developmental examination of how the child compares to his or her same-age peers. This is the normative developmental or vertical interpretation described by Bernstein (2000). As it is the nomothetic approach to interpretation, it serves to help us define the nature of the problem at a gross level. This is contrasted with the examination of Reitan's (1974) patterns of performance—the systematic analysis of intraindividual strengths and needs. This level of analysis is essential for developing hypotheses about cognitive characteristics and individualized interventions. The interpretation of left–right differences, as the term implies, requires examination of the hemispheric functions. We further this level of analysis by adding a posterior–anterior component. Pathognomonic signs are considered frank signs of brain damage, although there is some concern that not all pathognomonic signs are purely the results of brain damage. Instead, they may be better seen as gross signs of atypical brain development, organization, or function.

Levels of Performance

Although a levels-of-performance or nomothetic approach to interpretation is essential for understanding a child's developmental level, there are advantages and disadvantages associated with this type of interpretation. One advantage of nomothetic interpretation is that it is generally a simpler approach to understanding child performance; one score is easier to interpret than many. As a result, nomothetic scores are more familiar to both professionals and laypeople, and results are easier to communicate to others. We left-brain types want *the* answer, and nomothetic approaches allow concrete conclusions to be drawn. However, as discussed previously, there are certain problems associated with interpreting intellectual and other measures from a levels-of-performance perspective, especially when individual variability in performance is evident (Fiorello, Hale, McGrath, Ryan, & Quinn, 2001; Hale & Fiorello, 2001). For children with significant factor or subtest variability, global scores are essentially abstractions that represent a conglomerate of many different skills, making it virtually impossible to determine what cognitive or behavioral characteristic they actually represent (Lezak, 1995). However, rather than conclude that the nomothetic/normative approach is irrelevant, we need to see the scores for what they are worth. These normative scores provide a developmental benchmark to help determine how the child's performance is related to that of peers, and can be used to determine how performance changes over time (Rourke, 1994). Subtest or factor scores are readily interpreted by other professionals, and provide others with an opportunity to see how the child's performance differs on various measures.

For clarity of communication, we suggest you use standardized measures that provide a standard score (SS) that reflects performance in relation to the appropriate normative sample. Regardless of the derived score reported in the manuals, we prefer to put *all* scores in the same metric, because it is easier for others to interpret and provides for associated percentile ranks. Any normative score (e.g., *T* score, *z* score) can be converted to an SS via the equations listed in Application 3.2. However, ensure that you have the right value for the score, so that higher scores reflect better performance. For instance, if the Time score on the Trail Making Test (Trails Time) for a child is lower than the mean (i.e., faster performance), the child would have an SS below 100; however, using simple addition, the amount below 100 is how much the "real" SS would be above 100 (e.g., a calculated SS of 88 on Trails Time would equal an SS of 112).

In addition to putting scores in common metrics, we prefer to use normative descriptors rather than scores in reports. As discussed later, scores can be reported at the end of the report in a table and/or figure. It is distracting to have numbers and statistical concepts in the middle of your clinical impressions, and is meaningless for many people who read the report. We prefer the performance descriptors listed in Table 3.2, which are used for the results of many intellectual/cognitive tools (with some variation). We also advocate the use of confidence intervals, which provide readers with an understanding of the imperfect nature of measurement of human performance. You may be wondering about the use of age equivalents (AEs) or grade equivalents (GEs). We feel that these scores are some of the most dangerous scores available to us, because they are

---

APPLICATION 3.2. Converting to Standard Scores

Use the following equations to compute first a *z* score, and then a standard score (SS).

1. *z* score = (raw score – population mean)/population standard deviation
2. SS = 100 + (*z* score × 15)

Example: Let's say Sam is a 10-year-old boy who obtained 25/30 correct on a cancellation task. The mean number correct (*M*) for Sam's age is 25.68, with an associated standard deviation (*SD*) of 3.11. The following steps will give you the SS for Sam's performance:

1. z = (raw score – *M*)/*SD*
   z = (25 – 25.68)/3.11
   z = –.68/3.11
   z = –.219

2. SS = 100 + (*z* score × 15)
   SS = 100 + (–.219 × 15)
   SS = 100 + (– 3.29)
   SS = 97

Then you look up the percentile rank associated with an SS of 97 (found in most test manuals or statistics texts), and you see that this rank is 42, or the 42nd percentile. This metric also helps put things in perspective when *SD*s are high. For instance, let's say Sam earned a total of 14 right out of a possible 40 on the "List-Learning Test." The *M* for his age is 32.39, which at first glance suggests that Sam performed quite poorly on this measure. However, his SS is also based on the *SD*, and in this case, the *SD* for his age is 17.80. Although Sam got fewer than half the items on the test, his SS is an 85, which is just low average.

TABLE 3.2. Levels-of-Performance Descriptors

SS	Performance descriptor
130+	Significantly above average
120–129	Well above average
110–119	High average
90–109	Average
80–89	Low average
70–79	Well below average
69 or below	Significantly below average (intellectual/cognitive/ achievement) or impaired (neuropsychological)

often used by laypeople for a levels-of-performance interpretation, but they are psychometrically unsound (Sattler, 2001). Try to avoid reporting AE and GE scores, or if you do, make sure you add a note indicating that they are not valid for diagnostic purposes.

Even the reporting of SSs and percentiles should be undertaken with extreme caution. As discussed in Chapter 1, the results of our large-sample studies on the validity of IQ scores suggests that significant subtest or factor differences precludes the use of a Full Scale SS for any purpose (Fiorello et al., 2001; Hale, Fiorello, et al., 2001). These large-scale studies suggest that you should *never* report an IQ score whenever there is significant subtest or factor variability. Otherwise, you are reporting a score that is really composed of several different underlying abilities or skills (Lezak, 1995), and any interpretation of that IQ score would be considered inappropriate. How do you determine whether the factor or subtest scores underlying the IQ score are significantly different from one another? We do not recommend ipsative analysis, which involves collapsing the disparate subtest scores into a mean subtest score, and then determining whether any one subtest differs from that mean. As is the case with the global IQ, collapsing these subtest scores into any underlying mean score obscures important diagnostic information, because the very tests that are discrepant from one another are part of the mean score. Instead, we prefer to conduct pairwise comparisons of subtests or factors. The examiner must be aware that as the number of pairwise comparisons increases, the likelihood of a "false positive" or Type I error increases, and this fact has been used (appropriately) to criticize profile analysis (Macmann & Barnett, 1997). Therefore, planned comparisons such as within-factor and subscale comparisons make the most sense, as noted in Application 3.3.

Most test manuals have charts in the appendices to help you determine whether subtest–subtest or factor–factor differences are significant. If the critical values in the table are in decimals, always *round up* for every critical value. For instance, if the critical difference between Subtest A and Subtest B is 4.01 in the table, then you must have a 5-point scaled score difference for it to be significant. Make sure you use a $p < .01$ table (or, if necessary, a $p < .05$ table), or use the hand calculations described in Application 3.4. If there are significant differences between the subtests that make up a global factor or IQ score, we believe that the global score should not be interpreted—or even reported, for that matter. If you feel compelled (e.g., you have been told) to put invalid global scores in your report, indicate that they are invalid because of significant factor or subtest variability. Case Study 3.4 can help you address this issue.

What about tests or measures that do not have significance tables for determining score differences? What about comparisons across measures? Issues related to standardization of the in-

APPLICATION 3.3. Interpretation of Variable Profiles

Examine the following Differential Ability Scales (DAS) profile. It highlights the statistical concepts suggesting that we need to interpret scores beyond the global General Cognitive Ability (GCA) score.

<u>GCA = 106</u>

Verbal Ability = 103	Nonverbal Reasoning Ability = 99	Spatial Ability = 109
Word Definitions = 55	Matrices = 40	Recall of Designs = 54
Similarities = 50	Sequential and Quantitative Reasoning = 59	Pattern Construction = 58

Using what we call a "top-down/bottom-up" examination of this DAS protocol, we can determine whether a levels-of-performance interpretation is valid. Going "top down," we see that the GCA is composed of the three global Verbal Ability (SS = 103), Nonverbal Reasoning (SS = 99), and Spatial Ability (SS = 109) composite scores. When we examine the appendix in the test manual, we see that none of these scores are significantly different from each other at the .05 level, so at this point the GCA is still valid. Next, we look within each of these factors to determine whether the subtests are different. There is no significant difference between the Word Definitions (T = 55) and Similarities (T = 50) subtests, so we go "bottom-up" and find that the Verbal Ability factor SS of 103 is valid. Similarly, there is no difference between the Recall of Designs (T = 54) and Pattern Construction (T = 58) scores, so we find the Spatial Ability SS of 109 to be valid. At this point, nothing we have found suggests that we should interpret anything but the GCA. However, the 19-point difference between Matrices (T = 40) and Sequential and Quantitative Reasoning (T = 59) is highly significant; from a "bottom-up" perspective, therefore, the Nonverbal Reasoning SS of 99 does not truly reflect a unitary construct, and thus invalidates the GCA.

strument, such as type of normative sample, gender differences, cross-cultural representation, and the time when the norms were generated, will influence your interpretation of performance on different measures (Golden, Espe-Pfeifer, & Wachsler-Felder, 2000). While taking these factors into account, you must develop a method for comparison of generated SSs on different measures. There are several different methods for determining significant score differences, the best of which is probably a regression approach (see Flanagan, Ortiz, Alfonso, & Mascolo, 2002); however, this may not be feasible for you as a school practitioner, because few cross-instrument regression equations have been calculated and reported in the manuals. This is especially true if you have significant subtest/factor differences and you are asked to use the invalid global score. One approach that we find particularly useful and less cumbersome is the standard error of the difference (*SED*) (Anastasi & Urbina, 1997; Reynolds, 1985), described in Application 3.4; this provides you with a method for comparing SSs.

Where should you conclude your interpretation? The answer is relatively straightforward for us: If there are no significant subtest or factor differences, then interpret the global IQ score, as it appears to be a reliable and valid indicator of the child's current level of performance. This is, of course, an ideal situation—one where the child's assessment behavior and results suggest that he or she consistently exhibited at a certain level of performance. In a report for this type of child, you would merely report the global score and then provide general descriptions of the various subtests administered. Unfortunately, our results discussed earlier suggest that this "flat" profile is fairly uncommon among the children we see in the field (it is not found for approximately 80%–

The standard error of the difference (*SED*) takes into account the reliability of the measures being compared, and requires the same *SD* for each score. It does not take into account the correlation of the measures. It is defined as follows:

$$SED = SD\sqrt{2 - r_{xx} - r_{yy}}$$

The *SD* will be 15 for your analyses (all scores are converted to SSs). The r_{xx} is the reliability of the first subtest for the given age level, and the r_{yy} is the reliability of the second subtest at the same age level. Let's see whether a 20-point difference between an intelligence test and an achievement measure is significant. Twenty points seems significant, but let's see. On the "Ability Test," Fred earned an SS of 105 ($r_{xx} = .89$); on the "Reading Passages" test, he earned an SS of 85 ($r_{yy} = .72$). We plug these SSs into the equation:

$$SED = 15\sqrt{2 - .89 - .72}$$
$$SED = 15\sqrt{.39}$$
$$SED = 15\,(.624)$$
$$SED = 9.37$$

This is the critical value for *SED*, and the SS difference (105 − 85) must exceed this for it to be significant at the 68% confidence level. We prefer to use the 99% or 95% confidence level. To do so, the *SED* must be multiplied by 2.58 ($p = .01$) or 1.96 ($p = .05$) to obtain the critical value. If we do this, 2.58 × 9.37, we get a critical value of 24.16, and we would need a 25-point difference (we must always round up) between the Ability Test SS and Reading Passages SS for there to be a significant difference. Notice if we use the less stringent $p = .05$ level, our 20-point difference is significant because the *SED* is 19 (1.96 × 9.37 = 18.37). Again, we must always round up, so that a critical value of 17.0001 would require at least an 18-point difference for significance.

Although this method can be used to compare SSs on the same metric, the more appropriate (and complex) method takes into account the correlation between the two scores being compared. This is obviously the preferred method for comparison, but you must have the correlation coefficients between the two measures. Often you can find these coefficients for commonly used measures in test manuals (in the standardization section), but often you must use the simple difference approach described above if the correlations are not available. Again, the following regression-based approach (the standard error of the residual, or *SER*) is the preferred method for calculating whether two scores are different, but it requires the correlation between the two measures.

Let's say that there is a correlation of .55 between the Ability Test and Reading Passages. The first thing we need to do is to find the predicted Ability Test score. It is calculated by first computing a *z* score, which is easy enough; then multiplying this by the correlation to get the predicted score; and then changing back to a predicted SS from which the achievement score will be subtracted.

1. $z_{AT} = (\text{raw score} - M)/SD$

    $z_{AT} = (105 - 100)/15 = .33$

2. $z_{(AT\ predicted)} = r_{xy}\, z_{AT}$

    $z_{(AT\ predicted)} = .55(.33) = .1815$

(continued)

3. $SS_{\text{(AT predicted)}} = 100 + (z_{\text{(predicted)}} \times 15)$

$SS_{\text{(AT predicted)}} = 100 + (.1815)(15) = 102.72 = 103$

4. Discrepancy difference $= SS_{\text{(AT predicted)}} - SS_{\text{(RP)}}$

$$= 103 - 85 = 18 \text{ points}$$

So, if the *SER* we calculate is less than 18, we will reject the null hypothesis of no difference between the tests, and there will be a discrepancy. To calculate the *SER*, we first need to calculate the residual score reliability, which is defined by the following formula:

1. $r_{\text{residual}} = r_{yy} + (r_{xx})(r^2_{xy}) - 2r^2_{xy}/1 - r^2_{xy}$

2. $r_{\text{residual}} = r_{yy} + (r_{xx})(r^2_{xy}) - 2r^2_{xy}/1 - r^2_{xy}$

$$= .72 + (.89)(.55^2) - 2(.55^2)/1 - (.55^2)$$

$$= .72 + (.89)(.3025) - 2(.3025)/1 - .3025$$

$$= .72 + (.269225) - (.605)/.6975$$

$$= .55086$$

Now we can calculate the *SER*, which is defined by the following formula:

$SER = SD\sqrt{1 - r^2_{xy}} \sqrt{1 - r_{\text{residual}}}$

$$= 15\sqrt{1 - .3025} \sqrt{1 - 55086}$$

$$= 15(.83516)(.67018)$$

$$= 8.39560$$

We need to multiply this value by 1.96 for $p < .05$ ($1.96 \times 8.39560 = 16.455$) and round up to 17, which suggests that we need a 17-point difference for these scores to be significant. Our critical score was 18, so the scores are different. However, if we take the more rigorous route ($p < .01$), we obtain a value of 22 ($2.58 \times 8.39560 = 21.661$); this exceeds our 18-point difference between ability and achievement, so there is no significant difference at the .01 level.

Notice how these *SER* values are *lower* than the values we obtained using the simple *SED* formula described earlier. Therefore, you are more likely to reject the null hypothesis (i.e., there is a difference) with the *SER* than you are with the simple *SED* formula. Given that the *SED* is a much simpler formula, we'd suggest using the *SED* first and stopping there if you have significance, because you will also have significance if you use the *SER*. Similarly, if the difference between your test scores is much lower than the *SED* critical value, you could take a chance and suggest that there is no difference. However, keep in mind that the *SER* is related to the correlation between the two test scores, so "eyeballing" it may lead to error. If the difference between test scores is close to your *SED* critical value, but does not exceed it, you should calculate the *SER*. Keep in mind that you're more likely to make a Type II error (failing to reject the null hypothesis when it is indeed false) with the *SED*. In other words, when you use the *SED* formula, you are more likely to conclude that there is no difference between the scores when there actually *is* a difference, so in many ways it is the more conservative approach for determining whether two scores are different from one another. Using *SED*, you are more likely to have a false-negative result (no score difference when there actually is one) than a false-positive one (score difference when there isn't any).

CASE STUDY 3.4. Sara's Written Report

The following text from Sara's report will help you meet the need to report global scores that are not valid for interpretive purposes:

> On the Woodcock–Johnson III (WJ-III), a measure of intellectual and cognitive functioning, Sara obtained a General Intellectual Ability (GIA) score of 105, with 95% confidence of her true score falling between 99 and 111. This score is a standard score (SS), where the average score is 100 and the standard deviation is 15. This means that 68% of all children Sara's age score between 85 and 115. This score places her in the average range and at the 63rd percentile compared to her same-age peers. This global score suggests that she is performing at a level similar to, or greater than, 63% of her same-age peers. However, this score should be interpreted with caution, because there were significant differences among the subtests that are used to calculate this global score.

90%). Our research also confirms that there are high "base rates" for significant discrepancies (i.e., most children show factor differences), but our results suggest that even for typical children with variable profiles, the global IQ cannot be interpreted (Fiorello et al., 2001; Hale, Fiorello, et al., 2001). For children with variable profiles (i.e., significant subtest or factor differences), some have advocated interpreting subtest combinations (e.g., McGrew & Flanagan, 1998), but we feel that interpretation must go beyond nomothetic approaches to the idiographic level when significant subtest or factor scores are found. We must interpret patterns of performance—the difficult, controversial, and often maligned practice we have discussed in Chapter 1.

Patterns of Performance

As stated earlier, idiographic analysis should be avoided if possible, because interpretation of global factors is preferable to analysis of subtest scores (Anastasi & Urbina, 1997). However, if we have significant factor or subtest differences, we have no choice but to go to this level of analysis, especially in subtle cases in which we wish to understand the true nature of brain-related dysfunction (Golden et al., 2000). Interpreting patterns of performance requires clinical acumen— something that can only be acquired through considerable training and supervised experience. This book will help you build upon the skills already developed, but analyzing a child's patterns of performance requires discordant/divergent right-hemisphere processes, in addition to concordant/convergent left-hemisphere skills (both of which have been discussed in Chapter 2). Problem solving requires exploring multiple possibilities before formulating a plan (Allen & Graden, 1995), so frontal and right-hemisphere skills are critical. When examining children, we must look at all aspects of their behavior and environment, and establish the concurrent, ecological, and treatment validity of our test results, if our CHT model is to be fruitful.

An individual's test performance cannot occur in a vacuum (Lezak, 1995). Individuals are not scores, so we admonish you to avoid using a left-hemisphere, "cookbook" approach to subtest interpretation. Subtle qualitative differences in a child's performance across and within measures may be reflective of meaningful brain–behavior relationships, and these differences will be obscured if the focus is on test results only (Golden et al., 2000). Instead of focusing solely on scores, we advocate a process approach—one that emphasizes Luria's (1973) individualized assessment methodology and provides a strategy for maximizing the richness of clinical data (Bernstein, 2000). The Boston process approach, developed by Kaplan and colleagues (see Kaplan, 1997), attempts to objectify qualitative differences in child subtest data. Kaplan has argued that the problem with both fixed and flexible neuropsychological test batteries is that interpretation is based on correct or incorrect item performance, whereas the problem-solving process approach can provide insights into neuropsychological processes that have direct implications for intervention. To accomplish this, it is not enough just to examine the outcome of performance (i.e., right or wrong); rather, it is necessary to determine how the child arrived at a particular answer (Milberg, Hebben, & Kaplan, 1986). The process approach is inherently child-centered, sensitive to the unique characteristics of children and their environment. As stated earlier, we must recognize that the brain functions as a set of interdependent systems, with systems doing the best they can to process and respond to task demands in a gradiential fashion (Goldberg, 2001). Individual functional brain areas attempt to accomplish tasks that might typically be performed by a dysfunctional area, albeit not as successfully. This has been called the "complementary-contribution principle" (Bernstein, 2000): In the absence or dysfunction of one system, another system does the best it can to accomplish the task. How do these systems interconnect and cooperate or inhibit one another? It is your job to determine how the pattern fits together—a task that not only requires idiographic analysis of performance, but allows for verification of results by means of the CHT model.

When conducting CHT, you clinically examine a child's pattern of performance both within and between measures, because you cannot determine what one score suggests without analyzing other scores and data (Groth-Marnat, Gallagher, Hale, & Kaplan, 2000). You go beyond the typical input and output observations made by most psychologists, and focus on neuropsychological processes, which can shed light on important child strengths and weaknesses. Identification of strengths not only helps you avoid pathologizing the child; it also lays a foundation for subsequent intervention development (Spreen & Strauss, 1998). As argued earlier, exploring input and output demands led to misconceptions about hemispheric functions, and failed ATIs. The multifactorial nature of subtests requires fine-grained analysis of input, processing, and output demands, as well as systematic testing of the limits (TTL), if we are to realize the potential of our clinical tools to the extent necessary for evaluation of hypothesized strengths and needs (Kaplan, 1997).

Whereas the normative approach provides little insight into individual differences in academic performance and behavioral functioning, this idiographic orientation allows us to establish important linkages among cognitive, academic, and behavioral functioning. It can serve as an integrative framework for interpreting apparently disparate behaviors. However, we must be extremely cautious, because our own heuristics and biases can influence our interpretation (Bernstein, 2000). We must realize that subtest variability could be due to many factors, so interpretation should proceed only with the greatest of caution. We need to recognize that children with the same disorder may have different symptoms, and that similar symptoms can be caused by different disorders (Sattler, 2001). Variability among "cognitive phenotypes" is common, and even when these may look superficially alike, they may involve fundamentally different cognitive processes (Dennis, 2000). It is your responsibility to determine the nature of the expressed characteristics, and careful clinical analyses can clarify an otherwise confusing array of data (Lezak, 1995).

The key to successful CHT is recognizing the multifactorial nature of subtests, identifying the consistency among cognitive constructs tapped by the measures, and attempting to link them to brain functions. Demands analysis, as introduced in Chapter 1 and elaborated on in Chapter 4, provides you with the tool to recognize the similarities and differences among the subtests. We also provide you in this chapter with two appendices (Appendix 3.2 and Appendix 3.3) that you can reproduce for interpretive purposes. These forms allow you to take notes and generate hypotheses about a child's performance, based on the four-quadrant demands analysis approach described below. It is important to realize that demands analysis does not allow you to ignore the nomothetic or quantitative aspects of subtest performance. It requires you to recognize the limitations of qualitative analysis, and to consider the technical characteristics of subtests (e.g., sample space, unique and shared variance, and standard error of measurement), when drawing conclusions about child performance. Although poor technical quality has been a problem with neuropsychological assessment tools in the past (Reynolds, 1997), this is changing, and a majority of the instruments we list in Chapter 4 have excellent technical quality. Clinical and qualitative information is important, but neuropsychological assessment requires an examination of how test reliability and validity affect performance and interpretation (Groth-Marnat, 2000a). We agree that demands analysis is inherently more difficult and more prone to error if not undertaken with the greatest of care and empirical rigor. However, it can shed new light on seemingly random variations in subtest performance, especially if you consider the posterior–anterior and left–right axes discussed in Chapter 2.

Left–Right (and Posterior–Anterior) Differences

In addition to the left–right differences noted by Reitan (1974), we add the posterior–anterior axis as a concurrent level of analysis. Simply put, the posterior region is for understanding *input*, and the anterior region is for accomplishing *output*. The left and right hemispheres work side by side, with the right hemisphere responsible for discordant/divergent processes, and the left hemisphere carrying out concordant/convergent processing demands (Bryan & Hale, 2001). Recall that Luria's (1973) second functional unit is the one responsible for the interpretation of incoming sensory information, and the third functional unit is the one responsible for motor output and higher-order executive functions. These functions become increasingly lateralized as one ascends the hierarchy; however, as we have discussed, the left–right axis does not represent a verbal–nonverbal distinction, but rather a rote/crystallized–novel/fluid distinction. We can think of stimuli—regardless of whether they are auditory, visual, or somatosensory—as being processed by both hemispheres, with the division of labor directly related to whether there is a "descriptive system" available to process it (Goldberg & Costa, 1981).

This "descriptive system" idea can be related to Piaget's notion of a schema. If there is a schema or descriptive system to process the information, the left hemisphere is likely to carry out the task. The more rote, automatic, well-learned, or local a task is, the more likely the left hemisphere is to process it. The more novel, ambiguous, or global a task is, the more likely the right hemisphere is to process it. Most tasks will have some novel aspects, but novel problem solving requires the use of existing knowledge and skills, so bilateral performance is expected on most tasks. This rote–novel distinction does not suggest that findings supporting left- and right-hemisphere differences on the WISC Verbal–Performance scales are invalid (e.g., Riccio & Hynd, 2000). Instead, the model should help you recognize that interpretation must go beyond the typical verbal–nonverbal dichotomy, and that bilateral activity is rule rather than the exception.

Our new dichotomy can also be used to describe the posterior–anterior axis as well. The more a task requires fluid reasoning or novel problem-solving skills, the more the frontal executive system will be involved (Shallice, 1989). Given our understanding of hemispheric differences, it is the *right* frontal lobe that will be responsible for fluid reasoning and executive tasks, but recall that bilateral activity is likely. What about the left/storage–right/retrieval dichotomy? Recall that putting things into memory requires consolidation with existing knowledge (a left-hemisphere function), but retrieval requires considering multiple memories for words and concepts, as well as several possible responses (a right-hemisphere function). As the task becomes more automatic and crystallized, the posterior areas are more likely to respond to the task—especially in the left hemisphere, an area specialized for crystallized knowledge (knowledge gained through experience and education). Again, it is important to realize that all areas are likely to be involved in most tasks; only different degrees of involvement are required (Goldberg, 2001). This is highlighted in Application 3.5.

Because most brain areas are involved in many tasks we administer, we must exercise extreme caution in drawing inferences about particular brain areas' being affected or damaged (Taylor & Fletcher, 1990). For instance, a child may have difficulty with executive functions that could be related to the cingulate; limited motor skills because of poor dorsal stream feedback to the motor system; or problems with implicit language comprehension due to right temporal dysfunction that results in expressive language problems similar to "jargon aphasia." Keeping this important gradiential orientation in mind, we can begin to break down the posterior–anterior and left–right axes into four quadrants as depicted in Figure 3.1. Simply put, the right posterior hemisphere is specialized for global, coarse, or novel processing of stimuli, and the left posterior region is specialized for local, detailed processing of automatic or routinized information. Similarly, the right frontal region is important for brainstorming multiple ideas and carrying out complex motor programs requiring adaptation and change to environmental demands. Alternatively, the left frontal region would appear to be the area that brings closure, categorization, and compartmentalization of ideas, as well as the one that organizes concepts and develops motor programs to carry out complex actions (including familiar aspects of expressive language). Let's explore each of these quadrants in further detail.

APPLICATION 3.5. Brain Functions and Stages of Learning

For a better understanding of brain–behavior relationships in the classroom, it is important to relate brain functions to the stages of learning described by Smith (1981). During the initial *acquisition stage* of learning new information, regardless of the modality (e.g., auditory, visual), right-hemisphere resources are required. The more novel or unique the new information is, the more the right hemisphere will be required, and the activity will be more frontal, because executive demands will be high. The left hemisphere is working simultaneously with the right to develop a descriptive system or schema to process the information for the future. There's a gradual shift from right- to left-hemisphere processes as tasks become learned (Goldberg, 2001).

Left-hemisphere processes are necessary for both the *proficiency* and *maintenance* stages of learning. This is because the proficiency stage's objective is quick and efficient (fluent) performance, and the maintenance stage's objective is retention over time. Not only do both of these stages rely heavily on left-hemisphere processes, but posterior systems become more involved. *Proficiency* is the process of consolidating the skill into long-term memory and developing automaticity so that the task can be performed both accurately and quickly. Once proficiency is achieved, the skill must be stored in long-term memory for later use, so *maintenance* requires the left-hemisphere areas (mainly posterior) associated with long-term memory storage. This right-to-left shift in learning and retention of skills then changes again in the *generalization* and *adaptation* stages. To generalize skills, a child must use right-hemisphere skills to modify his or her behavior to cope with the novel application of the skill in new settings or situations. Finally, to capitalize on this knowledge in the *adaptation* stage and to recognize its use in novel problem-solving situations, substantial right-hemisphere involvement is required, and again executive demands are high. It is important to recognize that hemispheric activity in learning is not an either–or proposition. Instead, there is a gradual shift from right (especially right frontal) to left (especially left posterior), and back again as the child progresses through the learning stages.

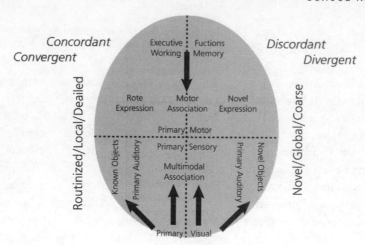

FIGURE 3.1. Four-quadrant analysis of brain function.

Right and Left Posterior Quadrants

At an input or primary cortex level, the right posterior region will be primarily responsible for left-side hearing, visual field, and somatosensory feeling, and the left posterior region will be responsible for these functions on the right side of the body. Finger agnosia (inability to recognize touch of fingers) and astereognosis (difficulty with recognizing objects by touch) may occur following damage to either the left or right parietal area. Damage to the left primary somatosensory area affects the right hand, and damage to the right area affects the left hand. However, this left–right dichotomy is not as simple as it seems (see In-Depth 3.3), because complex tasks require more right-hemisphere involvement, and simple, routine tasks require more left-hemisphere involvement.

IN-DEPTH 3.3. Simple versus Complex Sensory–Motor Tasks

Consistent with our reconceptualization of the two hemispheres, it may be the complexity of the task that determines the nature of a sensory–motor deficit: Right-hemisphere dysfunction may interfere with complex, novel tactile–motor skills, whereas simple, routinized tactile–motor skills may be more likely to occur with left-hemisphere dysfunction (Francis, Fletcher, & Rourke, 1988). These findings provide another clear example of how more complex or multimodal integration skills require right-hemisphere involvement. Because there is much more primary than association cortex in the left hemisphere, single-modality or simple, routinized somatosensory processing is likely to be attempted by the left posterior hemisphere.

   In this lateralization quest, we must recall that integrity of the corpus callosum and motor areas (i.e., frontal lobes–basal ganglia–cerebellum) plays a role in Francis and colleagues' (1988) conclusions as well. Surely damage to the left frontal cortex can cause right hemiparesis, but the motor tasks we use are likely to require contralateral activity as well; it is the amount that varies, based on the simple–complex dimension. As we can see, the dichotomy is not a simple one between the left hemisphere/right body and the right hemisphere/left body. Instead, you must examine the task performance in relation to other tasks, and determine whether performance deficits are due to input, processing, and/or output problems.

At a processing level, the right posterior region is especially good at recognizing unfamiliar or global relationships among stimuli parts, especially when multiple sensory modalities are involved. It is specialized for object recognition, especially when the objects are presented in a unique or novel perspective (ventral stream). As we have seen, processing novel faces and changes in facial expression requires the right ventral stream—hence the importance of this stream in social perception. Prosopagnosia, or inability to recognize faces, is likely to be caused by bilateral damage to the ventral stream; again, however, the details of facial recognition would be lost with left-hemisphere dysfunction, whereas right-hemisphere dysfunction would lead to global face recognition deficits. Common objects and faces may be more likely to be processed by the left ventral (temporal lobe) stream, but more abstract objects or unknown faces, or those consisting of new configurations, would be processed by the right inferior temporal lobe. For instance, if you encounter an octagon sign with the word "Alto" at an intersection, you will probably realize that this means "Stop," even if you do not know Spanish. Obviously, the two temporal lobes need to work together, via the commissures, to recognize the global/holistic (right) and local/detailed (left) characteristics of objects. The right temporal lobe works globally at a coarse level of processing to allow for generalization of the new object to other known objects, which would require the left temporal lobe functions. Apperceptive agnosia, or failure to perceive objects visually, could be due to right occipital–temporal lobe dysfunction (poor perception of whole objects) or to left occipital–temporal lobe dysfunction (poor perception of details or parts of objects). Associative agnosia, on the other hand, is an apparent disconnection between object perception (which is intact) and its semantic label. Whereas apperceptive agnosia may result from dysfunction occurring earlier in the ventral stream (i.e., the occipital lobe), associative agnosia may occur at a later point (i.e., the temporal lobe).

Spatial relationships, movement perception, and body awareness are primarily processed in the dorsal stream of the occipital–parietal areas. Dysfunction in the parietal lobe (especially the right) can lead to several additional types of agnosia, including limited awareness of self (asomatognosia) and the environment (neglect), usually in the contralateral hemispace. In addition, because this region is responsible for providing visual–spatial feedback to the motor system, constructional apraxia is often the result of right parietal lobe dysfunction, and may be more appropriately termed *constructional agnosia*. The right posterior ventral region is the area most likely to maintain ongoing perception of both facial affect and verbal prosody during social discourse. If the dysfunction is more superior, a prosodic agnosia could result; if it is more inferior, prosopagnosia and object agnosia could result. This right posterior area is also responsible for examining verbal incongruities, such as metaphor, idiom, sarcasm, and humor, as well as other types of implicit communication (both verbal and nonverbal). For these tertiary-level deficits, the occipital–parietal–temporal "crossroads" in the right hemisphere is likely to be affected. However, it is important to recognize that these novel higher-level interpretive processes are much more likely to require frontal involvement. Because these complex interpretive skills may not be needed at a young age, they may not be clinically manifested until the age at which they are required (Baron et al., 1995).

The homologous left-hemisphere regions play comparable roles, but they focus on different aspects of the stimuli. The left posterior quadrant is involved in local processing of detailed stimuli (making fine distinctions between one stimulus and another). It is also responsible for processing of well-known routinized information, so much of long-term memory is probably localized to this quadrant, in the areas that process that information (Gazzaniga, Ivry, & Mangun, 1998). Prior knowledge of places, objects, facts, details, and relationships will all be localized to this region, particularly to the temporal lobe. Gerstmann syndrome, characterized by finger agnosia, dysgraphia (problems with writing), dyscalculia (problems with math automaticity), and right–left confusion (due to body awareness and direction), is likely following left parietal lobe damage, and reading deficits can be caused by parietal dysfunction as well. It is not surprising that some types of apraxia (difficulty with carrying out motor activities) can be related to parietal lobe damage, because of limited body awareness or representation of posture (Sunderland & Sluman, 2000). Because phonemes are the basic sound units of language, the left posterior temporal lobe is probably responsible for phonemic awareness, analysis, and segmentation. Posterior and medial to this region, problems with receptive language, known as Wernicke's or fluent aphasia, are likely following damage to the parietal–temporal tertiary areas. The posterior ventral parietal (i.e., angular gyrus) and associated occipital regions are more likely to be involved in the written aspects of language. Obviously, any of these areas can be associated with comprehension deficits; however, because of the left hemisphere's propensity for fine, routine, and automatic processes, oral and written language comprehension are likely to be impaired. However, the rote–novel hemispheric distinction plays a role here, with left-hemisphere language areas responsible for explicit comprehension, and the right-hemisphere language areas responsible for implicit comprehension. We will return to these topics in Chapters 5–7.

Right and Left Anterior Quadrants

For the primary cortical areas, recall that the right frontal lobe is involved in motor control of the left side of the body, and that the left frontal lobe is responsible for right-side motor control. Recall that the secondary areas are differentiated by whether the motor skill is self- or other-oriented. The medial secondary area (the supplementary motor cortex) is responsible for self-directed movements, and the lateral secondary area (the premotor cortex) is responsible for movement in response to external stimuli. Because the supplementary motor area is responsible for internal motor scripts, it is not surprising that it is connected to the prefrontal cortex and basal ganglia. The premotor area has connections with the parietal cortex and cerebellum, because it is important in responding to environmental stimuli. Recall that during new skill learning, the premotor area is more active, but as skills become automatic or routinized, the supplementary motor area (in conjunction with temporal lobe and limbic structures) is best suited to perform the learned task. However, it is important to recognize that this distinction has been debated in recent times; the nature of the stimuli may be what determines the extent of premotor and supplementary motor area involvement, with both areas likely involved to some degree.

Because the left hemisphere is involved in fine, detailed, and routinized activities, it is not surprising that the apraxias, even though they are "visual–motor" difficulties, are more commonly associated with left-hemisphere dysfunction. They often go hand in hand (pun intended!) with aphasia (Springer & Deutsch, 1998). Damage to the supplementary motor area of the left frontal lobe can result in difficulty with developing a motor concept, and/or with carrying out a complex or routinized motor task. Although posterior left-hemisphere dysfunction can also cause ideational apraxia (in which the child cannot think of the concept/idea of what to do) or ideomotor apraxia (in which the child has the concept, but cannot carry out the steps) (Sunderland & Sluman, 2000), these problems can also occur following left medial frontal quadrant dysfunction. However, since these apraxias are the result of prior learning and knowledge, they are more common with left-hemisphere dysfunction, and are more rarely seen following right-hemisphere damage. Those with damage to the right parietal dorsal stream are more likely to have constructional apraxia because of visual–spatial, kinesthetic (due to poor feedback), and cross-modal processing deficits (Wilson & McKenzie, 1998).

As noted earlier, constructional apraxia is more difficult to evaluate and requires considerable clinical attention. Like the other apraxias, it could be due to problems with motor control (left premotor secondary cortex). However, it can also be caused by parietal dysfunction in either hemisphere. In the right hemisphere, dysfunction can lead to problems with spatial and motor movement feedback to the anterior motor system, and left parietal somatosensory problems (sensory feedback to the right hand) can lead to problems with somatosensory–motor feedback. Left posterior parietal dysfunction can also lead to orientation errors, resulting in reversal and/or rotation errors. Because these functions tend to be differentially processed by the two hemispheres (right, spatial/holistic feedback; left, motor and somatosensory control), cross-modal integration is required, and agenesis of the corpus callosum can also lead to constructional difficulties. You must try to determine whether a child's problem is with somatosensory functioning/orientation/movement (left parietal), global spatial feedback (right parietal), motor functioning (left frontal premotor area), or integration (corpus callosum), because you would attempt different remediation strategies for each type of deficit. Obviously, a child who has handwriting problems due to constructional apraxia should develop these skills by practicing handwriting, but different complementary intervention techniques for both handwriting and associated deficits are worth exploring. In addition, differential diagnosis is needed to determine whether occupational therapy services are required. We will return to interventions for handwriting in Chapter 7.

Differentiating between the higher functions of the right and left frontal lobes has been difficult, possibly because most "frontal" tasks require *correct* rather than *adaptive* responding (Goldberg, 2001). The limited empirical evidence for lateralized frontal lobe functions is less difficult to accept if we recall that both hemispheres are likely to be involved in most cognitive tasks; it is just the amount of involvement that varies. It would appear that the right frontal region is likely to be involved in many aspects of brain functioning, especially those that require novel problem-solving or fluid abilities. The right frontal region works with posterior regions to examine incongruities among stimuli, using divergent processes to examine discordant information. This area works to produce behavior that is flexibly consistent with the current situation, maximizing the likelihood of success.

The use of novel problem-solving skills/fluid abilities seems to follow an inverse-U pattern during child development, as depicted in Figure 3.2. Novel problem-solving skills are greatly

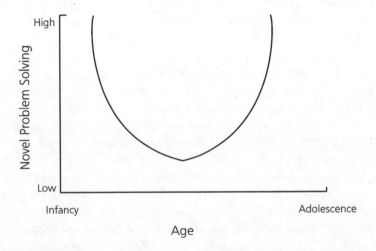

FIGURE 3.2. Changes in novel problem solving over time.

needed in infancy to learn sound–symbol associations and the nuances of functioning in the "real world." They are not needed as much during the early school years, when rote memorization and recall of facts and details predominate. As we will discuss further in Chapter 8, children with right frontal dysfunction are more likely to be recognized for their odd behavior and social alienation during these years than for their academic deficits. Academic, occupational, and social pursuits are more likely to be impaired during adolescence and adulthood, which can be frustrating for these children, because they were such "good students" in the early school years. As these children leave middle childhood, they have developed a very left-hemisphere, concrete understanding of the world; however, with the onset of adolescence and formal operational thought, the need for novel problem-solving/fluid abilities increases, as adolescents begin to question the validity of their earlier concrete beliefs.

Although most research does not differentiate between right and left frontal areas, this may be in part due to the limited attention the frontal lobes have received until very recently. Executive functions are all about self-regulation and control. They are likely to be bilaterally represented, but their dynamic nature suggests that the right hemisphere is probably more involved than the left. The right hemisphere is likely to be involved in executive strategizing, inhibiting, monitoring, evaluating, shifting, and changing performance—all important tasks in solving novel problems. Planning and organization skills, also considered executive tasks, are also likely to require right frontal functions, but because the left frontal region is associated with temporal relationships and categorization, these executive tasks may be more bilateral in nature.

Consistent with Luria's (1973) notions about the frontal lobes and memory, retrieval of information from long-term memory appears to be somewhat more closely related to the right frontal lobe than to the left. This is not because long-term memories are located there, but rather because retrieval requires a comprehensive (discordant/divergent) search pattern through the vast catalogs of information that are probably located in the left posterior regions. Working memory demands are high for long-term memory retrieval, because a person must keep the retrieval question in mind, find the appropriate long-term memories, and determine whether the ones located are the ones needed. Likewise, during novel problem-solving tasks, working memory requires retaining and acting upon novel information that has not yet been coded into long-term memory. Expressive linguistic skills (namely, in the area of affective prosody) and the implicit messages discussed in the right posterior section, are likely to be influenced by right frontal areas. If you see someone with a monotone, or someone who has difficulty modulating his or her voice (i.e., it is always too loud or too quiet), right frontal dysfunction could be the cause. Because visual attention requires a search strategy, the right frontal area, especially the frontal eye fields, may be more involved in visual selective attention and scanning.

The left frontal lobe is responsible for looking for concordant information and integrating information in a convergent, ordered fashion, so it is not surprising that it is involved in understanding of temporal relationships and consolidating information into long-term memory. For this reason, categorical thinking and behavior (e.g., determining how two words belong to a category) are likely to be left frontal tasks. Certainly, the left frontal region is responsible for expressive language, and Broca's or nonfluent aphasia is more likely following damage to this region. Broca's aphasia is known for halting speech and poor adherence to grammar—issues we will return to in Chapter 6. Why does Broca's aphasia lead to poor grammar? Because grammar is all about rules, and rule-governed behavior is what the left hemisphere thrives on.

Not only is the left frontal lobe the source of rules; it is also responsible for temporal (i.e., time-related) information processing. It helps the posterior regions organize information in a step-by-step, sequential, or successive fashion. Of course, all of these skills are necessary for language processes, but the left hemisphere's propensity for fine, detailed, and routinized processing is what makes symbolic communication lateralize to that hemisphere. Considering the left-hemisphere processes to be sequential or successive in nature is not wrong per se; it just fails to recognize the true nature of the left hemisphere, because it focuses on input and output demands. The left hemisphere likes rules, details, and prior knowledge, making it an ideal candidate to respond to most aphasia tests, and most achievement tests as well. In fact, it can be argued that *any* test requiring a "correct" response is really tapping left-hemisphere concordant/convergent functions.

"Red Flags" or Pathognomonic Signs

Pathognomonic signs are what we like to call "red flags," because they tell us that a child's processing is different from that of typical children the same age. Some make a distinction between "hard signs" and "soft signs," in that the former are clearly indicative of brain damage, and the latter are possibly indicative of brain dysfunction. There are some clear signs of brain damage that we should look for in our evaluations. For instance, a marked unilateral sensory or motor deficit, abnormal reflexes, changes in pupil size or eyelid function, visual field loss, and hearing loss can be considered clear signs of brain damage. As can be seen in Table 3.3, Lezak (1995) specifies several symptoms of brain damage, some of which you may have seen in your practice. It is important to recognize that discrimination of these signs is often difficult, so you must exercise caution when making inferences about these symptoms and brain damage. Some practitioners consider some of these symptoms "soft signs"—symptoms that are less predictive of brain damage and are quite common in children with disabilities. Soft signs such as motor overflow (different limb or finger movements from those the child is attempting to produce), motor incoordination, left–right confu-

TABLE 3.3. Possible Signs of Pathological Brain Function

Category	Signs and symptoms	Behaviors
Executive	Perseveration	Repetitive speech or other motoric behavior
	Impersistence	Inability to initiate/maintain behavior
	Confabulation	Distorted thoughts/incongruent associations
Motor	Lateralized differences	Motor speed and coordination/strength difficulties
	Gait/balance	Walking/standing difficulties
	Activity level	Hyperactivity or hypoactivity
Somatosensory	Lateralized differences	Touch sensitivity/symbol recognition difficulties
	Somatic complaints	Abnormal somatosensory experiences
Language	Dysarthria	Slurred speech
	Dysfluency	Articulation problems
	Verbal output	Rambling speech or poverty of speech
	Paraphasias	Letter/word substitutions
	Retrieval difficulties	Word-finding problems
Visual–spatial	Visual field problems	Loss of one or more visual quadrants
	Constructional apraxia	Problems with copying designs (both blocks and drawing)
	Spatial disorientation	Location problems/poor spatial judgment
	Right–left disorientation	Self/body part indentification wrong
	Neglect	Self or environment: Left > right side

sion, motor weakness on one side, distractibility, hypo- or hyperactivity, and emotional lability are better interpreted as signs of dysfunction than of damage.

Spreen, Risser, and Edgell (1995) differentiate between "developmental soft signs" (DSSs) and "soft signs of abnormality" (SSAs). DSSs are considered abnormal only if they persist or fail to develop within a developmentally appropriate time period. One DSS you regularly assess is a delay (compared to typical same-age children) in meeting developmental milestones. Several other DSSs we have seen include motor overflow, poor left–right orientation toward self or other, immature pencil grasp, poor fine or gross motor coordination, motor impersistence, poor gait/posture/stance, tactile extinction during simultaneous stimulation, and speech articulation problems. SSAs are considered abnormal if noted at any developmental level, and include many of the symptoms presented in Table 3.3. These SSAs include extreme sensory or motor asymmetries, reflex asymmetries, choreiform movements, dysgraphesthesia, dysdiadochokinesis, astereognosis, dysarthria, hypo- or hyperkinesis, labile affect, motor impersistence, oromotor apraxia, nystagmus, postural or gate abnormalities, significant incoordination, tremors, and word-finding difficulties. Since neither DSSs nor SSAs are frank pathognomonic signs, they should be seen more as signs of neuropsychological dysfunction than as signs of brain damage; indeed, some consider them nonfocal neurological signs (Hertzig & Shapiro, 1987). We must not forget that presenting problems such as developmental delay, learning difficulties, or immaturity, though commonplace may be among the first signs of a true neurological problem (Baron et al., 1995).

Common Interpretation Problems and Solutions

Before we leave our discussion of the neuropsychological approach to test interpretation, it is useful to explore where you might go wrong when implementing the CHT model. Despite your best intentions and efforts, you may make a mistake in your administration, scoring, or interpretation of neuropsychological and cognitive tests. Recognizing this possibility, you must be vigilant to reduce the chances of diagnostic error. One of the important characteristics of the CHT model is that the findings are incorporated within a larger problem-solving model, so that built-in corrections for error can take place during the intervention phase, when data-based decisions regarding efficacy are made (Allen & Graden, 1995). We must always remember that our hypotheses are just hypotheses until treatment validity is established. Nonetheless, we must still attempt to increase our self-awareness as clinicians and be on guard for common interpretation problems, as highlighted in In-Depth 3.4.

THE CHT APPROACH TO REPORT WRITING

Terminology Issues and Audience

As stated in the introduction to this text, using neuropsychological principles in practice does not provide you with the training and experience necessary to become a neuropsychologist. Therefore, it is critical that you ultimately discuss a child's *behavior*, not his or her *brain*, in your reports and conversations with parents and other professionals. Although we have come a long way in our understanding of brain–behavior relationships, we still know much more about developmental neuro*psychology* than about developmental *neuro*psychology (Rourke, 1994). Given our knowledge of the interrelationships among cortical systems, and the interplay among cortical and subcortical functions (Obrzut & Hynd, 1986), we must always recognize that children's problems

IN-DEPTH 3.4. Common Interpretation Errors and Possible Solutions

Lezak (1995) suggests that the following are the most common interpretation errors. We provide you with a brief discussion and our recommended solution for each one.

Problem 1: Overgeneralization of results

Discussion: Overgeneralization can happen within a child or across children. Some examiners have a tendency to draw broad-reaching conclusions from limited amounts of data, or to determine that the same conclusion should be drawn if the performance profile for one child is similar to that of another.

Solution: Avoid "cookbook" interpretations and the use of report templates.

Problem 2: Failure to find the problem

Discussion: Clinicians tend to miss problems when they rely on summary data that obscures diagnostically important differences, such as when they conclude from the summary score that there is or is not a problem.

Solution: Explore performance within and across subtests, and focus on neuropsychological processes, not subtest stimulus and response differences.

Problem 3: Confirmation bias

Discussion: In CHT, we develop and test neuropsychological hypotheses—but what if a child performs adequately on a measure we hypothesize the child will perform poorly on? Could this mean that we picked the wrong measure, or that it doesn't measure what we think it does, or that maybe we just have the *wrong* hypothesis?

Solution: When we have contradictory evidence, we may need to go back to the proverbial "drawing board" to develop a new hypothesis. We can't ignore contrary evidence, but must incorporate it within our diagnostic conclusions.

Problem 4: Misuse of data

Discussion: Sometimes we have a tendency to be overly cautious and underinterpret data, and at other times we draw dramatic conclusions with very little support.

Solution: Use the incremental validity of the objective results, and the outcome of your ecological validity investigation, to temper your interpretations.

Problem 5: Failure to consider base rates

Discussion: Significant performance differences are fairly common, both between and within measures. They are not in themselves diagnostic. Although our research findings suggest that significant differences must be analyzed at the subtest or factor level (Fiorello et al., 2001), it is critical that you determine why the differences occurred, and not automatically conclude that they represent underlying pathology.

Solution: To avoid false positives, you must ensure that the performance differences reflect a consistent problem (in both your testing results and your ecological validity sources) that interferes with academic achievement and/or psychosocial functioning.

are influenced by complex interactions of neuropsychological, behavioral, and environmental factors.

When you are writing reports and communicating results, use examples of child behavior you saw during testing, and comments that others have made, in an attempt to establish consensus among team members and parents. Engaging others in your feedback keeps them interested and invested in the findings. This type of interactive communication style during feedback helps maintain rapport and shared understanding—critical components of establishing a cooperative and collaborative parent relationship (Wise, 1995). Try to focus on the child's positive attributes, as well as his or her deficits and needs. Too often we focus on what is wrong with a child (Baron, 2000), instead of recognizing that the child can do something, even if it is below expected levels. The power of "positive reframes" in report writing can have a profound impact on how you write reports and communicate results, as noted in Case Study 3.5.

Most trainers suggest that you should avoid using psychological jargon and use standard terminology in reports, presenting the findings in a clear, succinct way, so that both professionals and nonprofessionals can understand them (Reynolds & Mayfield, 1999). Although you will hear similar beliefs echoed in almost every trainer's lecture on report writing and follow-up consultation, we believe that accomplishing all this is not that simple. Yes, it is a good idea for your reports to be understood, but we think you will be missing the proverbial boat if you try to write a brief report that truly conveys the complexity of a child in simple terminology. Many practitioners think they write reports that others can understand, but in reality most reports are not written so that an average adult can understand them. If the average adult doesn't know what you're talking about, think of what it must be like for a parent with an eighth-grade education or a disability. Either you can write a 15- or 20-page CHT report that conveys the child's performance in simple terms or defines all complex terms (but is too long for anyone to read), or you can write a brief report for professional use. We prefer the latter approach. After you write the brief professional report, take the summary paragraph and recommendations, and write a parent letter that describes the results in lay terminology. You are probably gasping, "What, more work, after all this hypothesis-testing stuff?" We'd like you to consider a few things before you dismiss this strategy outright:

CASE STUDY 3.5. Violet's Feedback Session

When we sat down to discuss the team's results and recommendations for Violet, a child with moderate mental retardation who had spent years in special education, no one expected the meeting to be very long. This was because Violet was a pleasant, compliant, and hard-working girl with significant intellectual and adaptive deficits. She always seemed to have a smile on her face, even when she was struggling. During the feedback session, I (Hale) primarily focused on what Violet *could* do and what was the next developmental step for her.

Approximately halfway through the presentation, the mother began to sob uncontrollably. We stopped the feedback to ask why and to provide support. Violet's mother reported that she had listened to these team meetings for years, and never once had anyone said anything good about her child. Although her global perception was probably skewed (I'm sure someone had said something positive about this nice child), it was a strong sentiment nonetheless. The positive approach obviously went a long way toward helping the mother understand her child, and gave her hope for her child's advancing beyond her current level of performance.

1. Writing 7-page reports takes a lot less time than writing 17-page reports.
2. Once a summary is written, modifying it does not take a lot of additional time (try this on your current reports; we have found that "stepping back" from complex presentation is relatively easy).
3. We have found parents to be highly appreciative of the letter approach, and they can receive the actual report if they want further information (which, of course, you must be willing to explain).
4. You will have additional time to write the parent letters, now that referrals have been reduced by the IAT.

In the feedback session, it is important to present results at a level that is understood by both the teacher and parents; you should note that the detailed report and letter (described earlier) will provide additional information for professionals and parents, respectively. Resist the temptation to provide a diagnostic label or make predictions about possible outcomes. During this time, it is important to use examples parents and teachers have provided, and to encourage descriptive statements from them in order to foster consensus. Parents may have difficulty accepting the results, and may experience a variety of emotions during the feedback session, so you must be attentive to their reactions (Mulick & Hale, 1996). By providing insight into the child's current functioning, and showing how this is related to the environment, you may be effectively disrupting a system of homeostasis (Whelan, 1999)—one that has been in place for some time and can be seen as adaptive, albeit dysfunctional. Also, recall that some parents you are talking with may have the same disorder as their child, which could affect their understanding and acknowledgment of the child's problem. The feedback session not only informs parents and teachers of the results, but it begins the intervention process as well.

Distinguishing between Certainty and Inference in Reports

One of the most daunting tasks for psychologists is turning observed behavior and test scores into an accurate interpretation that leads to effective interventions (Baron, 2000). Faced with an overwhelming amount of data, you may find yourself struggling to conceptualize how the results are related to brain functions, and how your interpretation is related to academics and behavior. It is important to recognize that test scores are not necessarily related to brain pathology, and also that a typical score does not necessarily mean there is no dysfunction (Lezak, 1995), because children perform tasks in different ways. Recall the complementary-contribution principle and the gradiental approach to interpretation: Children can use various intact brain structures in an attempt to adapt to different task demands. That is why your observations are so essential to CHT interpretation.

As noted in the previous section, you should be extremely cautious when test results are inconsistent, and avoid discussion of cause–effect relationships (Sattler, 2001). It is important to use qualifying terms when you write about behavior ("may," "could," "appears," "seems," "apparently," "reportedly," "likely," "probably," etc.). Unless you have neuroimaging or other neurological evidence, you cannot say with certainty that a single brain area is damaged or even dysfunctional. You can, however, use your knowledge of neuropsychological principles to understand which systems are dysfunctional, and how these systems are likely to influence academic achievement and psychosocial functioning. Even when there is direct evidence of brain damage, and it is consistent with your obtained data, you may want to minimize your discussion of the brain, because it only serves to increase the likelihood of "problem admiration." Instead, focusing on strengths and needs saves you from the uncomfortable position of responding to the question "Is this what causes my child's problem?"

Report Sections

This section of the chapter will remind you of some important report-writing considerations within the context of the CHT model. We all get into "writing ruts" that make our reports less informative and more "boilerplate," so that they do not reflect the truly unique nature of a child's functioning. In addition to the following material, Sattler's (2001) chapter on report writing is a fine source for refreshing your skills. In our opinion, the best reports require three things: revision, revision, and more revision. Although reports are objective, concise documents, there is an "art" to writing them well. Well-written reports convey information about children in interesting and compelling ways. Good report writers vary their sentence structure and word choice. They provide evidence to support conclusions, as well as examples that highlight ecological validity. Word choice is particularly important, because it conveys the strength of your diagnostic convictions. The stronger your conviction, the stronger the terms. The ramifications of using the words "could," "should," or "must" in recommendations are considerable.

If your report is written well, it will become an important document that follows a child for the rest of the child's life (or at least his or her academic career). Although report styles differ and will vary according to site needs and administrator demands, we recommend following these basic CHT sections, described below: the reason for referral; relevant background information; classroom observations and functional analysis; assessment observations; cognitive/intellectual assessment; cognitive hypothesis testing; academic functioning; psychosocial and behavioral functioning; summary; and recommendations.

Reason for Referral

As noted earlier, the reason for referral should address the concerns presented by those making the referral, but it should also consider other possible referral issues (such as the findings of the IAT prereferral interventions). It is important to be descriptive if possible, and to avoid overly general summative statements such as "behavior problems." The reason for referral is preferably brief—a short paragraph at most.

Relevant Background Information

The background information can provide you with both the foundation for establishing possible disorder causes, and data for establishing ecological validity. Good clinical interviews with the teacher, parent, and child will provide you with opportunities not only to develop hypotheses about a child's functioning, but to obtain concurrent validity evidence as well (Sbordone, 2000). The clinical interview is not only about gathering information; it helps establish important relationships with those who will eventually carry out the interventions and monitor their efficacy. We prefer to include three paragraphs in the history:

1. *Medical/developmental history.* This includes the gestation and birth history; any medical illnesses or accidents; vision and hearing status; and acquisition/delay of developmental milestones. If you do not recognize a medical condition, or are told of an accident involving possible

head trauma, explore these thoroughly. Even if doing so delays your report, you must obtain the necessary permissions and releases of information to fully understand a medical incident. If you do not understand terminology from the report, look it up in a medical dictionary. Apparently innocuous conditions or accidents can provide you with the evidence you need to understand the child's test performance and behavior in the environment.

2. *Family/social history*. Interpretation always occurs within a context; it varies depending on individuals, their life circumstances, and current environment (Lezak, 1995). Many school practitioners think that the home environment is not relevant for school diagnostic or intervention decisions. This is a serious omission. Not only can home circumstances affect current psychological functioning, but they can provide insight into the contingencies that shape a child's experience. In addition, many conditions discussed in Chapters 5–8 have a genetic basis. Understanding that a child may have a genetically based disorder not only aids in diagnosis; it also helps you tailor your feedback to family members and your recommendations for the child. This subsection can also include a list of the child's preferred free-time activities and social relationships, which can be seen as possible reinforcers and thus can serve to guide intervention efforts. You might also list any psychosocial stressors a child experiences outside the school setting.

3. *School/occupational history*. From the first educational experiences to the child's current placement, the school history provides the reader with information regarding the child's adaptation to the instructional environment. It should include a summary of both positive and poor academic performance, and peer and teacher relationships. Finally, this subsection should include information regarding the prereferral strategies previously attempted and the outcome of each.

Classroom Observations and Functional Analysis

As noted earlier, careful observation is critical not only for differential diagnosis, but for intervention development as well. The data collected will help you generate hypotheses about the child's interactions and coping strategies in the classroom (Sattler, 2001). At a minimum, classroom observations should include an anecdotal or narrative recording; a systematic observation using event, latency, duration, time-sampling, or interval recording (with a comparison peer); and a functional analysis, where the determinants of the target behavior are explored. Depending on the child, this section can be one to three paragraphs long.

Assessment Observations

Assessment observations should provide a synopsis of the entire evaluation; they are like a behavioral summary of the results, without extensive interpretation. If interpretation is offered during observations, observable and measurable behaviors that support the interpretation must precede or follow it. They should include the child's reliability as an informant, personal appearance, rapport with you, approach to both novel and routine tasks, cooperativeness and motivation, reaction to failure, frustration tolerance, need for encouragement, comprehension of instructions, oral expression characteristics, and general level of affect (Spreen & Strauss, 1998). It is important to describe the following in your assessment observation section:

1. The child's adaptation to testing.
2. Whether the child understood and complied with assessment demands.
3. The child's responses to visual, auditory, and motor demands.
4. The child's receptive and expressive language characteristics.

5. The child's attention, impulse control, motor activity, and executive behaviors.
6. The child's range of affect and frustration tolerance.
7. Need for testing accommodations, such as structure and redirection.

In these descriptions, it is best to focus on the child's behaviors, not on an absence of these (Sattler, 2001). In addition to reporting testing behaviors, be sure to indicate how the child responded to the testing situation, and whether performance was consistent between and within measures. Different behaviors may emerge during intellectual/cognitive, academic, and psychosocial assessment, and these should be noted. Finish this paragraph with a statement that reflects your thoughts as to whether the results are reliable and valid. Many assessors tend to say that results are valid regardless of testing behavior, but do not be afraid to report that a child's behaviors interfered with maximal performance, at least on some of your measures.

Cognitive/Intellectual Assessment

We usually begin this section with a nomothetic paragraph, reporting the various global scores and indicating whether they adequately represent the child's level of performance. Consistent with the example presented in Case Study 3.4, you should describe how the child's performance compares to that of the normative population for any global or factor score presented, reporting both confidence intervals and percentiles. At this point, you may wish to decide whether an additional factor score than those provided needs to be calculated. For instance, if successive processing appears to be an issue, you may wish to calculate a Sequential Processing factor score. Although this paragraph focuses on global scores, it is important to conclude with a statement that they are invalid if significant subtest variability is present (Fiorello et al., 2001). In such a case, global scores represent so many different constructs and are confounded by so many different issues that they are conceptually meaningless (Lezak, 1988).

After the nomothetic paragraph, we usually write one or more idiographic paragraphs. The idiographic paragraphs represent the various clusters of subtests, broken down by the factors reported in the manual, or a unique combination of subtests based on how scores cluster together. If the global scores are valid, then you should basically describe the subtests generally, so that the reader gains an understanding of the tasks that were administered. Otherwise, idiographic analysis is demands analysis; it requires careful examination of subtest input, processing, and output demands to determine the individual's pattern of performance. Because you have limited support for your clinical interpretation at this point, it is important to qualify your interpretive statements by adding terms such as "may," "seems," "could," and the like, as we have emphasized earlier. It is important to start the idiographic paragraphs with what the child does well (i.e., strengths) before addressing his or her purported deficits. Recognizing the child's strengths not only highlights the positives for your readers, but helps them begin to think about how these might be used for intervention purposes (Sattler, 2001). After discussing the child's possible deficits, conclude the idiographic analysis with possible reasons for the child's performance. These are the hypotheses you have generated via CHT, which are examined in the next section.

Cognitive Hypothesis Testing

Whether your results are consistent or not, CHT requires further examination of purported deficits, because most intellectual subtests are just too factorially complex to permit you to draw definitive conclusions from them. Support for hypotheses can come from subsequent measures, TTL, observations, interviews, and rating scales. Optimally, the results of all these hypothesis-testing strategies will be presented in this section, together with support for and against your hypotheses. The instruments you choose for hypothesis testing may be "neuropsychological" or other intellectual/cognitive subtests; the important consideration in choosing additional subtests is that the combination you choose adequately addresses your hypotheses about individual deficits. We usually include one paragraph for each hypothesis examined. One final consideration worth exploring has to do with your report presentation. When you are first using CHT, it is best to separate the intellectual (nomothetic and idiographic paragraphs discussed in the previous section) from the hypothesis-testing section. However, as you become more proficient at integrating assessment results, you may wish to report intellectual and hypothesis-testing data in one integrated section, which is the preferred method of presentation (Spreen & Strauss, 1998).

Academic Functioning

As noted earlier, it is best to administer some standardized academic achievement measures, and possibly curriculum-based measures, even if the educational diagnostician performs this task at your school. This allows you to determine how your interpretation is related to academic performance. At a minimum, try to assess word recognition/decoding, reading comprehension, math word problems, math computation, spelling, and written language. As with the use of neuropsychological tests for hypothesis testing, you may wish to use an additional achievement measure to further your impressions, such as using a pseudoword-reading subtest for a child with word recognition problems. In this section, you should discuss the similarities and differences between teacher- and/or parent-reported academic achievement and your findings. The relationship between neuropsychological functioning and academic performance is further addressed in Chapters 5–7.

Psychosocial and Behavioral Functioning

As discussed in Chapter 8, the relationship between neuropsychological functioning and psychopathology is becoming clearer with each passing year: Several childhood disorders once thought to be primarily the results of environmental determinants are now being linked directly to biological causes. Although these associations are becoming clear, the relationship between psychiatric disturbance and neuropsychological deficit is difficult to disentangle (Tramontana & Hooper, 1997), and examining it will require clinical vigilance on your part. For each child who presents with psychosocial or behavioral issues, we believe that you should entertain a possible genetic and neurobiological etiology for the child's problems. Even if the history, observations, and neuropsychological patterns of performance are not reflective of a biologically based psychopathology, a child's cognitive patterns may reflect a processing or an expression preference during social discourse, and this propensity could lead to social or behavioral problems. It can also reveal that the child uses certain cognitive strengths to compensate for academic or psychosocial deficits. As in Bandura's (1978) model of reciprocal determinism, the relationships among cognition, behavior, and environment are interrelated and inseparable. In this section, it is important to address both signs of internalizing and externalizing disorders, as many people consider only the latter in determining whether a child has a psychosocial problem. We will return to the relationship between neuropsychological functioning and psychopathology in Chapter 8.

Summary and Recommendations

The report summary conveys all the pertinent information embodied in the report, synthesizing the major aspects of the child's behavior in relation to the environment. Some practitioners have questioned the utility of including a summary in psychological reports, because some readers may skip over pertinent report sections and instead read the final summary. A summary should include at least one sentence covering each of the areas presented above, and several sentences related to the data. In school settings, the report summary should not include diagnostic and/or placement recommendations, but you can discuss what a child needs. Your job is not to fix the problem or label the child, but rather to offer flexibility in eligibility, placement, and intervention decisions (Sattler, 2001).

Because the goal of clinical assessment is to optimize a child's development in all domains, we believe that recommendations should address all aspects of the child's life. Although report recommendations should be specific enough to be useful, they should not be mandates regarding intervention, since generating these is a team responsibility. We prefer to offer multiple possible interventions to help parents and teachers begin the intervention-brainstorming phase of problem solving, which is addressed further in the next chapter. Some have suggested that compensatory strategies are more effective than remediation approaches (Rourke, 1994), but this issue is not so straightforward. We see the compensation–remediation relationship to be directly related to age and severity of condition, as depicted in Figure 3.3. For older children or those with severe deficits, a compensatory strategy should predominate, and remediation should be less prominent. However, for younger children, or those with less severe conditions, remediation should be the focus of intervention efforts. Whereas both strength-based compensation and/or remediation of neuropsychological weaknesses may be individualized for each child, it is important to recognize that interventions must occur within the context of academic instruction, not in isolation (Teeter, 1997). Recommendations should include both instructional and behavioral components tailored to each child's unique needs, as well as classroom accommodations to help the child maintain performance in less impaired areas.

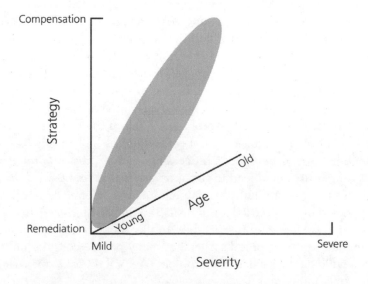

FIGURE 3.3. Tailoring teaching strategies for individual children.

Don't think that you must know everything about intervention, or that every intervention you recommend must be implemented and effective. Traditional psychometric assessments do not provide the necessary information to facilitate intervention (Sattler, 2001), and neuropsychologists typically don't have much training in intervention (Obrzut & Hynd, 1986); this makes your instructional and behavioral knowledge especially useful during intervention planning, implementation, and evaluation. Since you have determined the child's unique characteristics and documented these in the report summary, you now have overcome one of the greatest difficulties in linking assessment to intervention: accurate identification of the child's unique characteristics (Rourke, 1994). Recognizing the child's strengths and needs from a neuropsychological perspective is the first important step in developing individualized interventions (Groth-Marnat et al., 2000), and recommendations are only a first "brainstorm" of possible strategies that could help the child. Throughout the remainder of this book, we examine the linkages among assessment findings, recommendations for intervention, and ways to help children succeed in various academic and behavioral areas.

APPENDIX 3.1. Ecological Validity Examples of Brain Dysfunction

Brain area	Left-hemisphere damage	Right-hemisphere damage
Occipital lobe	• Slow reading and substitution of letters • Poor spelling • Limited picture details	• Difficulty with visual imagery • Poor drawing/coloring • Misreading of facial expressions
Dorsal stream	• Difficulty with left–right orientation • Reverses letters/numbers • Directional confusion in drawings and writing • Poor sound–symbol association • Limited association between quantity and number symbols • Poor local processing	• Poor spatial skills in letters, words, and drawings • Difficulty with math column alignments and attention to operands • Difficulty with bumping into objects • Poor awareness of self and the environment: Inattention • Poor global processing
Ventral stream	• Difficulty with recognizing and naming known objects • Poor recognition of familiar faces • Difficulty with sight word learning and efficient reading (no automaticity) • Poor fine processing	• Difficulty with learning new objects and faces • Poor perception of facial affect • Difficulty with sight word learning—tendency to decode everything • Poor coarse processing
Lateral/medial temporal lobe	• Difficulty with long-term memory for objects, words, and general knowledge • Poor memory for known or famous faces • Possible dislike of social studies and preference for science • Preference for abstract and flexible tasks that require creativity • Desire to explore complexities of the world, but difficulties in making decisions	• Difficulty understanding multiple perspectives and meanings of objects, words, and general knowledge • Difficulty with recognizing facial affect • Preference for routinized and specific tasks • Possible preference for reading, social studies, and language arts (especially in early grades) • Preference to avoid complexities of world for safe, predictable, and conventional behaviors
Superior temporal lobe	• Poor phonemic awareness and auditory processing • Possible "mishearing" of comments or directions • Frequent requests for repetition or clarification • Possible repetition of words that sound similar	• Poor prosody awareness and limited understanding of rate and pitch of language • Possible "mishearing" of emotional valence of words (e.g., hearing anger when speaker excited) • Possible difficulty modulating own prosody
Anterior parietal lobe	• Difficulty in grasping objects with right hand • Writing that is too soft or too dark • Complaints that hand hurts when writing • Poor hand coordination in sports	• Difficulty in grasping objects with left hand • Poor bilateral motor coordination • Difficulty in catching a ball with a baseball mitt

(continued)

Occipital–temporal–parietal "crossroads"/ Wernicke's area	• Reliance on sight word approach and learning math facts to automaticity because of poor sound–symbol association • Difficulty with explicit language, reading, and math comprehension • Focus on general status of relationship to understand interaction dynamics • Greater likelihood of understanding humor, metaphor, and indirect messages	• Possible use of phonemic approach to decode all words, but poor comprehension • Difficulty with implicit language, reading, and math comprehension • Focus on facts and details to understand interactions • Greater likelihood of understanding concrete, explicit, and direct messages
Posterior frontal lobe	• Difficulty with right-handed motor functions • Likelihood of ideomotor or constructional apraxia • Difficulty with drawing and writing • Difficulty with dressing or carrying out tasks requiring multiple motor behaviors in sequence • Possible ambidexterity or left-handedness • Difficulty in performing learned motor programs • Possible poor articulation	• Difficulty with left-handed motor functions • Poor learning of motor scripts • Limited motor reaction to environmental stimuli • Difficulty with bimanual motor activities • Possible poor prosody
Medial frontal lobe/ Broca's area	• Limited verbal fluency • Low mean length of utterance • Semantic and phonemic paraphasias • Halting speech and word-finding problems • Poor syntax in speech and writing	• Fluent expression and high mean length of utterance • Poor verbal prosody, mechanistic manner of speech • Semantic paraphasias due to inflexible word choice • Poor humor and overly concrete oral and written expression
Dorsolateral prefrontal cortex	• Poor encoding of new information • Preference for flexible schedules and requirements • Executive dysfunction likely, including problems with planning, organizing, sequencing, implementing, and monitoring behavior • Poor routinization of learned behavior • Poor concordant/convergent thought	• Poor retrieval of existing information • Preference for routines and detailed requirements • Executive dysfunction more likely, including problems with strategizing, evaluating, shifting, and changing behavior • Poor novel problem solving • Limited discordant/divergent thought • ADHD, inattentive type (?)
Orbital prefrontal cortex	• Pseudodepression: Avoidance and inhibition (?) • Negative affect (?) • Excessive emotional regulation (?)	• Pseudopsychopathy: Approach and impulsivity (?) • Indifferent affect (?) • Lack of emotional regulation (?)

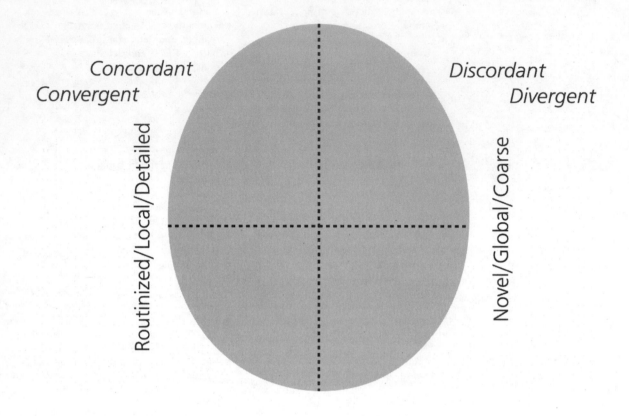

Concordant
Convergent

Discordant
Divergent

Routinized/Local/Detailed

Novel/Global/Coarse

Appendix 3.3. Blank Brain: Lateral View

CHAPTER 4

⌞⌞⌞⌞⌞⌞⌞⌞⌞⌞⌞⌞⌞⌟

Linking Assessment to Intervention

THE COGNITIVE HYPOTHESIS-TESTING MODEL

Prereferral Issues

In our cognitive hypothesis-testing (CHT) model, emphasis is placed on helping a majority of children through systematic prereferral services. As a psychologist, you must *intervene to assess*: You must develop an effective prereferral intervention program, using a team approach such as an intervention assistance team (see Ross, 1995) and problem-solving consultation, to reduce the number of referrals for formal evaluation. A large majority of children can be helped via an indirect service delivery model, and consultative approaches can effectively reduce the number of referrals for formal standardized evaluation. This is the only way in which the comprehensive CHT evaluations we argue for will be feasible; reducing referrals means gaining more time to conduct both interventions and more comprehensive evaluations.

Of course, there have been calls for more emphasis on prereferral interventions, or a move to interventions instead of referrals, for many years. Since Public Law 94-142 originally mandated serving children with disabilities rather than excluding them, school psychology has tried to emphasize interventions. The National Association of School Psychologists issued a volume titled *Alternative Educational Delivery Systems* (Graden, Zins, & Curtis, 1988), which called for more consultation, more teacher assistance teams, and more interventions. The 25th-anniversary issue of the *School Psychology Review* (Harrison, 1996) called for the same, as did *Best Practices in School Psychology IV* (Thomas & Grimes, 2002). Despite these numerous calls for professional change, however, school psychologists continue to spend the majority of their time in determining eligibility for special education (Hosp & Reschly, 2002). Why is this? There are probably several reasons. Intervention resources often depend on special education eligibility. Also, the funding to pay school psychologists may come from special education money. High student–psychologist ratios, as well as a high number of required assessments, may contribute to a lack of time to spend in alternative roles (e.g., Wilczynski, Mandal, & Fusilier, 2000). How can we increase the perceived value of interventions? In many schools, special education is seen as the only way to get help for a child who is experiencing difficulties. Systems change efforts must include resource allocation for supporting children in general education. Then the school psychologist's ability to help design and monitor those interventions will be seen as a valuable role, and the consultation role can increase. And when evaluations are truly useful for intervention design, rather than focusing entirely on eligibility, they will be valued as well. Only with a mix of both these roles can school psychologists completely fulfill the promise of their training.

As noted earlier, a child's behavior and his or her environment are inextricably related. The environment—including teachers, peers, the curriculum, and the classroom structure and routine—exerts a great influence on the child's behavior. But the child's characteristics—biological constraints, temperament, past learning history, and current skills—also influence both the child's behavior and, in turn, the environment. Practitioners can use information about *both* parts of the cycle to intervene and develop individualized interventions that will work with the environment to meet the child's unique needs. We suggest paying attention to both sides of the equation, since we feel that an exclusive focus either on external, environmental factors or on within-child factors neglects half the picture. This approach combines the two most powerful strands of the school psychology profession: individual psychoeducational assessment (e.g., Kamphaus, 2001; Sattler, 2001), and intervention development and monitoring from the behavioral intervention and problem-solving consultation models (e.g., Erchul & Martens, 2002; Thomas & Grimes, 2002).

CHT in Assessment and Intervention

Initially, standard problem-solving consultation is used in CHT to develop data-based interventions at the prereferral level. But a child who does not benefit from these initial interventions is referred for a formal CHT evaluation. The referral question, history, and previous interventions are examined to develop a theory of the problem (see #1 under "Theory" in Figure 4.1). If cognitive functioning is thought to be related to the academic or behavioral deficit areas in question (see #2 under "Hypothesis" in Figure 4.1), the intelligence/cognitive test is used as one of the first-level assessment tools (see #3 under "Data Collection/Analysis"). Via demands analysis, the findings are interpreted (see #4 under "Data Interpretation") to determine possible cognitive strengths and weaknesses (#5 under "Theory"). This is where many psychologists stop the process. Because of time demands, psychologists in the schools typically write their reports and pres-

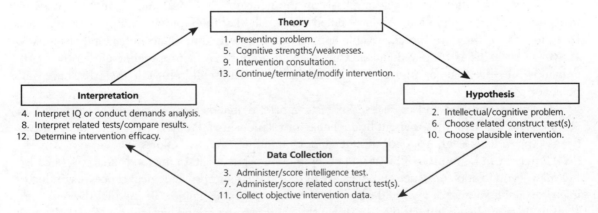

FIGURE 4.1. The cognitive hypothesis-testing (CHT) model.

ent their findings in a team meeting; they have little contact with the child, parents, or teacher thereafter (unless individual therapy is offered). But our CHT model goes beyond this to choose additional measures (#6 under "Hypothesis") to confirm or refute the intellectual test data (#7 under "Data Collection/Analysis"). The results are examined in light of the record review/history, systematic observations, behavior ratings, and parent/teacher interviews to gain a good understanding of the child (#8 under "Data Interpretation").

Completing the initial assessment is where the CHT process *begins*, not ends. Interventions are subsequently developed using the understanding of the child and the environment during collaborative consultative follow-up meetings with teachers and/or parents. Possible intervention strategies are explored in consultation with the teacher (#9 under "Theory"), and an intervention plan likely to succeed is developed (#10 under "Hypothesis"). The systematic intervention is then undertaken (#11 under "Data Collection/Analysis") and evaluated to determine intervention efficacy (#12 under "Data Interpretation"). If the intervention does not appear to be effective, it is revised or recycled until beneficial results are obtained (#13 under "Theory"). Like brief experimental analysis (Chafouleas, Riley-Tillman, & McGrath, 2002), the CHT model we describe uses a problem-solving approach and single-subject methodology to examine child performance over time. We are strong advocates for behavioral technology and single-subject methodology. The difference between our model and other behavioral approaches is that we use information about cognitive functioning in developing our interventions.

Conducting Demands Analysis

Demands analysis is a core component of the CHT model. It is the key both to accurate identification of childhood disorders and to development of interventions that are sensitive to individual needs. The demands analysis process that we present here is derived from two assessment traditions. The first tradition is the "intelligent testing" approach, which examines global, factor, and subtest scores based on clinical, psychometric, and quantitative research (e.g., Flanagan & Ortiz, 2001; Kamphaus, 2001; Kaufman, 1994; McGrew & Flanagan, 1998; Sattler, 2001). When formulating your clinical demands analysis, you must be careful to examine all relevant technical and cross-battery subtest information. Heavily influenced by the Luria (1973) approach to neuropsychological assessment, the second tradition consists of the developmental and process-oriented neuropsychological assessment approaches (e.g., Bernstein, 2000; Kaplan, 1988; Lezak, 1995). Although demands analysis may seem similar to other versions of profile analysis (e.g., Kaufman, 1994), the major difference is the emphasis on the neuropsychological and cognitive processes necessary for task completion. We have noted previously that the input and output demands are straightforward; they are the observable and measurable test stimuli and behavioral responses. However, research is clearly demonstrating that the underlying neuropsychological processing demands are essential for understanding and helping many children with their learning and behavior problems.

For many children and most tests/subtests, a brief demands analysis should be sufficient to examine and test hypotheses about brain–behavior relationships. We have provided you with two forms (Appendix 4.1 and Appendix 4.2) to guide you in interpretative efforts. The form in Appendix 4.2 may even be more helpful as you become more accustomed to demands analysis, because this allows you to add constructs as necessary to reflect the neuropsychological processes underlying a particular subtest or if a child responds in an idiosyncratic manner. To conduct the demands analysis, identify tests/subtests that represent the child's strengths and weaknesses. Enter them in the appropriate spaces in Appendix 4.2, and for each measure conduct a task analysis of the *input*, *processing,* and *output* demands. *Input* refers to the stimulus materials as well as the directions, demonstrations, and teaching items. Think about what modality or modalities are needed for the input—for example, whether there are pictures or verbal directions, whether the content is meaningful or abstract, and what other aspects of the content are relevant (e.g., level of English language used or amount of cultural knowledge required). *Processing* refers to the actual neuropsychological processing demands of the task, as discussed in Chapters 2 and 3. Think about the primary requirement (often suggested by the test's developers), but also secondary requirements, such as the executive and working memory skills needed to keep a stimulus in mind while processing it. *Output* refers to the modalities and skills required for responding to the task. Is the output a complex verbal response, a simple pointing response, or a complex motoric response? If oral expression is needed, is syntax important, and is word choice an issue? These are some of the questions you must answer in demands analysis. The form we provide in Appendix 4.1 is merely a tool for you to begin thinking about underlying psychological processes. We have included blanks in the last column for you to provide additional subtest input, processing, and output demands. Once you have listed the input, processing, and output demands for all of the child's strengths and weaknesses, it is important to look for commonalities and contradictions among the data.

After completing the sheets for each subtest, you attempt to identify patterns in the child's performance. If you find that one particular processing demand is required on all low-score tests, and it is not needed for the high-score tasks, you would hypothesize that this demand is a weakness for the child. Information from your observations of the child during testing, as well as information provided by the teacher, should also be consistent with any hypotheses. The weakness may be a cognitive processing weakness, but it may also be a sensory or motor weakness, a result of emotional interference, or a consequence of limited exposure or background. Enter this information on the worksheet provided in Appendix 4.3. Although these sheets and interpretive texts (e.g., Groth-Marnat, Gallagher, Hale, & Kaplan, 2000; Kamphaus, 1993; Kaufman, 1994; McGrew & Flanagan, 1998; Sattler, 2001) can be helpful in conducting demands analysis, you should not be lulled into a "cookbook" approach when interpreting subtest data—a tendency that often results in erroneous interpretation. To guard against this and to foster accurate interpretation, we have provided a checklist in Appendix 4.4. This checklist is primarily for you to complete to aid in clinical judgment, but it could possibly be used as an informant rating scale as well.

Let's walk through a demands analysis of the Wechsler Intelligence Scale for Children—Fourth Edition (WISC-IV) Block Design subtest to see what the process looks like. First, consider the input. The task has oral directions, and the task is modeled for younger children and those who have difficulty on the first item. The stimulus materials (booklet with visual model and two-color blocks) are abstract colored shapes, so that verbal encoding is difficult. The task will be novel for most children (although perhaps not on reevaluation or as the testing progresses). The processing demands are quite complex and involve both hemispheres and executive/frontal demands. Primarily, Block Design is a right-hemisphere task, since it is visual–spatial (i.e., involves the dorsal stream), is novel, and does not depend on crystallized prior knowledge. However, there is some bilateral processing because of the bimanual sensory and motor coordination, as well as the part (directional orientation of the blocks—left parietal) and whole (gestalt/spatial—right parietal) coordination (see Kaplan, 1988). There is a heavy frontal component, due to the executive and motor requirements of the task. The frontal demands include planning and organization, self-monitoring and evaluation of the response, inhibition of impulsive responding, and fine motor and bimanual coordination. This is particularly true if the child uses a trial-and-error approach. Note particularly if the child has more difficulty after the lines are removed from the stimulus book, as this may suggest right posterior (i.e. configuration problem) or frontal (delayed responding due to novelty) difficulties. Considering the output, Block Design requires fine motor and bilateral motor coordination, and adequate processing speed. Bilateral sensory–motor coordination requires the corpus callosum, so look for midline problems or a tendency to use just one hand. Slow responding may be due to difficulties in frontal–subcortical circuits (i.e., prefrontal–basal ganglia–cingulate) or the sensory–motor system (constructional praxis)—inattention/disorganization (symptoms resembling attention-deficit/hyperactivity disorder [ADHD]), low cortical tone or lethargy (motivation problems or depression-like symptoms), or perfectionistic tendencies (symptoms resembling obsessive–compulsive disorder [OCD] or other anxiety disorders).

Although conducting demands analysis may be helpful in understanding patterns of performance, remember that multifactorial tasks can be solved in more than one way, so that the demands analysis may differ from child to child. For instance, a child who uses good executive and psychomotor skills to compensate for a right posterior spatial problem may still do well on Block Design, but you would err if you concluded that the child had adequate visual–spatial–holistic processing skills. This is where we psychologists have often gone wrong in the past: concluding that the same subtest measures the same thing for all children. For instance, concluding that poor WISC-IV Information subtest performance is due to a limited "fund of information" may not be correct if a child has retrieval problems or difficulty due to limited knowledge in just one area, such as science. Concluding that a child has adequate attention, working memory, and executive function because he or she has an average WISC-IV Digit Span scaled score, but a Digits Forward score of 10 and a Digits Backward score of 2, would clearly be inappropriate (see Hale, Hoeppner, & Fiorello, 2002). Table 4.1 provides you with some sample demands analyses on a few additional subtests, so you can see how the process works. As you become more familiar with using demands analysis to task-analyze subtests you will eventually become quite comfortable with determining the demands on any subtest. In my (Hale's) graduate child neuropsychology assessment class, I have a final exam item that requires students to do a "mystery test" demands analysis on a test they have not been exposed to in class. Though students find this challenging, they typically find that they can identify the key input, processing, and output demands on the test. Try this activity yourself. Generalizing these skills to other measures will allow you to expand your use of demands analysis to just about any instrument you are trained to administer.

We now turn to a discussion of neuropsychological tests for use in the CHT model. Although many of these tests may be new to you, it is important to realize that the demands analyses you perform on cognitive and intellectual measures apply to neuropsychological measures as well. Do not let yourself be overly concerned that these measures are "neuropsychological"; many of them are easier to administer and score than the measures you are used to. For instance, the Stroop Color–Word Test requires approximately 5 minutes to administer (a stopwatch is needed to time 45 seconds for each subtest), and it has brief, simple instructions. Even though it is easy to administer, it is highly sensitive to executive functions and to frontal–subcortical circuit dysfunction.

ASSESSMENT TOOLS FOR CHT

Fixed versus Flexible Batteries in Hypothesis Testing

One of the biggest debates in neuropsychological assessment is whether to use a fixed test battery (a standard set of tests) or a flexible battery (a set of tests chosen for an individual child) (Bornstein, 1990). Fixed batteries predominated early in the field's history, but flexible batteries have become increasingly popular, especially since they tend to be more time- and cost-effective. Fixed batteries tend to lead to more testing than is needed to address unique child characteristics.

TABLE 4.1. Sample Demands Analysis of Selected Subtests

<u>WISC-IV Block Design</u>

Input

- Models and abstract visual pictures
- Oral directions—moderate English-language knowledge
- Demonstration/modeling
- Low cultural knowledge and emotional content

Processing

- Visual processing (spatial relations, visualization)
- Perception of part–whole relationships
- Discordant/divergent processing (analysis)
- Constructional praxis
- Bimanual coordination/corpus callosum
- Concordant/convergent processing (synthesis)
- Attention and executive demands: Moderate
- Planning and strategy use
- Inhibition of impulsive/wrong responding
- Novel problem solving: Low to moderate

Output

- Fine motor response, arrangement of manipulatives
- Timed score with speed bonus; process score without time bonus
- Visual–motor integration

<u>SB5 Picture Absurdities (Levels 4, 5, and 6—Nonverbal Knowledge)</u>

Input

- Large color pictures
- Oral directions
- Sample item
- High cultural and English-language knowledge

Processing

- Visual scanning
- Perception of objects (ventral stream)
- Crystallized ability for prior knowledge (left temporal)
- Discordant/divergent processing (analysis)
- Attention and executive demands: Low to moderate
- Persistence/inhibition of impulsive responding
- Novel problem solving/reasoning

Output

- Brief oral or pointing response
- One right answer (convergent responding)

<u>WJ-III Visual–Auditory Learning</u>

Input

- Brief oral directions, teaching items, feedback
- Semiabstract figures/symbols
- Moderate cultural and English-language knowledge

(continued)

TABLE 4.1. *(continued)*

<u>WJ-III Visual–Auditory Learning</u> *(continued)*

Processing

- Visual perception of figures/symbols (dorsal and ventral streams)
- Sound–word/symbol–rebus association
- Working memory/learning
- Encoding and retrieval of associative/semantic memory
- Benefiting from feedback
- Inhibition of impulsive/wrong responding
- Syntax knowledge: Helpful
- Attention and executive demands: Moderate to high
- Memory: primary; novel problem solving: secondary

Output

- Brief oral response
- Oral formulation/retrieval

<u>CAS Nonverbal Matrices</u>

Input

- Brief oral directions; sample and teaching items
- Abstract/nonmeaningful figures
- Low cultural knowledge and English-language knowledge

Processing

- Visual scanning and discrimination
- Color processing
- Visual–spatial processing (dorsal stream)
- Part–whole relationships
- Discordant/divergent processing (perceptual analysis)
- Novel problem solving and inductive reasoning/fluid abilities
- Attention and executive demands: Moderate
- Inhibition of impulsive/wrong responding

Output

- Pointing response
- Multiple-choice format (can solve by elimination/match to sample)

In addition, a fixed battery gives examiners the impression that the battery assesses all relevant neuropsychological domains (Lezak, 1995). We too prefer a flexible-battery approach in the CHT model, because different measures and techniques can be used to address hypotheses developed after initial data gathering. You may need one or more measures that look at a particular domain in depth. For instance, if you're interested in an apparent visual–sensory–motor integration deficit, you really need to pick and choose measures that tap each of these four possible causes to get a better understanding of the problem and direction for intervention.

This is not to say that a fixed-battery approach should be completely avoided. Some neuropsychologists prefer such approaches, because all the children tested are administered the same tests in the same order. This can serve both research and practice needs. Obviously, many children who receive the same measures would be needed for a group-design research project. For clinicians, fixed-battery approaches not only help standardize performance expectations across children, but also allow practitioners an opportunity to develop "head norms" about child performance. It is much easier to interpret a measure after dozens of regular administrations than if it is used sparingly to test hypotheses for individual children. In addition, once demands analyses have been done on the fixed-battery subtests, they may only need to be changed slightly for children who perform them in a unique way. Finally, the use of a fixed battery does not preclude additional hypothesis testing with other instruments. Actually, using an intellectual/cognitive measure (e.g., the Woodcock–Johnson III [WJ-III]), a fixed battery (e.g., the Halstead–Reitan), and additional hypothesis-testing measures (e.g., subtests from the Comprehensive Test of Phonological Processing [CTOPP]) might be the ultimate approach for conducting CHT. However, it is important to remember that as the number of measures increases, the likelihood of child performance variability and of Type I error increases as well.

Intellectual Tests for Hypothesis Testing

You may be surprised to find that you are already familiar with many of the tools available for CHT—including the intelligence/cognitive tests discussed in Chapter 1, such as the subtests found on the Differential Ability Scales (DAS), Stanford–Binet Intelligence Scale: Fifth Edition (SB5), WISC-IV, and WJ-III. Although intelligence test subtests are typically factorially complex (McGrew & Flanagan, 1998), there is often a wealth of information published about these measures; their technical quality can be thoroughly evaluated; and you are familiar with their scoring and interpretation. The manuals on these measures come with many statistics to support interpretation, such as reliability, standard deviations, standard error of measurement, correlations, factor analyses, and validity studies.

To aid in your demands analysis of these and other measures, it is worthwhile to consult *The Intelligence Test Desk Reference* (McGrew & Flanagan, 1998), which specifies subtest technical characteristics from a *Gf-Gc* cross-battery approach perspective, and Sattler's (2001) *Assessment of Children: Cognitive Applications* text. Similarly, CHT of the skills necessary for academic performance can utilize subtests from several achievement batteries. For instance, on the WJ-III Tests of Achievement, the Story Recall subtest can be used to assess long-term memory encoding and retrieval of semantic information in addition to receptive and expressive language. Another valuable text for use in CHT is *The Achievement Test Desk Reference* (Flanagan, Ortiz, Alfonso, & Mascolo, 2002) which provides readers with technical information and guidance in administering and interpreting many achievement measures.

Although these intellectual and achievement instruments are useful in CHT, let us now examine several test batteries that are often considered "neuropsychological" instruments. It is important to realize that many neuropsychological tests are easy to administer and score, and that they tap many of the constructs already discussed in this book. We do not claim to present an exhaustive list of measures, just those that we have found to be useful in our practice of CHT. We do not suggest that these measures are better than others, or that measures not included here cannot be adopted in the CHT model. However, recall that it is your responsibility to evaluate whether a measure has adequate technical quality for use in CHT. In addition, you should complete a demands analysis for each measure you use and review the extant literature on new tests before you use them. Do not automatically assume that a test measures what we suggest, or what the test authors report in the manual. Although our interpretive information is limited, you can consult the test manuals and other interpretive texts to aid in your understanding of the measures (e.g., Groth-Marnat, 2000b; Golden, Espe-Pfeifer, & Wachsler-Felder, 2000; Reynolds & Fletcher-Janzen, 1997; Spreen & Strauss, 1998). Your background, training, and experience will determine your need for individual training and supervision on these measures.

Traditional Neuropsychological Test Batteries

We begin our review of instruments by discussing two of the most commonly used neuropsychological test batteries (NTBs): the Halstead–Reitan NTB (Reitan & Wolfson, 1993) and the Luria–Nebraska NTB (Golden, Purisch, & Hammeke, 1985). Though we aren't advocating that every school psychologist use one of these batteries, a brief description follows to familiarize you with them. These batteries are often used as "fixed" batteries, and both have a long tradition of use in neuropsychological assessment and research, so there are many supplemental resources and publications to aid in their interpretation.

Halstead–Reitan NTB

Table 4.2 provides an overview of the constructs tapped by the Halstead–Reitan NTB (Reitan & Wolfson, 1993) subtests, and of possible brain areas responsible for performance. The Category Test requires the child to view simple objects on a screen and press a button coinciding with the numbers 1 to 4. The child is not told how to perform the task, but instead receives feedback after each response. (A more recent version of the Category Test is mentioned later in Table 4.10.) For the Tactile Performance Test, the child is blindfolded and presented with an upright formboard and shapes. The child places the different shapes in the corresponding holes as quickly as possible, first with the dominant hand, then with the nondominant hand, and then with both. The Trail Making Test is a connect-the-dots task, where the child draws a line connecting numbers in order (Trails A), and then alternating between numbers and letters (Trails B), as quickly as possible. For the Sensory-Perceptual Examination, a brief screening of visual, auditory, and somatosensory functioning is followed by three somatosensory tasks: finger touching, writing of numbers (older children) or symbols (young children) on fingers/hands, and recognition of shapes, all hidden from the child's view. The Finger Tapping test is a simple measure of motor speed and persistence. The Halstead–Reitan provides an Impairment Index of brain dysfunction/damage, which ranges from 0 to 10. Although the original norms may have been limited, more recent normative data and in-

TABLE 4.2. Characteristics of Halstead–Reitan Neuropsychological Test Battery (NTB) Subtests

Subtest	Constructs purportedly tapped	Brain areas involved
Category Test	Concept formation, fluid reasoning, learning skills, mental efficiency	Prefrontal area, cingulate, hippocampus, temporal lobes (?) (associative and categorical thinking)
Tactile Performance Test	Tactile sensitivity, manual dexterity, kinesthetic functions, bimanual coordination, spatial memory, incidental learning	Lateralized sensory and motor areas, parietal lobes, corpus callosum, hippocampus
Sensory-Perceptual Examination	Simple and complex sensory functions	Lateralized sensory areas (more complex, bilateral?)
Finger Tapping	Simple motor speed	Lateralized motor areas
Trail Making Test, Parts A and B (Trails A and B)	Processing speed, graphomotor coordination, sequencing, number/letter facility (Trails B also requires working memory, mental flexibility, set shifting)	Trails A: Dorsal stream, premotor area, primary motor area, corpus callosum; Trails B: also prefrontal–basal ganglia–cingulate

terpretive strategies have been developed. For a recent review of the Halstead–Reitan NTB, see Nussbaum and Bigler (1997).

Luria–Nebraska NTB

The Luria–Nebraska NTB (Golden et al., 1985) consists of 12 scales derived from Luria's (1973, 1980a, 1980b) approach to neuropsychological assessment, which emphasizes flexible administration and interpretation of measures. Therefore, it is not a true fixed battery per se, but practitioners may have a tendency to administer it as such. The 12 Luria–Nebraska subscales are labeled Motor, Rhythm, Tactile, Visual, Receptive Language, Expressive Language, Writing, Reading, Arithmetic, Memory, Intelligence, and Delayed Memory. Because the traditional examination may take up to 2 days to complete (Golden, Freshwater, & Vayalakkara, 2001), this instrument may not be practical for use in the schools. As we will see in the next section, several contemporary neuropsychological assessment tools are available to assess skills similar to those tapped by the Luria–Nebraska domains, and many were designed solely for use with children. For a recent review of the Luria–Nebraska NTB, see Golden (1997).

Neuropsychological/Cognitive Tests for Hypothesis Testing

We now review instruments that assess multiple as well as specific areas of neuropsychological functioning. You may wish to use an entire test at times, but for the most part, you will pick and choose subtests from these batteries for CHT. They are listed in alphabetical order.

Children's Memory Scale

Since we are often asked to give an indication of a child's capability of learning in the classroom, it is somewhat surprising that more educational administrators don't mandate assessment of learning and memory skills. Designed for use with children aged 5–16, the Children's Memory Scale (CMS; Cohen, 1997) is an excellent measure of learning and memory designed for clinical assessment. It was carefully standardized on a representative sample. It is not surprising that the CMS demonstrates adequate internal consistency for a memory measure, and comprehensive validity studies support the instrument's construct validity. It has six core subtests, two each in the Auditory/Verbal, Visual/Nonverbal, and Attention/Concentration domains; the last domain is probably the least useful in CHT. In addition, there are three supplemental subtests, one for each domain. The subtests we typically use are presented in Table 4.3. The reported subtests all have delayed portions for further examination of long-term memory retrieval—an advantage of this measure. A disadvantage is relying on the Auditory/Verbal–Visual/Nonverbal dichotomy for organizing the battery.

Cognitive Assessment System

Designed for ages 5–17, the Cognitive Assessment System (CAS; Naglieri & Das, 1997) is a relatively new measure of cognitive functioning that represents the authors' planning, attention, simultaneous, and successive (PASS) model (Das, Naglieri, & Kirby, 1994). It is purportedly based on Luria's model of neuropsychological processing and assessment, but as we have seen in Chapter 2, there is no PASS acronym in Luria's model. In addition, although the authors' confirmatory

TABLE 4.3. Characteristics of Children's Memory Scale (CMS) Subtests

Subtest	Constructs purportedly tapped
Auditory/Verbal	
Stories	Auditory attention, semantic long-term memory encoding and retrieval, sequencing/ grammar, verbal comprehension, expressive language
Word Pairs	Paired-associate task; auditory attention, learning novel word pairs
Word Lists	Selective reminding task; long-term memory encoding, storage, and retrieval of unrelated words
Visual/Nonverbal	
Dot Locations	Visual–spatial memory encoding and retrieval (dorsal stream), susceptibility to interference
Faces	Visual–facial memory encoding and retrieval (ventral stream)
Attention/Concentration	
Sequences	Rote recall of simple information followed by mental manipulation/executive function items

factor analysis has been used to support a four-factor model, cross-battery analyses have raised doubt about the model, with findings suggesting that the Planning and Attention factors should be combined (Carroll, 1995; Keith, Kranzler, & Flanagan, 2001; Kranzler & Keith, 1999). This would certainly fit with Luria's (1973) model, as attention and executive functions are intimately related to the integrity of the third functional unit or frontal lobes (except for cortical tone, which would be the responsibility of Luria's first functional unit). Of course, for an individual child, planning and attention may differ and lead to different recommendations, so their separation may be relevant for individual children.

Another issue has to do with purported relationships between the hemispheres and CAS measures. Whereas the association between simultaneous processes and right-hemisphere functions makes sense, the association of the left hemisphere with successive processes needs further examination. As we have seen in Chapters 2 and 3, this representation is not entirely correct— leaving the construct validity of the PASS model in question, at least as a neuropsychological test. Two of the successive tasks rely heavily on grammatical structure, and all use verbal information, so they are not truly tests of successive processing. It is interesting to note that the test authors' own predictive validity study, using the WISC-III, CAS, and WJ-R achievement scores, revealed that the WISC-III Verbal scale consistently predicted achievement domains better than the CAS factors.

Given these criticisms, why do we advocate use of the CAS in CHT? We like to use several of the CAS subtests for hypothesis testing. The scale was adequately normed, and most subtests show good technical characteristics. In addition, the test authors have provided us with the first substantial treatment validity studies of any cognitive measure, presented in the PASS Remedial Program (PREP; see Das, Carlson, Davidson, & Longe, 1997). The PREP has focused primarily on reading, with training of successive and simultaneous skills leading to improved word recognition and decoding skills. There is also evidence that strategy-based instruction can improve math achievement in students with poor planning skills. We do not think, however, that the CAS should be used to measure global intellectual functioning, even though it provides a Full Scale standard score (SS). Absent from the CAS, moreover, is a measure of crystallized intelligence (*Gc*). Although the lack of *Gc* measurement makes the CAS a fair test for people for people of linguistic and cultural difference, it doesn't adequately tap left-hemisphere processes as a result. Therefore, though we feel that the CAS is not adequate as a baseline measure of global functioning, it is a good tool for hypothesis testing. Given these caveats and criticisms, we present the CAS subtests we typically administer in Table 4.4. Please note that our interpretation is somewhat different from that presented by the test authors.

Comprehensive Test of Phonological Processing

The CTOPP (Wagner, Torgesen, & Rashotte, 1999) is a unique measure of the cognitive constructs most commonly associated with reading and language disorders. Designed for use with children and youth aged 5–24, it measures phonological awareness, phonological memory, and rapid automatized naming, which have been linked with word recognition, word attack, and other basic reading skills (Wolf, 2001). The CTOPP is composed of 13 subtests, several of which we find useful in CHT. It was recently normed on a fairly large representative sample, and subtests have good to excellent good technical characteristics. Validity studies show the phonological awareness and rapid naming tasks have strong relationships with reading skills.

TABLE 4.4. Characteristics of Cognitive Assessment System (CAS) Subtests

Subtest	Constructs purportedly tapped
Planning	
Matching Numbers	Sustained attention, visual scanning, psychomotor speed
Planned Connections	Substitute for Halstead–Reitan Trails A and B (see Table 4.2), but no separation
Attention	
Expressive Attention	Substitute for Stroop Color–Word Test (see Table 4.10); inhibition of automatic response (reading words) to name ink color of printed word
Number Detection	Cancellation task; sustained attention, visual scanning, visual discrimination, inhibition, psychomotor speed
Simultaneous Processing	
Nonverbal Matrices	Typical *Gf* measure of inductive reasoning; multiple-choice format
Verbal/Spatial Relations	Similar to Token Test for Children (see Table 4.10); receptive language, verbal working memory, grammatical relationships, visual scanning/discrimination
Figural Memory	Similar to DAS Recall of Designs (see Chapter 1, Table 1.1); visual perception, spatial relationships, visual memory, graphomotor reproduction, constructional skills, figure–ground relationships (?)
Successive Processing	
Word Series	Word span; rote recall of unrelated words
Sentence Repetition	Rote recall of meaningless sentences; grammatical structure important
Sentence Questions	Similar sentence stimuli to Sentence Repetition, but child answers questions (e.g., "The brown is purple. What is purple?" Answer: "The brown.")

Table 4.5 outlines the CTOPP subtests and what they measure. The Nonword Repetition subtest is an interesting task that taps phonemic processing and expression skills for nonsense words (e.g., "lidsca"), similar to other visually presented pseudoword tasks. However, it includes an auditory model (so the child hears the nonword first) and an auditory working memory component (because the child has to recall what he or she heard). This task can be combined with the Blending Nonwords (e.g., "raq" + "di") subtest to help determine whether the phonological breakdown is occurring at the individual-phoneme level or the assembly level. An additional concern with the CTOPP is the limited assessment of rapid naming. Including rapid naming of more complex letter combinations (e.g., digraphs, diphthongs) and simple words presented two grades below reading level would have been helpful. Although phonological processes have been linked to left temporal lobe functions, and rapid naming is typically associated with frontal structures, you should recognize that several areas are involved in reading competency, as discussed in Chapters 2 and 5.

Delis–Kaplan Executive Function System

The Delis–Kaplan Executive Function System (D-KEFS; Delis, Kaplan, & Kramer, 2001) is a measure of key components of executive function, mediated primarily by the frontal lobe. It was recently developed and normed on a large representative national sample to assess ages 8–89. Unlike many neuropsychological measures, the D-KEFS has extensive information about technical quality presented in the manual, which facilitates interpretation. Any of the specific tests can be administered separately, making it ideal for use in CHT. Many of the tasks have rich histories in neuropsychological assessment, and research is likely to support the validity of these measures. Table 4.6 describes the individual D-KEFS tests and the constructs purportedly assessed by each.

Kaufman Adolescent and Adult Intelligence Test

Although the Kaufman Adolescent and Adult Intelligence Test (KAAIT; Kaufman & Kaufman, 1993) provides good measures for hypothesis testing of *Gc* and fluid intelligence (*Gf*), it is pri-

TABLE 4.5. Characteristics of Comprehensive Test of Phonological Processing (CTOPP) Subtests

Subtest	Constructs purportedly tapped
Phonological Awareness	
Elision	Phonological perception, segmentation, individual phonemes
Blending Words	Phonological assembly; similar to WJ-III Sound Blending (see Chapter 1, Table 1.4)
Phonological Memory	
Nonword Repetition	Phonemic analysis, assembly, auditory working memory
Rapid Naming	
Rapid Object Naming	Object recognition, naming automaticity, processing speed, verbal fluency
Rapid Digit Naming	Number automaticity, processing speed, verbal fluency
Rapid Letter Naming	Letter automaticity, processing speed, verbal fluency

TABLE 4.6. Characteristics of Delis–Kaplan Executive Function System (D-KEFS) Subtests

Subtest	Constructs purportedly tapped
Sorting Test	Problem solving, verbal and spatial concept formation, categorical thinking, flexibility of thinking on a conceptual task
Trail Making Test	Mental flexibility, sequential processing on a visual–motor task, set shifting
Verbal Fluency Test	Verbal fluency
Design Fluency Test	Visual fluency
Color–Word Interference Test	Attention and response inhibition
Tower Test	Planning, flexibility, organization, spatial reasoning, inhibition
20 Questions Test	Hypothesis testing, verbal and spatial abstract thinking, inhibition
Word Context Test	Deductive reasoning, verbal abstract thinking
Proverb Test	Metaphorical thinking, generating versus comprehending abstract thoughts

marily designed for children 11 years of age and older, so this limits its use in CHT to older children. For *Gc*, the Word Knowledge subtest is a measure of word knowledge and verbal concept formation; Auditory Comprehension taps understanding of oral information; and Double Meanings measures categorical responding (i.e., the child must determine the word that best fits two different meanings). For *Gf*, the Rebus Learning subtest is similar to the WJ-III *Glr* task; Logical Steps taps logical reasoning and problem solving; and Mystery Codes requires detecting relationships and applying them to solve novel problems. It also has four extended-battery subtests: Famous Faces, Memory for Block Designs, Rebus Delayed Recall, and Auditory Delayed Recall. Although the KAAIT cannot be used for younger children, it is easy to administer and score, and has fairly good technical characteristics (Sattler, 2001). Consider using this battery in CHT if you work with older children, as we feel it is a much more theoretically sound instrument than the Kaufman Assessment Battery for Children (Kaufman & Kaufman, 1983), which suffers from the same problem as the CAS (the simultaneous/right-hemisphere–successive/left-hemisphere dichotomy).

NEPSY

The NEPSY (Korkman, Kirk, & Kemp, 1998) is the first *truly* developmental neuropsychological measure designed for children aged 3–12. There are 27 subtests designed to provide a comprehensive evaluation of five functional domains: Attention/Executive Functions, Language, Sensorimotor Functions, Visuospatial Processing, and Memory and Learning. The NEPSY subtests and flexible administration format are primarily based on Luria's (1973, 1980a, 1980b) model. However, like similar measures, the test does not break tasks down into primary, secondary, or tertiary skills; nor does the manual readily identify the relationships between subtest performance and the first, second, and third functional units. With many years in development, the NEPSY has all the advantages of being published by a major test developer, including an adequate normative sample, subtest technical quality, and ample validity studies. Not all of the NEPSY subtests show comparable technical quality, however, so Table 4.7 presents the subtests we have found to be most beneficial in CHT. In addition, though the Language subtests serve as a measure of *Gc*, the NEPSY does not adequately measure *Gf* or novel problem-solving skills.

TABLE 4.7. Characteristics of NEPSY Subtests

Subtest	Constructs purportedly tapped
Attention/Executive Functions	
Tower	Planning, inhibition, problem solving, monitoring, and self-regulation
Auditory Attention and Response Set	Sustained auditory attention, vigilance, inhibition, set maintenance, mental flexibility
Visual Attention	Visual scanning, self-organization, processing speed
Design Fluency	Visual–motor fluency, mental flexibility, graphomotor responding in structured and unstructured situations
Language	
Phonological Processing	Similar to WJ-III *Ga* subtests (see Chapter 1, Table 1.4); auditory attention, phonological awareness, segmentation, assembly
Comprehension of Instructions	Similar to token test for Children (see Table 4.10); receptive language, sequencing, grammar, simple motor response
Repetition of Nonsense Words	Auditory presentation of nonsense words; phonemic awareness, segmentation, assembly, sequencing, simple oral expression
Verbal Fluency	Similar to Controlled Oral Word Association Test (see Table 4.10); rapid long-term memory retrieval in structured (semantic cue) and unstructured (phonemic cue) situations
Sensorimotor Functions	
Fingertip Tapping	Simple motor speed, perseverance
Imitating Hand Positions	Visual perception, memory, kinesthesis, praxis
Visuomotor Precision	Visual–motor integration, graphomotor coordination without constructional requirements
Finger Discrimination	Simple somatosensory perception, finger agnosia
Visuospatial Processing	
Design Copying	Visual perception of abstract stimuli, visual–motor integration, graphomotor skills
Arrows	Spatial processing, visualization, line orientation, inhibition, no graphomotor demands
Block Construction	Similar to WISC-III Block Design (see Tables 1.3 and 4.1)

Process Assessment of the Learner: Test Battery for Reading and Writing

To look in more detail at the processes involved in reading and writing, the Process Assessment of the Learner: Test Battery for Reading and Writing (PAL; Berninger, 2001) is available to complement regular standardized achievement testing. Individual subtests can be administered and interpreted, making this test ideal for CHT. There are also intervention materials available for both individual and classroom implementation. The PAL includes measures of phonological processing; orthographic coding; rapid automatized naming; and integration of listening, note taking, and summary writing skills. Although the PAL is used for examining academic skills, it focuses on processes associated with these skills, making it especially useful for linking assessment to intervention.

Test of Memory and Learning

The Test of Memory and Learning (TOMAL; Reynolds & Bigler, 1994) is in many ways a more comprehensive measure of learning and memory than the CMS. Designed for children aged 5–19, the TOMAL consists of 10 core and 4 supplemental subtests, and 4 delayed-recall subtests. It was carefully standardized, and the norms are representative of the 1990 U.S. census population. Reliabilities tend to be quite strong across ages, especially for the composite scores. Unfortunately, the validity studies are not as comprehensive as those for the CMS. However, further support for its use in memory assessment can been found in subsequent studies reported in the literature. Table 4.8 provides an overview of the TOMAL subtests we find useful in CHT. The Delayed Recall Index includes delayed recall from the Memory for Stories, Word Selective Reminding, Facial Memory, and Visual Selective Reminding subtests. As with the CMS, one of the difficulties with the TOMAL is its breakdown into verbal and nonverbal memory domains.

Wide Range Assessment of Memory and Learning

The Wide Range Assessment of Memory and Learning (WRAML; Sheslow & Adams, 1990) was the first child memory scale on the market, having been developed in the 1980s. Like the other measures reviewed here, it examines verbal and visual memory, and includes a learning index score. Additional examination of delayed recall is possible. For verbal memory, rote, sentence, and story memory are tapped. For visual memory, both abstract and meaningful memory are assessed, and visual–sequential memory is assessed via an interesting Finger Windows subtest, which is difficult to mediate with verbal skills. There are also a list-learning task, a memory-for-designs task (in which the child tries to find matching designs), and a sound–symbol association task. These tasks are challenging yet interesting for children, making the WRAML a possible alternative to the CMS and TOMAL. It is fairly easy to administer and score. It has a large normative sample

TABLE 4.8. Characteristics of Test of Memory and Learning (TOMAL) Subtests

Subtest	Constructs purportedly tapped
Verbal Memory Index	
Memory for Stories	See CMS Stories (Table 4.3 lists this and other CMS subtests)
Word Selective Reminding	Similar to CMS Word Lists, but no interference task
Paired Recall	See CMS Word Pairs
Digits Backward	Similar to WISC-III/WJ-III versions; more demands on attention, working memory, executive functions
Nonverbal Memory Index	
Facial Memory	See CMS Faces; good ventral stream measure
Visual Selective Reminding	Visual analogue to word selective reminding, with dots; dorsal stream, visual–motor coordination, praxis without visual discrimination
Abstract Visual Memory	Visual discrimination of abstract symbols, recognition memory
Visual–Sequential Memory	Visual discrimination of abstract symbols, sequencing, praxis
Memory for Location	See CMS Dot Locations; good dorsal stream measure
Manual Imitation	Short-term visual–sequential memory, praxis

and adequate technical characteristics. However, some have questioned the construct validity and structure of the test (for a review, see Spreen & Strauss, 1998).

WISC-IV Integrated/WISC-III Processing Instrument

We conclude this section with the unique WISC-IV Integrated and its predecessor, the WISC-III Processing Instrument (WISC-III PI; Kaplan, Fein, Kramer, Delis, & Morris, 1999). These instruments are unique because they help examiners test the limits and derive both qualitative and quantitative data for interpretive purposes. Designed to objectify many of the qualitative neuropsychological interpretation methods posited by Kaplan and colleagues in their Boston process approach (see Chapter 3), these measures are easily incorporated into your assessments, especially if you use the WISC-III or WISC-IV as your initial intellectual assessment tool. Because the WISC-IV and WISC-III subtests are factorially complex, tapping several cognitive processes, further evaluation is often needed to pinpoint individual strengths and weaknesses. Designed primarily for children aged 8–16, the WISC-IV Integrated and WISC-III PI have additional measures and procedures for hypothesis testing, so it may be helpful to administer only the sections that are relevant to the areas of concern (Sattler, 2001). Some procedures are administered during the WISC-IV or WISC-III, while others are administered immediately following the assessment. Several of the WISC-IV Integrated/WISC-III PI procedures are designed to provide a more comprehensive way to look at scoring WISC-IV/WISC-III responses, while several other stand alone subtests can aid in CHT. Although some reliabilities are low and more validity information would be helpful, the WISC-IV Integrated and WISC-III PI have satisfactory concurrent validity, and they are unique instruments for obtaining qualitative and quantitative information about a child's cognitive functioning (Sattler, 2001). An overview of the WISC-IV Integrated/WISC-III PI measures and procedures we prefer, and the constructs purportedly measured by each, are presented in Table 4.9.

Supplemental Neuropsychological Measures for Hypothesis Testing

Table 4.10 presents a number of other neuropsychological measures we have found useful in CHT. Although some are specifically for use with children, others listed in this table have a long history of use in neuropsychological assessment of adults, and most have been adequately extended downward for use with children. These instruments measure a variety of cognitive or neuropsychological constructs, and many have been found to be sensitive to brain functions and dysfunctions. They can be used to test initial hypotheses or validate hypotheses derived from previously discussed measures. Some measures, such as the Rey–Osterreith Complex Figure (a visual–spatial–graphomotor task) and the California Verbal Learning Test (a language task), could be listed under other table subheadings. However, we have put the measures in the domains that are most likely to serve our CHT purposes.

BEHAVIORAL NEUROPSYCHOLOGY AND PROBLEM-SOLVING CONSULTATION

Utilizing Assessment and Consultation Skills

Now that we have reviewed the assessment part of our model, let's integrate it with consultation technology. Notice the heading above. Isn't *behavioral neuropsychology* an oxymoron? No, because we believe that these two technologies should become one, not be seen as antithetical. Con-

TABLE 4.9. Characteristics of WISC-III Process Instrument (WISC-III PI) Subtests and Procedures

Subtest	Constructs purportedly tapped
Verbal scale/Verbal Comprehension and Working Memory Indices	
1. Information Multiple Choice 2. Vocabulary Multiple Choice (WISC-IV Integrated also includes Similarities and Comprehension Multiple Choice)	Long-term memory retrieval of prior learning (1) and word knowledge (2); compares free-recall and recognition memory
Picture Vocabulary	Taps receptive word knowledge for comparison with expressive word knowledge in #2 above
1. Arithmetic Addendum 2. Written Arithmetic	1. Mental problem solving of items read simultaneously with examiner; paper/pencil for failed items; reduces attention/executive/working memory demands, and eliminates auditory processing requirements 2. Presents equations on paper; helps determine math skills in absence of Arithmetic processing demands
Sentence Arrangement (WISC-III PI)	Verbal analogue to WISC-III Picture Arrangement; semantic/grammatical knowledge and sequencing, but not temporal relationships
Digit Span Forward/Backward	Separates rote auditory memory (Forward) from attention, working memory, and executive functions (Backward)
1. Letter Span Rhyming and Non-Rhyming 2. Letter Number Sequencing—Embedded Words	1. Letters of sequence rhyme or do not rhyme, with the former resulting in phonological/auditory processing demands, reducing rote aspect of encoding and retrieval 2. Letters form words, which helps encoding, but working memory still relevant; may be more difficult breaking known word into alphabetical order
Performance scale/Perceptual Reasoning and Processing Speed Indices	
1. Block Design PI 2. Block Design Multiple Choice	1. Part A (Unstructured): six additional designs; Part B (Structured): failed Part A designs; helps determine configuration (right-hemisphere) vs. orientation (left-hemisphere) errors 2. Visual discrimination, spatial perception; removes visual–motor integration and processing speed demands
1. Visual Span Forward/Backward 2. Spatial Span Forward/Backward	Visual–spatial analogues to digit span forward/backward; with Digit Span, can compare auditory with visual sensory and working memory, sequencing, mental flexibility, and ability to shift cognitive sets 1. Visual attention, numeric memory, and verbal response 2. Spatial–holistic or visual–sequential memory, praxis
1. Coding Incidental Learning Recall 2. Coding–Symbol Copy	1. Paired-associate symbol recall, free recall, paired-associate digit recall (visual memory and graphomotor reproduction of symbols and numbers, retrieval of number–symbol associations) 2. Visual–motor integration, graphomotor skills, and processing speed
Symbol Search	Child marks matching symbol in array or no box; ensures "guessing" is not occurring; better measure of discrimination and sustained attention
Elithorn Mazes	Maze-like task; assesses executive functions such as planning, organization, monitoring, working memory, and inhibition better than WISC-III Mazes, still requires graphomotor skills

TABLE 4.10. Supplemental Measures for Hypothesis Testing

Subtest	Constructs purportedly tapped
Attention/memory/executive function	
Children's Category Test (Boll, 1993)	See Halstead–Reitan Category Test (Table 4.2)
Wisconsin Card Sorting Test (Heaton, Chellune, Talley, Kay, & Curtis, 1993)	Executive functions, problem solving, set maintenance, goal-oriented behavior, inhibition, ability to benefit from feedback, mental flexibility, perseveration
Tower of London (Shallice, 1982)	See NEPSY Tower (Table 4.7)
Stroop Color–Word Test (Golden, 1978)	See CAS Expressive Attention (Table 4.4)
Rey–Osterrieth Complex Figure (Meyers & Meyers, 1995)	Visual–motor integration, constructional skills, graphomotor skills, visual memory, planning, organization, problem solving
Conners Continuous Performance Test II (CPT; Conners & MHS Staff, 2000)	Computerized measure of sustained attention, impulse control, reaction time, persistence, response variability, perseveration, visual discrimination
Gordon Diagnostic System (Gordon, 1991)	Similar to Conners Test (see above) for vigilance task; delay task includes problem solving, learning temporal relationships, impulse control, self-monitoring, ability to benefit from feedback
California Verbal Learning Test—Children's Version (Delis, Kramer, Kaplan, & Ober, 1994)	Verbal learning, long-term memory encoding and retrieval, susceptibility to interference
Comprehensive Trail-Making Test (CTMT; Reynolds, 2002)	Attention, concentration, resistance to distraction, cognitive flexibility/set shifting
Behavior Rating Inventory of Executive Function (BRIEF; Gioia, Isquith, Guy, & Kenworthy, 2000)	Parent and teacher rating scales of behavioral regulation, metacognition; includes clinical scales assessing inhibition, cognitive shift, emotional control, task initiation, working memory, planning, organization of materials, and self-monitoring; includes validity scales assessing inconsistent responding and negativity
Sensory–motor/nonverbal skills	
Developmental Test of Visual–Motor Integration (Beery, 1997)	Visual-perceptual skills, fine motor skills, visual–motor integration
Grooved Pegboard (Kløve, 1963)	Complex visual–motor–tactile integration, psychomotor speed (compare to simple sensory–motor integration)
Judgment of Line Orientation (Benton & Tranel, 1993)	See NEPSY Arrows (Table 4.7)
Language measures	
Oral and Written Language Scales (Carrow-Woolfolk, 1996)	Listening comprehension, oral expression, written expression; not limited to single-word responses, as the PPVT-III and EVT (see below) are
Comprehensive Assessment of Spoken Language (Carrow-Woolfolk, 1999)	Language processing in comprehension, expression, and retrieval in these categories: lexical/semantic, syntactic, supralinguistic, pragmatic; the supralinguistic and pragmatic categories show promise in the assessment of right-hemisphere language skills

(continued)

TABLE 4.10. *(continued)*

Subtest	Constructs purportedly tapped
Language measures *(continued)*	
Clinical Evaluation of Language Fundamentals—Fourth Edition (CELF-4; Semel, Wiig, & Secord, 2003)	Assesses receptive and expressive language with the core subtests, but also allows assessment of language structure, language content, and memory; includes standardized observations in the classroom and assessment of pragmatic language skills, in addition to individual assessment
Test of Language Development—TOLD-3, Primary and Intermediate; Newcomer & Hammill, 1997)	Primary version assesses phonology, semantics, and syntax; Intermediate version assesses semantics and syntax
Receptive auditory/verbal skills	
Wepman Auditory Discrimination Test—Second Edition (Wepman & Reynolds, 1987)	Auditory attention, phonemic awareness, phonemic segmentation, phoneme position (primary/medial/recent)
Peabody Picture Vocabulary Test—Third Edition (PPVT-III; Dunn & Dunn, 1997)	Receptive vocabulary (visual scanning/impulse control); conormed with EVT (see below)
Token Test for Children (DiSimoni, 1978)	See NEPSY Comprehension of Instructions (Table 4.7)
Expressive auditory/verbal skills	
Controlled Oral Word Association Test (Spreen & Benton, 1977)	See NEPSY Verbal Fluency (Table 4.7)
Boston Naming Test (Goodglass & Kaplan, 1987)	Expressive vocabulary, free-recall retrieval from long-term memory versus cued-recall retrieval (semantic/phonemic)
Expressive Vocabulary Test (EVT; Williams, 1997)	Expressive vocabulary (picture naming); conormed with PPVT-III (see above)

sultation is often described as something a school psychologist will do before a standardized assessment, or instead of a standardized assessment. However, data collection is important in consultation too, and the fact that you are doing standardized assessments doesn't mean you can't do problem-solving consultation. All we are suggesting is that these two functions of school psychologists can be combined to make both stronger. You can bring assessment data into the consultation data-gathering phase when this is appropriate, linking interventions to the child's strengths and needs. And instead of being the mysterious "WISC jockey" who borrows a child for a couple of hours and then produces a useless report, you can ensure that the assessment you do is linked to the teacher's concerns and the child's performance in the classroom. The CHT emphasis on *ecological validity* and *treatment validity* is what sets our model apart from other test interpretation models. Most referrals for consultation concern academic problems, and most of those academic problems are reading difficulties (Bramlett, Murphy, Johnson, Wallingsford, & Hall, 2002). Although general consultation on reading instruction may be helpful, combining this knowledge with information about the multiple determinants of the child's problem can have important effects on the intervention you and the teacher choose, and on the success the child experiences as a result of your efforts.

Consultation is intended to be collaboration between equals, but the fact that the consultant is there to help the consultee solve a problem has the potential to make the power relationship unequal. Consultants tend to make requests at a high rate, and consultees are generally likely to respond by agreeing with these requests (Erchul & Chewning, 1990). It seems that many consultees agree with consultants during meetings, but don't really feel ownership of the interventions developed during consultation, because many of these interventions are not fully implemented (Wickstrom, Jones, LaFleur, & Witt, 1998). We believe that the power issues within the consultative relationship must be acknowledged and dealt with directly. Both school psychologists and teachers feel that expertise and informational power are essential in making changes with teachers (Erchul, Raven, & Whichard, 2001). You are using your expertise and knowledge to help solve a problem, influence a teacher to make changes, and support and develop the teacher's skills (Erchul & Martens, 2002). You can be directive and informative, such as telling a teacher about intervention research, without being coercive (Gutkin, 1999).

Consultation begins with the premise that the consultant works with the consultee (usually the classroom teacher) to solve a client's (the teacher's student's) problem. Although the two professionals are presumed to be equals, working together to help the child, it is also assumed that both professionals have specific expertise to bring to bear on the problem. In our view, your knowledge of neuropsychological and cognitive functions, neuropsychological assessment, the academic and behavioral intervention literature, and intervention-monitoring methodology should be the core of expertise that you as the consultant bring to the relationship. The teacher's knowledge of the student's classroom performance, awareness of effective and ineffective teaching techniques for this child, and professional expertise as a teacher form the core of his or her expertise as the consultee. Fully acknowledging the expertise of the consultee is one part of building rapport, but this knowledge is also necessary if an appropriate problem solution is to be found. An intervention plan that takes into account what resources are available and what interventions the teacher is already trying in the natural environment should have greater applicability and effectiveness (Riley-Tillman & Chafouleas, 2002). The following problem-solving consultation model is a summary of models presented by Erchul and Martens (2002) and Kratochwill, Elliott, and Callan-Stoiber (2002), combined with our CHT model.

Stages of Problem-Solving Consultation

Problem Identification

During the initial interview, the consultant (you) and the consultee identify a target behavior for intervention. The behavior must be defined in an observable, measurable way. In addition, information is needed about how often and when the behavior occurs, and a data collection method should be devised. Baseline data should begin to be collected. Problem identification in CHT is somewhat more complex than in other problem-solving models, as it includes data collected from prereferral interventions, permanent products, observations, interview, and preliminary assessment results that you need to check out with the teacher to ensure that your findings have ecological validity. This stage covers the initial theory and hypothesis steps in the CHT model (refer back to Figure 4.1).

Problem Analysis

During the second interview, a more in-depth study of the target behavior is made, including a functional assessment. An excellent resource for conducting a functional assessment is a handbook written by O'Neill and colleagues (1997) that includes reproducible forms. This assessment should include a review of the baseline data that have already been collected, and an interview with the teacher to identify possible causes, establish events, and determine consequences of the behavior. Most functional assessments focus on obvious causes for the behavior, such as seeking attention or escaping from a task. The CHT process will provide information about the student's cognitive processing strengths and weaknesses to use in developing hypotheses, such as processing difficulties, memory problems, language deficits, or difficulty with unstructured situations. As part of the problem analysis, a review of interventions that have already been attempted and their effectiveness is also helpful. Although CHT includes functional analysis in this stage, it relies on much more information from numerous data sources. Hierarchical ordering of preferred target behaviors is undertaken at this stage, but the nature of CHT may require more than one intervention for a particular child (e.g., reading fluency intervention, speech–language therapy for expressive language, occupational therapy for graphomotor skills). This stage is covered in the initial data collection/analysis and data interpretation steps of CHT, which provide a more detailed theory as to why the child is having difficulty.

Plan Development/Implementation

After the problem analysis, the *theory* is used by the consultant and the consultee to develop an intervention plan together (i.e., an effective intervention hypothesis). This plan takes into account not only the student's characteristics and behavior, but also the classroom ecology and the teacher's style and preferences. Working together, they brainstorm all possible interventions, then choose the intervention that is likely to be effective and can be plausibly implemented. Goals will be set, participants will be determined, and data collection will be initiated and continued during implementation of the intervention.

Plan Evaluation/Recycling

After an agreed-upon period of time, the consultant and consultee meet to review the collected data and evaluate the intervention (i.e., data collection/analysis and data interpretation). There are numerous methods for evaluating interventions via within-subject experimental designs, several of which we will review later in the chapter. If the intervention is successful, either the intervention is extended, or it is discontinued if the target has been reached. If minor revisions appear necessary, the consultee makes them at this time, and they decide on an additional meeting to evaluate the revised intervention. If different or more intensive interventions appear necessary (i.e., a new theory or hypothesis), a new intervention can be attempted, or additional special education support services may be needed. This process is also important as the instructional supports begin to be removed and the child begins to function completely within his or her natural environment with natural consequences. The theory–hypothesis–data collection/analysis–data interpretation cycle continues until the problem appears to be under natural stimulus–consequence control. As you can see, the CHT model is not really about testing per se; it is about a way of practice that combines the best technologies of problem-solving consultation with comprehensive evaluations.

Practicing Behavioral Neuropsychology

Since we are suggesting that you combine neuropsychological assessment with behavioral methods, In-Depth 4.1 and Table 4.11 review the basics of behavioral interventions for those readers

IN-DEPTH 4.1. Review of Behavioral Psychology Principles

RESPONDENT CONDITIONING TECHNIQUES

Respondent conditioning is a method of eliciting behavior by manipulating a stimulus. An example of a conditioned stimulus is the teacher's turning on and off the light to cue a child's transition behavior. Behavioral examples might include anxiety about tests or speaking in class, or fear when the teacher raises his or her voice. Common interventions, including relaxation training and systematic desensitization, may be used to treat anxiety responses in students. However, more broadly conceived, variations in stimuli can lead to different behaviors (e.g., varying spacing or size of letters during reading, using simultaneous visual and auditory teacher instructions, using an adapted pencil for sensory problems for writing, tapping on a desk to cue on-task behavior, etc.). Modeling and discriminative stimuli designed to elicit operant behaviors, though not considered respondant techniques, can both be related to stimulus–response psychology.

OPERANT CONDITIONING TECHNIQUES

Operant conditioning is a method of affecting behavior by manipulating the consequences of that behavior. Behaviors that are followed by reinforcing consequences (either presentation of something positive or removal of something negative) will tend to recur. Behaviors that are followed by punishing consequences (either presentation of something negative or removal of something positive) will be less likely to recur, as indicated in Table 4.11. One of the best uses of operant technology is the "Premack principle," in which a less reinforcing behavior is reinforced by a more reinforcing one (e.g., providing computer time after a certain level of reading accuracy is obtained). Positive reinforcement can include natural consequences (these are preferable) or secondary ones (e.g., tokens, points). A good use of negative reinforcement is reducing the workload if a child demonstrates mastery on an assignment.

People are often confused about the difference between *positive reinforcement* (presenting something positive) and *negative reinforcement* (removing something negative). Why do children have tantrums? Not only because they are positively reinforced for having tantrums, but their parents are negatively reinforced as well—they get peace and quiet by giving in to the children. Most interventions in school should use *positive reinforcers*, and these can even be used to teach children *not* to do something, so (we hope) you don't have to use punishment. You identify an alternative behavior, preferably one that is incompatible with the negative behavior, and reinforce that behavior (i.e., differential reinforcement of other/alternative/incompatible behavior). For example, Taniqua is always running in the halls. Instead of punishing her for running, reinforce her for walking. In some cases, a child may not be able to do the target behavior. In these situations, reinforcing successive approximations of target behaviors, or "shaping," is what we have to do with academic and behavioral deficits.

Is there a place for punishment in the schools? If a child is always being punished at school, it becomes aversive, something to avoid; it may even eventually lead him or her to drop out. A particular teacher who, or a subject that, is punishing may also be seen as aversive. There is another problem with punishment, though: The child isn't actually learning a replacement behavior. We prefer to use school interventions to teach children how to do something, rather than just to suppress negative behavior. If you must use punishment, we recommend that you use negative punishment that involves taking away something positive (either *time out from reinforcement* or *response cost*) combined with differential reinforcement. For example, if Kyle is aggressive on the playground, you can use negative punishment by having him sit on the sidelines and miss 5 minutes of recess, but you must also use positive reinforcement when you see Kyle playing nicely.

As you will recall from training, the schedules of reinforcement influence how a skill will be learned and maintained. Continuous reinforcement is good for skill acquisition, but this acquired skill will also be extinguished quickly, so intermittent reinforcement on a variable-ratio or interval scale is more appropriate. Think about slot machines; infrequent payoffs can maintain betting behavior for a long time! The same thing can happen in a classroom. If a teacher slips and accidentally reinforces an unwanted behavior, that behavior will be maintained longer.

TABLE 4.11. Reinforcement and Punishment

	Provide	Remove
Positive consequence	Positive reinforcement	Negative punishment (response cost)
Negative consequence	Positive punishment	Negative reinforcement

Note. Shaded boxes *increase* the preceding behavior; unshaded boxes *decrease* the behavior.

who may not recall the details. As part of the problem-solving model, you need to recognize that antecedent and consequent actions affect the child's learning and behavior, and that cognitive processes interact with these determinants. Having this understanding allows you to use what cognitive psychologists have called *stimulus–organism–response* (S-O-R) psychology, in which stimulus and response are still important, but the organismic variables (i.e., child neuropsychological processes) help you determine what the best intervention is and how to carry it out. The behavior technologies become especially useful in designing the intervention, determining intervention efficacy, and managing contingencies.

Developing and Evaluating Interventions

After cycling through the first four steps of CHT, and refining a theory as to what will help the child, you and the consultee need to use behavioral strategies combined with specific instructional methods to help the child learn—through either remediation, accommodations, or both. In Chapters 5–7, we offer a number of interventions for academic skills problems. Some problems transcend academic domain boundaries, and the comorbidity among academic learning disorders is quite high. To help you understand the relationship between neuropsychological functioning and academic domains, we have provided a worksheet in Appendix 4.5. This worksheet may be useful in your examination of the academic issues associated with a child's neuropsychological functioning. This ensures that when you identify the cognitive pattern of performance, you are relating it to the academic pattern of performance seen on testing and the classroom, which should help guide intervention planning and implementation. Taking what you know about the child's current level and pattern of performance, academic interventions, problem-solving consultation, and behavioral technologies, you can design, implement, and evaluate an intervention for him or her. In CHT, we recommend using single-subject (within-subject or single-case) research designs to evaluate the effectiveness of interventions. We believe that practitioners should collect child performance data on a regular basis to ensure that interventions are effective (Fuchs & Fuchs, 1986; Lindsley, 1991; Skinner, 1966; Ysseldyke, 2001). We recommend that similar models be used to evaluate any intervention, whether it is behavioral, academic, cognitive, or socioemotional. In this section, we review the most useful designs for evaluating school-based interventions, illustrating each intervention model with hypothetical examples.

All of the research designs we discuss require two basic concepts. One is that you must have some way of *measuring the outcome* you want. Behaviorists generally call this "taking data," but you can think of it as "evaluating progress" or "checking up on the intervention." You can't simply say, "Yep, Jimmy's doing better"; you must have some way to *show* that the child is doing better. The outcome measure you choose depends on the target behavior and the goal of the intervention. You can use information that the teacher already collects (i.e., authentic data—homework completed, spelling test score, office referrals or detentions, absences, etc.). You can collect information as part of the intervention itself (e.g., math worksheets, curriculum-based measurement [CBM] probes of reading fluency, flashcards placed in correct and incorrect piles). You can also develop a data collection plan that interferes very little with the teacher's routine (e.g., child self-monitoring, using a wrist counter, completing end-of-the-period or end-of-the-day checklists). Finally, you can use systematic observation to observe the target behavior directly, using event, duration, latency, partial-interval, or whole-interval recording. With observational data collection, it is important to use a randomly selected peer at baseline to establish a discrepancy with the target child. Table 4.12 presents some suggestions for outcome measures that can be useful in the classroom.

The second basic concept is that you must have a *baseline* measurement, in addition to measuring the behavior during the intervention. Teachers are generally used to just measuring the outcome of teaching, such as giving a test at the end of a chapter. But to evaluate how effective an intervention is, you have to measure the child's performance at the start (without the interventions), and then keep measuring as you implement the intervention to see how the child's performance changes. Without having a baseline for comparisons, you won't know whether the child's improvement is really due to the intervention. In describing some of the intervention models below, we use the letter A to refer to the baseline condition. The other letters (i.e., B, C) represent whatever interventions you implement.

TABLE 4.12. Examples of Outcome Measures for School-Based Interventions

Outcome area	Possible measures
Several behaviors	Pre- and postratings on a brief behavior rating form. Daily report card with ratings for day. Systematic observation using event, duration, latency, partial-interval, or whole-interval recording.
Negative classroom behavior (e.g., calling out, getting out of seat, yelling, aggression)	Measurement of rate via tally marks, golf wrist counter, or pennies/paper clips transferred from pockets. Student self-monitoring of behavior on sheet or card.
Serious negative behavior	Count of office referrals or detentions.
Positive classroom behavior (e.g., raising hand, giving correct answers)	Measurement of rate or student self-monitoring as above. Observational data as above.
Attention, on-task behavior	Periodic classroom observations. Child self-monitoring of skills.
Academic work completion	Worksheets or other permanent products. Measurement of accuracy, rate, or both.
Homework completion	Completed homework. Daily report card signed by parent and/or teacher.
Academic skills accuracy	Correct–incorrect flashcards kept in separate piles by student or peer. Worksheets graded in percentages correct and recorded in grade book.
Academic skills fluency (speed and accuracy)	CBM probes (Shinn, 1989).
Academic skills comprehension	Pre- and posttest with alternate forms.

ABAB/ABAC Designs

The ABAB design is used when you have picked one intervention and you want to see if it works better than the baseline condition (i.e., better than what the teacher would normally do). It is also sometimes called a "reversal design," because you do the intervention, then reverse to baseline for a short while, then do the intervention again. It's a good way to show that the intervention is really what's affecting the child's performance, but it doesn't work well for a situation where your intervention actually teaches the child something new. For example, if you teach a child to break a word into syllables to sound it out, you can't "unteach" that for the reversal phase. It also is not appropriate to do a reversal phase if the behavior you are trying to reduce is harmful to the child or others. For instance, if you are using time out to reduce hitting, it would be unethical to do a reversal phase. As a result, this design is best for situations where you want to change the *rate* at which a child does something that he or she already knows how to do. For an example of an ABAB design, please see Case Study 4.1 and Figure 4.2.

The ABAC design allows you to compare two different interventions to see whether they are different from the baseline, and to see which is better at changing the child's behavior. Similar to the ABAB design, you first collect baseline data, then implement the first intervention (B), then reverse to baseline, and finally implement the second intervention (C). For instance, after taking baseline data on multistep math addition item accuracy (A), you can determine whether a child is more accurate if he or she draws lines between columns (B), or follows a step-by-step algorithm

CASE STUDY 4.1. Jared's Impulsive Calling Out

An 8-year-old boy diagnosed with ADHD, Jared, was described by his teacher as extremely impulsive. The behavior that she identified as most problematic was Jared's calling out in class. Systematic observation data suggested that the teacher typically accepted Jared's answer when he called out, but then she often reminded him to raise his hand the next time. After discussing the baseline data with the teacher, we decided that she would use a wrist counter to count whenever Jared called out during whole-group instruction.

Figure 4.2 presents the results for the ABAB intervention designed to reduce his inappropriate call-out behaviors. During the first week, the teacher collected the baseline data. She counted Jared's call-outs without doing anything different about them, and this information was charted. The next week, the teacher continued to count Jared's call-outs, but she ignored him immediately after each call-out, practicing negative punishment. She only acknowledged Jared if he raised his hand first and did not call out, which was differential reinforcement. Notice that at first, Jared's call-outs increased. This is called an *extinction burst*—a very common finding when a previously rewarded activity is being ignored. After that, Jared's call-outs began to decline. The teacher then returned to baseline for a short time (accepting call-out answers and reminding him to raise his hand), and the call-outs became frequent again. After a few days of this, the intervention was reintroduced. As you look at Figure 4.2, you should notice a few things. Each phase is separated by lines and labeled, so the baseline and intervention phases are clear. Within the baseline phase, Jared was calling out very frequently; the average was about 20 times per day. During the first intervention phase, his call-outs increased at first and then began to decline. As soon as the reversal to baseline took place, they increased again to about 20 times per day. During the second (and final) intervention phase, call-outs declined to an average of only 8 times per day. You can clearly see that the intervention was what was affecting Jared's behavior (this is called *establishing functional control*), because every time the intervention was implemented, he changed his behavior.

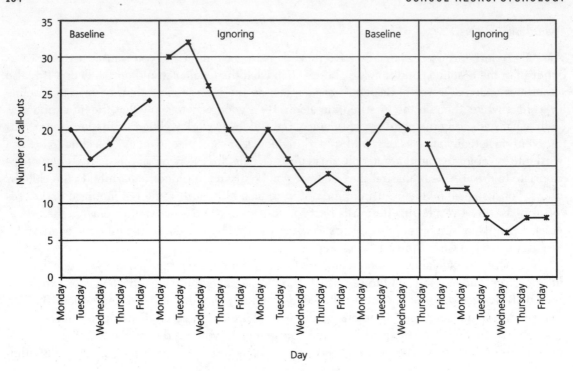

FIGURE 4.2. Jared's calling out.

sheet on how to complete the problems (C). Case Study 4.2 and Figure 4.3 provide an example of an ABAC design.

Multiple-Baseline Design

A multiple-baseline design is useful when you expect the child's learning to be cumulative, so you don't want to reverse success. This design can teach children to display target behaviors across settings, people, or behaviors. For instance, if staying on task is the target behavior, you first seek on-task behavior in one class, then another, and so forth. In this design, you collect baseline data in two or more subjects or at two or more times during the day. Then you start the intervention in one subject or at one time during the day, while continuing to take baseline data at the other time(s). Later, you introduce the intervention in the other subject or at the other time. If the child's performance changes in each setting only when the intervention is in place, you will know that the intervention is responsible for the change. An example of this design can be found in Case Study 4.3 and Figure 4.4.

Pre- and Posttest Design

A pre- and posttest design is useful when you can't collect data every day, but you want to measure the effectiveness of an intervention via direct observation, test, or rating scale. Although it is more difficult to establish functional control, it is an easier method of data collection and is more likely to be acceptable to teachers. For this design, it is important to choose a test (preferably one with alternate forms) or a rating scale that can be given repeatedly with minimal practice effects.

CASE STUDY 4.2. Increasing Marcie's Reading Speed

Marcie was a 9-year-old girl who was pleasant, cooperative, and hard-working. However, she was a slow, choppy reader, and her teacher sought support in helping Marcie to read more fluently. Marcie was in a small reading group with three other children, and the teacher worked individually with Marcie for 15 minutes every day, but she was still struggling. The teacher now had an aide in class and wanted to know what the aide could do with Marcie. Based on the CHT evaluation information, I found that Marcie had good phonemic awareness skills, and her phonemic segmentation and blending were not problems, but her word finding and rapid naming skills were quite poor. I met with the teacher, and we thought of two possible interventions for Marcie: one where the aide would use flashcards to improve Marcie's speed at identifying words, and one where the aide would read orally with Marcie to increase the fluency of her reading. We decided that CBM of reading fluency, using daily 1-minute probes, would be a good outcome measure. As can be seen in Figure 4.3, her fluency was quite low at baseline (A). During the first intervention phase (B), the aide pronounced each word for Marcie; Marcie repeated it; Marcie and the aide then practiced with the flashcards for about 10 minutes; and they finished with another 1-minute CBM probe. After this intervention, the teacher returned Marcie to the baseline condition (A), but the aide continued to take CBM probes during this time. Finally, the second intervention phase was introduced (C). This intervention involved the aide's reading the passage to Marcie one time with expression and fluency, and then their reading it together in tandem for about 10 minutes. Again, the sessions ended with another 1-minute CBM probe. As you can see from looking at Marcie's chart, the flashcard drill improved her fluency over baseline, but the tandem reading was much more effective. This is not to say that tandem reading is a better intervention for all children; it just appeared to be better for Marcie.

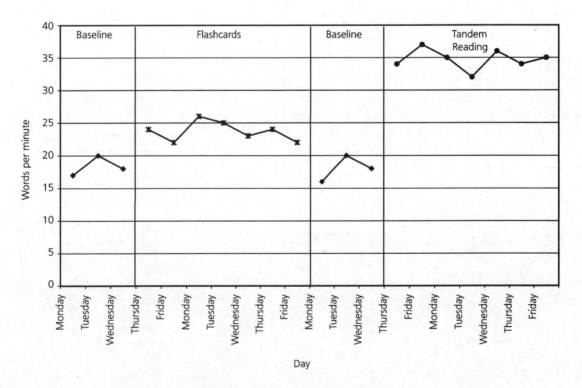

FIGURE 4.3. Marcie's reading fluency.

CASE STUDY 4.3. Ellen's Accuracy Problem

Ellen was a 7-year-old girl who presented as a fast, careless worker. She reportedly completed her seatwork as fast as possible, without worrying about the accuracy of her responses. I (Fiorello) met with Ellen's teacher, and we decided to try to increase Ellen's accuracy by using rewards for correct respond-ing. The teacher used Ellen's number correct on her seatwork papers to measure the outcome. She made sure that there were exactly 10 questions on each worksheet in math and spelling, and noted in her grade book the number correct for each day. For the first week, the teacher collected baseline data in both subjects for each day, and these data were charted on a multiple-baseline graph (see Figure 4.4). After collecting a week of baseline data, the teacher explained to Ellen that she could earn 1 point for each spelling word she copied correctly during seatwork, and the points could be traded for free time at the end of the morning classes. At the same time, Ellen's math work was kept in the baseline condition, with no rewards offered. As you can see from Ellen's chart, her spelling accuracy improved when re-wards were added, but her math remained inaccurate. The next Monday, the teacher explained that the point system would apply to math as well, and as you can see from the figure, Ellen's accuracy in math improved thereafter.

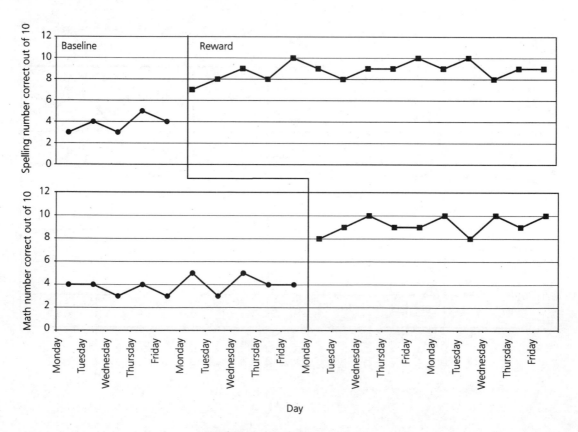

FIGURE 4.4. Ellen's accuracy.

The pretest results become your baseline, and then you test again after implementation of the intervention to judge its effectiveness. Observations and brief rating scales can be used repeatedly if you choose to gather multiple data points during the intervention. Case Study 4.4 and Figure 4.5 provide an example of how to use a pre- and posttest design.

CBM Progress Monitoring

CBM is useful for evaluating the effectiveness of instructional interventions on reading, mathematics, and writing. A brief probe is completed for several days during baseline, and then repeated every 1–2 days following the intervention session. These data are plotted to gauge progress over time. An *aimline* shows the goal that has been set for the student. The beginning of the line is determined by the child's baseline performance or behavior; the end of the line is determined by where the child should be, compared to his or her peers, and how long it will take for the child to "catch up" once the intervention is in place. Unfortunately, there are no explicit guidelines for "how long it should take." For instance, if the child is 2 years behind, saying that he or she will make it up in a month is unrealistic. Conversely, it is inappropriate to give a child too long to catch up. After you establish an aimline, a *trendline* is drawn, which shows the rate of improvement in the skill. If the trendline is below the aimline for several days, the intervention should be adjusted or changed, or possibly you have set too high a goal for the child. Case Study 4.5 and Figure 4.6 highlight the use of CBM progress monitoring.

Multiple-Intervention Design

Before we leave our section on behavioral neuropsychology and problem-solving consultation, it is important to recognize that not all intervention designs discussed will fit nicely with the needs of a child, teacher, or parent. Certainly you want experimental control and good outcome data, but beyond that, you have to be sensitive to the needs of all parties, or the intervention effort will not be effective. Interventions that are easy are preferred, but they may not be effective. Others may be labor-intensive and have good experimental control, but because they are so cumbersome, treatment adherence or integrity is limited. This is where you, as the consultant, must work with the consultee to take into account the nature of the problem, the environmental determinants of the problem, and the resources available to affect behavior change. Case Study 4.6 and Figure 4.7 provide an example of alternative treatments for a child who does not respond easily to interventions.

CASE STUDY 4.4. Herman's Auditory Processing

Herman was a boy with a common problem: a history of frequent ear infections (otitis media) and poor auditory processing. He was having difficulty learning the letter sounds in his kindergarten class. His teacher referred him to the reading specialist, who arranged for Herman to complete a 6-week computer-based auditory processing and phonics program. Before Herman began the program, I (Fiorello) was called in to develop a method for monitoring the efficacy of the program. We agreed that I would administer the CTOPP and CBM of the alphabet sounds and would chart his scores, as depicted in Figure 4.5. After 6 weeks, I administered both tests again. Since the CTOPP has age-based SSs, you can see that Herman's auditory processing improved over the course of the program. In addition, charting his improvement in letter sound knowledge helped the teacher compare Herman to other children, to guide her expectations for his curricular progress.

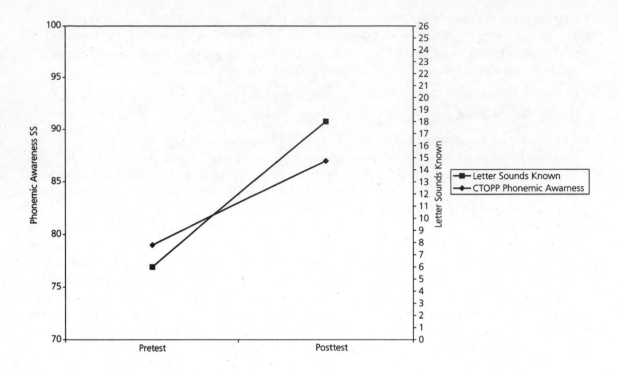

FIGURE 4.5. Herman's auditory processing and letter sound knowledge.

CASE STUDY 4.5. Beverly's Limited Expressive Language

When I (Fiorello) was called in to consult with Beverly's teacher, Beverly was having considerable difficulty with expressive language, primarily because she spoke very little during conversations with her teacher and peers. CHT results revealed difficulty with word retrieval, oral fluency, and expressive syntax. Data collection with an audiotape recorder began, and Beverly's oral fluency at baseline was found to be only 23 words per minute on average (see Figure 4.6). Her teacher set a goal of 45 words per minute, and we decided that a peer tutoring program would be implemented. The teacher picked a child who was not only friendly with Beverly, but also talkative, social, caring, and supportive. Each time the two children would get together, they would discuss a topic of interest. To facilitate this process, the teacher brainstormed possible topics with them before the intervention. As you can see, the peer tutoring improved Beverly's oral fluency at first, but on Days 10, 11, and 12, Beverly's fluency scores fell below the aimline. When three data points fall below the aimline, a decision point is reached. This means that it is time either to adjust or change the intervention, or to readjust the aimline. In Beverly's case, this ensured that goals would be set at a level where they could realistically be attained, while still ensuring that Beverly was making appropriate progress. It was decided that Beverly's goal might have been a little ambitious; however, she was making progress in the program and was developing a good relationship with the peer.

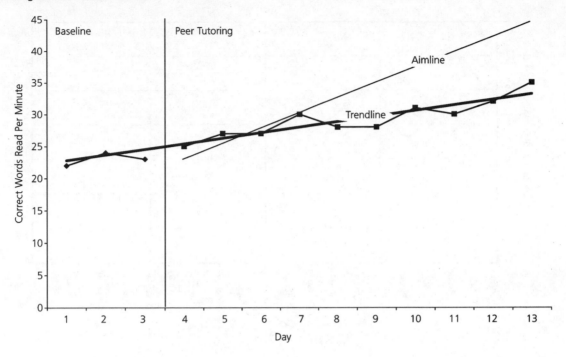

FIGURE 4.6. Beverly's CBM chart.

CASE STUDY 4.6. Coping with Gary's OCD

Gary was a student diagnosed with OCD. His classroom teacher's main concern was Gary's incessant questioning about assignments during seatwork. Gary typically asked for clarification of the directions, and the meaning of individual items. The teacher wanted to decrease Gary's questioning and increase his on-task behavior. She agreed to count Gary's questions with a wrist counter during the seatwork period in her class. As can be seen in Figure 4.7, Gary's baseline average was a little over 10 questions per period. We decided to try a number of interventions, starting with the easiest to implement and gradually adding more intrusive ones. This called for a variation on the ABAC design, where the interventions were cumulative (it might be called an A-B-BC-BCD design). First, the teacher developed a checklist for completing seatwork, and she taught Gary to use it to answer his own questions. She then laminated it and let him check off each item for himself. During this intervention, Gary's questions decreased slightly, to an average of about eight per period. The next intervention added was a set of five tokens that Gary had to use to ask questions. He would turn in one token every time he asked a question; any question after that would not be answered. Gary's questions decreased again, eventually settling at five per period. At this point, the teacher added one more intervention: She provided Gary a reward—a choice of activity during the last 5 minutes of class—if he had one token left at the end of the period. This lowered Gary's questions to four immediately. If the teacher had felt that even fewer questions would be allowed (based on what was normally acceptable in class, perhaps one or two), she could have gradually increased the number of tokens necessary for a reward.

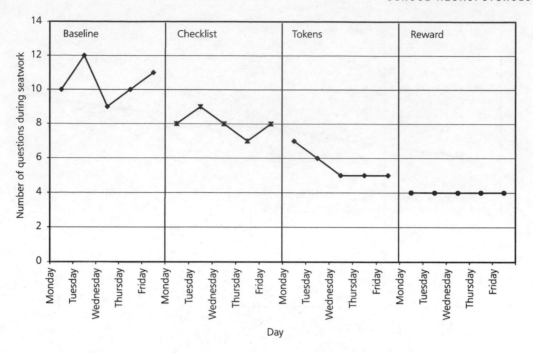

FIGURE 4.7. Gary's teacher questions.

LINKING ASSESSMENT TO INTERVENTION: A CASE STUDY

Considerations and Caveats

Now that we have given you a good understanding of assessment practices and measures, brain–behavior relationships, and consultation and intervention technologies, the next step is to bridge the gap between these apparently disparate areas of psychology. We provide you with one more case study, and detailed information in Chapters 5–8, in an attempt to make assessment information meaningful for individualized interventions for children with unique assets and deficits. As noted previously in this book, this is a tall order; it is a path that some have chosen, but few have found success in their quest. You may be disappointed to find that we don't offer you diagnostic–prescriptive advice in the following chapters. We feel that this is where the early researchers on aptitude–treatment interactions went astray: Not all children learn the same way, even if they show similar neuropsychological profiles, so we don't oversimplify things by saying, "If you have this disorder, then do this intervention."

To paraphrase an old adage, some interventions work for some children some of the time, but no interventions work for all children all of the time. You may feel confident that you have a good understanding of a child's neuropsychological strengths and weaknesses, but if you don't have ecological and treatment validity, then your results are of questionable value. Even if you have a good handle on the problem and the findings have ecological validity, the intervention you and the teacher choose may be ineffective. Don't dismiss the original findings; rather, try to understand why the intervention you thought would be effective was not, and try to modify it or try another intervention. This recycling of interventions is necessary, whether you use a CHT approach or a regular behavioral consultation method. We provide you with assessment and intervention information about various learning and behavior disorder subtypes, but it is up to you to use CHT with the technologies presented in this chapter to individualize interventions for the children you serve.

Cognitive Hypothesis Testing for Scott's Motor Problem

Case Study 4.7 and Figure 4.8 present the completed CHT worksheet (see Appendix 4.3) for Scott, a student referred for "motor problems" in the classroom. We have purposely picked Scott's case because it highlights the use of CHT without the use of "neuropsychological" tests. We do this so that you can become familiar with the CHT procedure while using tests you already know. This also demonstrates that CHT and neuropsychological analysis of the data can occur with typical cognitive/intellectual measures. In Chapters 5–8, we will provide you with several reading, mathematics, written language, and emotional/behavior disorder case study examples that use CHT and the neuropsychological tests described earlier in the chapter.

As you can see from Scott's case, the original "theory" about motor problems was not quite right, as the deficit appeared to be related to visual–spatial dorsal stream functions, or poor perceptual feedback to the motor system. The process would have continued with this case had all results come back negative. For instance, we may have wanted to check out left parietal somatosensory functions, but Scott didn't show differences in writing pressure. He could have also had difficulty with integration of information across the midline or bimanual functions, suggesting problems with the corpus callosum. We could have done additional neuropsychological tests to look at these, but found enough testing and ecological validity evidence to support our hypothesis.

Although Case Study 4.7 and Figure 4.9 suggest that Scott's intervention was effective, it should be noted that Scott was receiving occupational therapy during this time, so the positive results could have been related to this intervention. Obviously, as time went on, both interventions may have had a positive and complementary effect. This is not a good empirical practice per se, as we don't want two interventions going on at the same time. However, our experience suggests that the experimental rigor required of articles published in, say, the *Journal of Applied Behavior Analysis* may not always be feasible in the field. The bottom line is that we need to help children, and if they get better and we have data that show it, we are better off as a result. Now that we have the methods to link assessment to intervention, the remainder of this book will focus on the neuropsychological aspects of specific academic and behavior problems experienced by the children we serve.

CASE STUDY 4.7. CHT for Scott's Motor Problem

Scott, aged 9-9, had attention, social, and handwriting problems. The teacher referred him for "fine motor problems," because his work was always messy, and there were many erase marks and smudges on the work he turned in. His poor alignment of columns resulted in many math calculation errors on multistep problems. After prereferral strategies were unsuccessful at improving the quality of this work, he was referred for a comprehensive CHT evaluation. As can be seen in Figure 4.8, the initial assessment with the WISC-IV suggested strengths in auditory working memory, and three possible weaknesses: spatial visualization, visual–motor coordination, and/or visual memory. Having developed a theory as to what was difficult for Scott, I (Fiorello) needed to test my hypotheses one by one to see which ones were correct.

To examine these possible problems, I wanted to use untimed visual processing tasks that did not require motor output. I picked the WJ-III Spatial Relations and Picture Recognition subtests to look at spatial visualization and visual memory. Then I decided to choose a task measuring motor coordination and speed without significant visual processing to look at motor functioning. For this, I picked the motor portion of the Beery Developmental Test of Visual–Motor Integration (VMI). Based on the overall profile and results of these hypothesis testing subtests, only the Spatial Relations subtest was impaired; this suggested that Scott's difficulty was more of a dorsal stream problem than a ventral stream or frontal motor problem.

However, these findings would be considered tentative until I checked to make sure that the results had ecological validity. The information from the teacher interview and ratings, classroom behavior observations, and work samples provided the necessary confirmation that Scott had difficulty with spatial processing and perceptual feedback to the motor system. At this stage, it is important to remember to check for possible alternative explanations to the hypothesis, in order to avoid confirmation bias. For Scott, you will notice that work samples showed problems with spatial organization on the page and poor column alignment in math. In addition, the teacher interview indicated that Scott had problems during recess and gym with respecting peers' personal space. As a result, these apparently disparate findings were entered in the ecological validity section.

At this point, I felt I had a fairly clear understanding of Scott's strengths and weaknesses. My understanding of neuropsychology helped to clarify why Scott was having attention and social problems as well, since right parietal lobe dysfunction can lead to neglect of self and environment. I now had a "theory" as to why Scott was having problems with learning and social functioning, and I could now meet with the teacher to discuss interventions, developing hypotheses about what interventions might work, implementing the most probable one, and determining whether it was successful.

To begin this process, I completed the assessment of academic skill problems and cognitive weaknesses. Next, I examined resources available and cognitive strengths for possible use in the intervention. For Scott, the team referred him for occupational therapy, and I made classroom recommendations to improve his current academic functioning. I met with the teacher, and we decided to focus on his messy work/handwriting problem. The teacher liked the idea of using graph paper, and we decided that Scott would be rewarded for staying within the lines on his writing assignments first, and on his math assignments second. After completing his assignments, Scott completed a checklist that indicated how many times his writing went outside the prescribed lines. For each word or problem Scott stayed within the lines on, he received a token reinforcer that could be traded in at the end of the day for a computer time reward. This setup called for a multiple-baseline design as described earlier. In Figure 4.9, notice how Scott showed some improvement in writing, but math difficulties were still prominent. After the intervention was implemented during math class, Scott began to improve in both areas.

Student's name: _Scott_____ Age: _9-9__ Grade: _4_____
Reason for referral: _Messy written work, poor handwriting_____

Preliminary hypotheses—Based on presenting problem and initial assessment, the following cognitive strengths and weaknesses are hypothesized:

Strengths:

Auditory working memory

Possible weaknesses:

Spatial visualization
Motor coordination
Visual memory

Hypothesis testing—Follow up with related construct tests:

Areas of suspected weakness:

Spatial visualization
Motor coordination
Visual memory

Follow-up tests:

WJ-III Spatial Relations
Beery VMI inc. motor section
WJ-III Picture Recognition

Strengths/weaknesses:

Spatial relations on WJ-III well below average—Weak spatial visualization
Motor coordination on VMI average—No motor weakness
Picture recognition on WJ-III average—No visual memory weakness

Associated with academic and/or behavior problems?:

Yes—Spatial visualization weakness can lead to poor handwriting (spacing and letter formation) and messy work layout on page.

(continued)

FIGURE 4.8. Completed Cognitive Hypothesis-Testing Worksheet (see Appendix 4.3) for Scott.

Ecological validity—Information from observations and teacher ratings:

Strengths:

Participating in class discussion

Possible weaknesses:

Spatial organization—layout on page, trouble aligning columns in math, difficulty with peers in recess and gym re: "space"

Evaluation summary—Based on analysis of all evaluation information, the following cognitive strengths and weaknesses are identified, and concordance or discordance is calculated if necessary:

Cognitive strengths:

Oral language
Auditory memory

Concordant with academic and/or behavioral strengths?:

Yes—class discussion relies on oral language and auditory skills.

Weaknesses:

Spatial visualization and organization in space

Concordant with academic and/or behavioral weaknesses?:

Yes—spatial visualization is related to work layout, handwriting, and interpersonal space issues.

Discordant with cognitive strengths?:

Yes—spatial visualization is mediated by right occipital lobe, while oral language and auditory memory is primarily mediated by left hemisphere.

(continued)

FIGURE 4.8. *(continued)*

Summary of evaluation information for intervention development	
Academic/behavioral presenting problems: Messy work Poor handwriting	**Cognitive weaknesses:** Spatial organization and processes
Resources for intervention in environment: Consultant available Special education and OT consult and materials	**Cognitive strengths:** Oral language Auditory memory
Potential interventions: Use paper with raised lines and graph paper for written work. Allow dictation for lengthy written assignments. Teach keyboarding skills. Work with psychologist on interpersonal space issues.	

FIGURE 4.8. (continued)

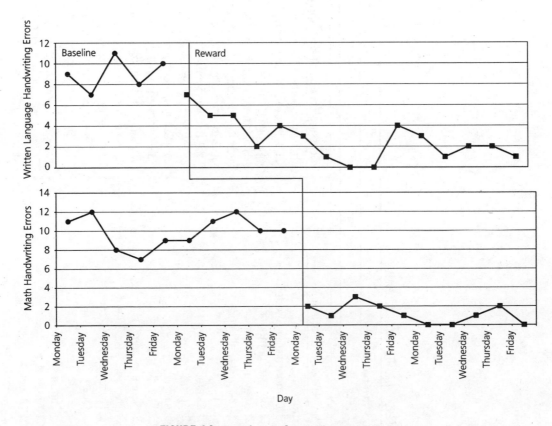

FIGURE 4.9. Scott's graph paper intervention.

165

APPENDIX 4.1. Demands Analysis

Student's name: _____ Age: _____ Grade: _____

Test/subtest: _____

Input (check all that apply)	Processing (check all that apply)	Output (check all that apply)
Instructions ☐ Demonstration/modeling ☐ Gesture/pantomime ☐ Brief oral directions ☐ Lengthy oral directions Timing ☐ Overall time limit ☐ Speed bonus Teaching ☐ Sample item ☐ Teaching item(s) ☐ Dynamic assessment ☐ Feedback when correct ☐ Querying Visual stimulus ☐ Pictures/photos ☐ Abstract figures ☐ Models ☐ Symbols (letters, numbers)	Left hemisphere ☐ Concordant/convergent ("explicit") Right hemisphere ☐ Discordant/divergent ("implicit") Executive functions (frontal–subcortical circuits) ☐ Sustained attention/concentration ☐ Inhibition/impulsivity ☐ Working memory (specify _____) ☐ Flexibility/modify/shift set ☐ Performance monitoring/benefit from feedback ☐ Planning/organization/strategy use ☐ Memory encoding/retrieval ☐ Novel problem solving/reasoning ☐ Temporal relationships/sequential processing ☐ Expressive language (L R) Neuropsychological functional domains ☐ Sensory attention (T O P) (L R) ☐ Primary zones (T O P) (L R) ☐ Secondary/tertiary zones (T O P) (L R)	Oral ☐ Brief oral ☐ Lengthy oral ☐ Report of strategy use Motor ☐ Fine motor–point ☐ Fine motor–graphomotor ☐ Fine motor–manipulatives (e.g., blocks, pictures) ☐ Visual–sensory–motor integration ☐ Gross motor Written language ☐ Brief written response ☐ Lengthy written response Response format ☐ Open/free-response ☐ Constrained/multiple choice

□ Written language
□ Large–small
□ Color important
Auditory stimulus
□ Brief verbal
□ Lengthy verbal
□ Spoken
□ Tape/CD (headphones used? Y N)
□ Background noise
Content
L M H Cultural knowledge
L M H English-language knowledge
L M H Emotional content

□ Prior learning/long-term memory
□ Sensory–motor coordination
□ Multimodal integration
□ Dorsal stream (occipital–parietal)
□ Ventral stream (occipital–temporal)
□ Receptive language (L R)
CHC abilities and narrow abilities
Higher-level processing
□ Gf–fluid reasoning _____
□ Glr–long-term storage and retrieval _____
□ Gv–visual processing _____
□ Ga–auditory processing _____
Lower-level processing
□ Gs–processing speed _____
□ Gsm–short-term memory _____
Acquired knowledge and achievement
□ Gc–crystallized intelligence _____
□ Grw–reading/writing _____
□ Gq–quantitative ability _____

Other
Input: _____
_____
_____
Processing: _____
_____
_____
Output: _____
_____
_____
Comments: _____
_____
_____

In the "Input" column: Y N, yes or no; L M H, low, medium, or high. In the "Processing" column: L R, left or right; T O P, temporal, occipital, or parietal; CHC, Cattell–Horn–Carroll.

APPENDIX 4.2. Brief Demands Analysis

Student's name: _____   Age: _____   Grade: _____

	Test/subtest	Input	Processing	Output
Strengths				
Weaknesses				

APPENDIX 4.3. Cognitive Hypothesis-Testing Worksheet

Student's name: _____ Age: _____ Grade: _____

Reason for referral: _____

_____

_____

Preliminary hypotheses—Based on presenting problem and initial assessment, the following cognitive strengths and weaknesses are hypothesized:

Strengths:

Possible weaknesses:

Hypothesis testing—Follow up with related construct tests:

Areas of suspected weakness:

Follow-up tests:

Strengths/weaknesses:

Associated with academic and/or behavior problems?:

(continued)

Ecological validity—Information from observations and teacher ratings:

Strengths:

Possible weaknesses:

Evaluation summary—Based on analysis of all evaluation information, the following cognitive strengths and weaknesses are identified, and concordance or discordance is calculated if necessary:

Cognitive strengths:

Concordant with academic and/or behavioral strengths?:

Weaknesses:

Concordant with academic and/or behavioral weaknesses?:

Discordant with cognitive strengths?:

(continued)

Summary of evaluation information for intervention development	
Academic/behavioral presenting problems:	**Cognitive weaknesses:**
Resources for intervention in environment:	**Cognitive strengths:**
Potential interventions:	

APPENDIX 4.4. Neuropsychological Assessment Observations Checklist

Student's Name: _____ Age: _____ Grade: _____

1. Pays close attention to task.	1 2 3 4 5	Has difficulty with selective or sustained attention.
2. Attention is consistent despite distraction.	1 2 3 4 5	Is easily distracted by external stimuli.
3. Shows good impulse control.	1 2 3 4 5	Is overly impulsive.
4. Shows appropriate activity level.	1 2 3 4 5	Has inappropriate activity level (specify: low or high).
5. Affect/mood is appropriate.	1 2 3 4 5	Affect is not appropriate (specify:).
6. Works quickly when appropriate.	1 2 3 4 5	Pace is too slow.
7. Can hold information in working memory to respond to questions.	1 2 3 4 5	Has difficulty retaining information in working memory to answer questions.
8. Can switch easily from one task to another.	1 2 3 4 5	Has difficulty switching tasks.
9. Plans/organizes before responding.	1 2 3 4 5	Responds without planning or organization.
10. Evaluates performance/modifies behavior.	1 2 3 4 5	Does not evaluate performance or modify behavior.
11. Comprehends orally presented information.	1 2 3 4 5	Does not comprehend orally presented information.
12. Follows directions or answers questions without repetition.	1 2 3 4 5	Requires frequent repetition of directions and questions.
13. Has adequate syntax and grammar.	1 2 3 4 5	Has difficulty with syntax and grammar.
14. Completes directions with one or more steps.	1 2 3 4 5	Has difficulty with sequential processing of directions.
15. Expresses self fluently.	1 2 3 4 5	Has difficulty expressing self fluently.
16. Does not exhibit word-finding difficulty.	1 2 3 4 5	Has word-finding difficulty.
17. Verbalizations are logical and organized.	1 2 3 4 5	Verbalizations are rambling and tangential.
18. No difficulty with nonliteral, metaphoric, or figurative language.	1 2 3 4 5	Language is overly literal and concrete.
19. Articulation is clear.	**1 2 3 4 5**	**Has poor articulation or phonemic paraphasias.**
20. Can easily recall information from long-term memory.	1 2 3 4 5	Has difficulty recalling information from long-term memory.

(continued)

21. Learns new material without repetition.	1 2 3 4 5	Needs many repetitions to learn new material.
22. Can learn new associations with few errors.	1 2 3 4 5	Makes frequent errors when learning new associations.
23. Can perceive and differentiate colors.	1 2 3 4 5	Appears to be partially or completely color-blind.
24. Easily discriminates/perceives visual stimuli.	1 2 3 4 5	Has poor visual acuity or visual perception.
25. Perceives visual stimuli throughout visual fields.	1 2 3 4 5	Has visual neglect. (Side? _)
26. Easily understands body language.	1 2 3 4 5	Has difficulty understanding body language.
27. Perceives spatial/holistic/global relationships.	1 2 3 4 5	Does not readily identify spatial/holistic/global relationships.
28. Shows no spatial configuration breaks.	1 2 3 4 5	Shows configuration breaks.
29. Shows no directional confusion.	1 2 3 4 5	Has directional confusion/orientation problems/reversals.
30. Perceives objects and faces.	1 2 3 4 5	Has difficulty perceiving objects and faces.
31. Can easily perceive auditory stimuli.	**1 2 3 4 5**	**Has difficulty perceiving auditory stimuli in the R _ and/or L _ ear.**
32. Hears and uses prosody effectively.	1 2 3 4 5	Has difficulty with receptive or expressive prosody.
33. Perceives tactile stimuli well.	1 2 3 4 5	Has difficulty discriminating tactile stimuli.
34. Handles materials smoothly.	1 2 3 4 5	Is clumsy when handling materials.
35. Has good pencil control/graphomotor skills.	1 2 3 4 5	Has poor pencil control/graphomotor skills.
36. Has established handedness (side? _).	1 2 3 4 5	Has not established handedness.
37. Has good bimanual control.	1 2 3 4 5	Has difficulty with bimanual control or crossing the midline.
38. Has good gross motor skill.	1 2 3 4 5	Has poor gross motor skill (clumsy or awkward).
39. Has good balance.	1 2 3 4 5	Has poor balance.
40. Has good muscle tone.	1 2 3 4 5	Has tone problems (too floppy, too rigid).

APPENDIX 4.5. Psychological Processes Worksheet

Client's name: _____ Date of birth: _____

Clinician's name: _____ Date: _____

Identify the psychological processes associated with the student's identified learning deficits with a (–) sign, and the strengths with a (+) sign. Remember that more than one psychological process should be involved for identified deficits.

Attention and Executive Frontal Lobe Processes

	Basic reading	Reading comp.	Basic math	Math reasoning	Spelling	Written lang.	Oral exp.	Listening comp.
Sustained attention								
Selective attention								
Overall tone								
Planning								
Strategizing								
Sequencing								
Organization								
Monitoring								
Evaluation								
Inhibition								
Shifting/flexibility								
Maintenance								
Change								
Motor overactivity								
Motor underactivity								
Constructional apraxia								
Ideomotor apraxia								
Ideational apraxia								
Visual scanning								
Sensory–motor integration								
Expressive language								
Long-term memory retrieval								
Working memory								
Perseveration								
Grammar								
Syntax								
Math algorithm								
Problem solving								
Fluency/nonfluent aphasia								
Dysnomia								

(continued)

Attention and Executive Frontal Lobe Processes *(continued)*

	Basic reading	Reading comp.	Basic math	Math reasoning	Spelling	Written lang.	Oral exp.	Listening comp.
Paraphasia								
Circumlocution								
Confabulation								
Concept formation								

Comments: _____

Concordant/Convergent Left-Hemisphere Processes

	Basic reading	Reading comp.	Basic math	Math reasoning	Spelling	Written lang.	Oral exp.	Listening comp.
Sensory memory								
Discrimination								
Perception (meaningful)								
Phonemic awareness								
Phonemic segmentation								
Phonemic blending								
Sound–symbol association								
Morpheme comprehension								
Lexicon/word comp.								
Sentence comprehension								
Literal/concrete/explicit comp.								
Math fact automaticity								
Long-term memory								
Declarative memory								
Automaticity								
Simple/rote sensory–motor integration								
Detail perception								
Sight word recognition								
Local/part/fine processing								
Dysphonetic								
Convergent thought								
Concordant thought								
Fluent aphasia								
Paraphasia								
Neologism								
Left–right confusion								

Comments: _____

(continued)

Discordant/Divergent Right-Hemisphere Processes

	Basic reading	Reading comp.	Basic math	Math reasoning	Spelling	Written lang.	Oral exp.	Listening comp.
Sensory memory								
Discrimination								
Perception (abstract)								
Spatial processing								
Perceptual analysis								
Visualization								
Ambiguity								
Asomatognosia								
Prosopagnosia								
Agnosia								
Neglect								
Object visual perception								
Spatial visual perception								
Grapheme awareness								
Sensory integration								
Complex sensory–motor integration								
Constructional apraxia								
Prediction								
Inference								
Metaphor/idiom/humor								
Nonliteral/figurative/implicit comp.								
Social perception/judgment								
Prosody								
Word Choice								
Holistic/global/gestalt processing								
Whole/coarse processing								
Novelty/new learning/encoding								
Pragmatics								
Facial/body gestures								
Problem solving								
Dyseidetic								
Divergent thought								
Discordant thought								
Fluent aphasia								
Paraphasia								
Neologism								

Comments: _____

CHAPTER 5

|ㅣㅣㅣㅣㅣㅣㅣㅣㅣㅣㅣㅣㅣ|

The Neuropsychology of Reading Disorders

HISTORICAL PERSPECTIVE ON LEARNING DISABILITIES

Searching for Children with Learning Disabilities

Before we discuss specific types of learning disorders (LDs), we begin this chapter with a historical overview of the field of learning disability research and practice. We distinguish between "LDs," a *clinical* label, and "learning disabilities," a *legal* label. As we review the history of learning disabilities, keep this distinction in mind; it may be related to controversy regarding learning disability identification and intervention practices. Nearly half of the children served by the Individuals with Disabilities Education Act (IDEA) are children with learning disabilities (National Center for Education Statistics, 1999), but we are still debating what learning disabilities are, how we assess them, and how best to determine eligibility for learning disability services (Kaufman & Kaufman, 2001). Although most educators and researchers now recognize that children with learning disabilities are a heterogeneous population, few have attempted to examine this diversity until recently. There is still no clear agreement on the etiology of learning disabilities. Various researchers and practitioners advocate conceptualizing learning disabilities as developmental delays, developmental deficits, or environmental problems. Researchers are certainly concerned about the diagnostic validity of learning disabilities, but there is even more concern about learning disability identification in the schools (e.g., Lyon et al., 2001; MacMillan, Gresham, & Bocian, 1998; B. A. Shaywitz, Fletcher, Holahan, & Shaywitz, 1992). In addition, most researchers and clinicians still operate under the assumption that there are verbal and nonverbal subtypes of learning disabilities—a conceptualization first described over three decades ago (Johnson & Myklebust, 1967), which confounds diagnostic accuracy and intervention efficacy.

With no clear consensus on the cause of learning disabilities, could psychologists have obscured important differences among these different types of learning problems? Should children with developmental *deficits* be the only ones classified with learning disabilities? Isn't it better to think of learning disabilities as developmental *delays*? The short answer is that for children with "true" learning disabilities, longitudinal research confirms that the *delay* model is inadequate for explaining the nature of their specific *deficits* (Francis, Shaywitz, Stuebing, Shaywitz, & Fletcher, 1994).

However, the question remains: How do you discriminate between children with learning deficits and learning delays? And if a deficit model represents children with learning disabilities, how do you identify the deficits, and are they amenable to different interventions? These are important questions, and we will return to them when we present the latest research findings on the neuropsychological characteristics of children with LDs; first, however, we want to provide you with a historical perspective on learning disabilities. This historical perspective can shed light into the limitations associated with previous research and service delivery, which can then provide you with an incentive to dispel preconceived notions about LDs/learning disabilities, and to develop innovative assessment and intervention strategies—the focus of the remainder of this book.

Beginning in the late 1800s, following the seminal aphasia findings of Broca and Wernicke, there was a renewed interest in brain-based problems, and in different treatments for individuals with learning problems. In the early 20th century, children who were apparently "normal," but otherwise had difficulty learning to read, were thought to have a condition termed "congenital word-blindness" (see Wong, 1996). Because their symptoms were similar to those of adults with known cerebral infarcts or other brain injuries (acquired alexia), they were assumed to have a congenital brain defect that impaired their visual processing of letters, necessitating a phonetic approach to reading instruction. Orton's (1937) idea that cerebral dominance was not fully established in these children—causing *strephosymbolia*, or reversals of letters and words—also received much attention. Based on Goldstein's work with soldiers who had sustained brain damage, Werner and Strauss (1940) identified perceptual and attention difficulties associated with brain injuries, providing individualized interventions for children with such injuries outside the regular classroom environment. These and similar efforts led to the then-popular term *minimal brain dysfunction* (MBD), which assumed a neurological basis for learning problems (Clements, 1966).

Thinking that medical-type labels such as MBD had little to do with educational intervention, Samuel Kirk provided us with the term *learning disabilities* in the 1960s (Kirk & Bateman, 1962). He advocated for special education services, and focused on the cognitive processing components of learning disabilities, moving the field away from the focus on a neurological basis. Kirk began research that focused on language difficulties rather than perceptual processing difficulties as the cause of learning disabilities, and was one of the developers of the Illinois Test of Psycholinguistic Abilities (ITPA; Kirk, McCarthy, & Kirk, 1968). Although the ITPA was a good idea from a historical perspective, it was not a psychometrically sound measure, and attempts to link ITPA results to intervention were not fruitful (Ysseldyke & Sabatino, 1973). As noted in Chapter 1, early efforts to establish aptitude–treatment interactions (ATIs) probably failed for a number of reasons, including poor measurement of constructs, definition of groups, and attempts to maintain treatment integrity. However, these early studies are often considered pivotal in moving both researchers' and practitioners' emphasis away from linking etiology to intervention, and instead focusing on remediation of educational deficits. Whereas Kirk is often referred to as the "father of learning disabilities," Ysseldyke, who failed in his early attempts to establish ATIs, could be considered to be the father of the "paradigm shift" position—one that calls for eliminating the use of intelligence testing in the identification of children with learning disabilities.

Defining Learning Disabilities

Learning disabilities were included in the predecessor of IDEA, the landmark Public Law 94-142, which was passed by the U.S. Congress in 1975. There are many different definitions of learning disabilities, presented by individual researchers or organizations serving people with such disabilities. The basic definitions have historically included a stipulation that a learning disability is a *processing disorder* that causes academic deficits, and that it is not due to another disability or disadvantage (the *exclusionary* criterion). Although a *severe discrepancy* between intellectual ability and achievement has been included in most definitions, many have argued for the elimination of this criterion (e.g., Berninger & Abbott, 1994). The numerous limitations of the severe-discrepancy model are well known (e.g., Aaron, 1997), with opponents of the model often citing evidence suggesting that "garden-variety poor readers" and children with reading disabilities are remarkably similar (B. A. Shaywitz et al., 1992; Siegel, 1992).

Although these findings have been used to suggest that all children learn the same way, we know that there are many learning disability subtypes with and without comorbid conditions (Wong, 1996), whereas a vast majority of the group studies have treated learning disabilities as homogeneous. Another problem with inclusion criteria in these studies is that some children may have another type of disability or may not even have a disability at all, but are classified as having a learning disability (MacMillan et al., 1998). In addition, children thought to be "garden-variety poor readers" may actually have undetected learning disabilities, possibly because of referral bias or differential identification practices resulting from the measures used (Sofie & Riccio, 2002). These issues suggest that we need to do a better job at identifying the neuroanatomical, neurophysiological, and functional relationships among learning disability subtypes, which could lead to more effective interventions for these children (Spreen, 2001). Nonetheless, individuals have fervently called for elimination of the discrepancy formula and intellectual assessment (e.g., Pasternack, 2002). One product of this position is the currently popular "resistance to intervention" model for identifying children with learning disabilities. Basically, the idea is that children who are failing are given help, and if they still fail, they are then considered eligible for special education. However, this model is fraught with problems, including the lack of uniform training and resources for teachers, questionable reliability and validity of the measurement tools, and no consistent method for ensuring treatment integrity within or across conditions (Hale, Naglieri, Kaufman, & Kavale, 2004). In addition, Hale, Naglieri, and colleagues (2004) argue that the model does not require evaluation of the basic (neuro)psychological processes—a *fundamental* component of the federal definition of learning disabilities.

Probably our biggest limitation in effectively meeting the needs of children with learning disabilities is finding out who these kids really are. Collapsing different types of children into a single group only undermines accurate identification of and interventions for their difficulties. Take one group of children with high verbal and low nonverbal skills, and another group with high nonverbal and low verbal skills, and put them in one big "learning disability" group. What is the result? A group that has average skills. Noting these widespread concerns of the discrepancy model, Flanagan, Ortiz, Alfonso, and Mascolo (2002) argue that the use of cross-battery assessment techniques can help identify specific processing deficits associated with academic deficits; this is gaining recognition as an alternative model (Torgesen, 2000). This is a position we advocate in our own cognitive hypothesis-testing (CHT) model, where processing deficits are identified and confirmed, and then are linked to deficient academic performance. At the same time you establish a *concordance* between processing deficits and academic problems, we also believe that you should establish a *discordance* between processing areas unrelated to the academic area and the deficient academic area, as suggested in In-Depth 5.1. Consistent with the ideas put forth by Kavale and Forness (1995), we believe that discrepancy (discordance) is an important criterion for determining whether a child has a learning disability, but it is not a *sufficient* one! Using the concordance–discordance model adds weight in determining eligibility, and it makes good clinical sense, but even these criteria need additional support if children with learning disabilities are to be accurately identified.

IN-DEPTH 5.1. The Concordance–Discordance Model of Learning Disability Determination

Rather than using the much-maligned discrepancy model, we promote the use of a *concordance–discordance model*, which has three criteria that should be met for learning disability identification. Not only does this model represent a more accurate way to identify children with learning disabilities, but it could lead to more effective interventions, because it helps the team recognize each child's unique cognitive strengths and needs. When determining whether a child meets these criteria, we first look for a *concordance* between the deficient achievement area and the neuropsychological processes associated with that area, and attempt to rule out other possible causes for the disorder. Second, we attempt to establish a *discordance* between the deficient achievement area and neuropsychological processes *not* related to the achievement area in question. Third, we look for a *discordance* between processing strengths and weaknesses. For example, as we discuss later in this chapter, a word-reading disorder can be due to deficits in phonemic awareness, orthographic coding skill, rapid automatic naming, processing speed, temporal sequencing of sensory input, or processing automaticity, or any combination of these (Miller & Tallal, 1995; Wolf, 2001). A comprehensive CHT evaluation may reveal deficits on measures of auditory processing and sequencing (the processing weakness cluster), and good performance on measures of nonverbal reasoning and visual-perceptual skills (the processing strength cluster). These subtest scores could be used to create composite weakness and strength cluster scores for the child. Based on these scores, the child should demonstrate a significant difference (in terms of standard error of the difference [*SED*]; see Chapter 3, Application 3.4) between the strength cluster and the weakness cluster, and a significant difference between the strength cluster and the achievement deficit score, but no significant difference between the weakness cluster and the achievement deficit score. Once you identify the deficit area in both processing and achievement, you need only to find a processing area unrelated to the achievement deficit (demonstrated by research), and you have both concordance and discordance—a process graphically represented in the following diagram:

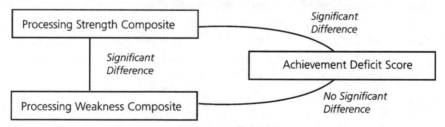

The following example highlights the use of the concordance–discordance model, using the standard scores (SSs) from the Cognitive Assessment System (CAS) and the Wechsler Individual Achievement Test—Second Edition (WIAT-II) for a 9-year-old boy:

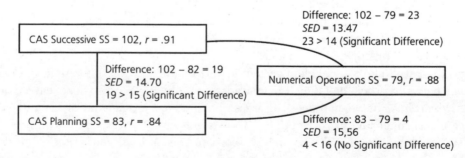

Note. There were no significant differences between CAS subtests within each scale; therefore, the SSs were reliable and valid.

(continued)

IN-DEPTH 5.1. *(continued)*

In the CHT model, if *no* processing weaknesses associated with academic deficits are identified, this suggests that the difficulties may be primarily the results of other causes. Consistent with this line of reasoning, if other processing areas thought to be unrelated to the deficient academic area are also deficient, then the child would be considered a low achiever, as all skills would be low. Although we generally adhere to the National Association of School Psychologists' position that children should be served without the need to label them, we believe that the concordance–discordance model can be used to identify children with learning disabilities more accurately.

We are currently undertaking research designed to establish and validate different processing clusters for use with this model, so that statistical tests can be performed to establish both concordance and discordance for individual children. The example presented above is possible only because there were no significant differences between subtests within each CAS scale, and because reliability data are available (in manuals) for each score. Had there been significant differences within a scale, we would have had to determine a different composite score—one that reflected the child's unique processing strengths and weaknesses. Since subtest reliabilities are available in manuals, you can do comparisons for individual subtests. If this is attempted, try to use only subtests that have high technical quality, and use the more rigorous $p = .01$ criteria for the *SED* calculation. You can create composite scores by averaging subtest scores that cluster together clinically, but averaging their reliability coefficients for *SED* calculation is questionable. However, that is probably better than using a composite score where the subtests are significantly different from one another. Once our research provides multiple composite scores and their reliabilities are established, we believe that the concordance–discordance model will not only aid in determining eligibility, but can also help establish areas of strength and need for intervention planning. However, we admonish practitioners not to become overly focused on statistical comparisons of data to determine eligibility for learning disability services. As noted throughout this book, you must use multiple assessment tools and collect data from multiple sources if you are to recognize a child's unique strengths and needs, and to ensure that your diagnostic and treatment decisions have ecological and treatment validity.

Interventions for Children with Learning Disabilities

When researchers have identified specific types of learning disabilities, with and without comorbid conditions, individual differences in both identification and intervention begin to emerge (Keeler & Swanson, 2001; Lyon et al., 2001; Miller & Tallal, 1995; Prifitera & Dersh, 1993; Rourke, 1994; B. A. Shaywitz et al., 1992; Wolf, 2001). However, most studies have used undifferentiated "learning disability" groups of children, even though we know that such children differ widely. Before we leave our historical overview of learning disabilities, it is worth noting what we know about LD interventions to date. In a meta-analysis of LD treatments, Swanson, Hoskyn, and Lee (1999) found that direct instruction and strategy instruction were both effective interventions, and that a model combining the two was most effective. As noted in Appendix 5.1, Swanson and colleagues also identified specific instructional components that were found to be effective overall, and those that were found to be effective with different types of LDs. Of the findings, it is interesting to note that interactive small-group instruction was more effective than one-on-one instruction. In reviewing these findings, it is important to note that Swanson and colleagues reported on few subtype studies, because there was little agreement on how to subtype children with LDs, and almost no studies examined differential intervention effectiveness for subtypes.

Swanson and colleagues used a typical discrepancy definition for identification of LDs, so there is no clinical information about students' strengths and weaknesses.

Knowing the limitations of previous research on the characteristics and treatment of children with LDs/learning disabilities provides us with a foundation for understanding the issues affecting service delivery to these children. We have come a long way since Samuel Kirk coined the term "learning disabilities," and with the advent of neuropsychological approaches to LDs, a new door has been opened for practitioners and researchers to recognize and treat the unique needs of these children. In the remainder of this book, we begin by discussing subtypes of reading disorders (RDs) in this chapter, and then provide you with similar information about subtypes of math, written language, and psychosocial disorders, including information that can help you design interventions to ameliorate the difficulties of children with these disorders.

CHARACTERISTICS OF CHILDREN WITH READING DISORDERS

The Comorbidity Issue

Before we explore the different types of RDs, and of other disorders you will find in your practice, a brief discussion on comorbidity is in order. During my (Hale) special education training for dual certification, I found it somewhat surprising how little overlap there was between the learning disabilities and behavior disorders curricula. In the learning disabilities classes, there was much discussion of academic problems, but little discussion of socioemotional issues. The opposite was true in the behavior disorder classes, as if these two groups of children were completely different. They were thought to be alike in one respect: They were both thought to benefit from behavioral interventions. When I first entered the field as a special education teacher, I believed that all children were pretty much the same and learned the same way. However, it wasn't until I was in the "trenches," trying to teach children with reading and other problems, that I realized the old adage "one size fits all" does not apply to children with LDs (see In-Depth 5.2). Treating all children as if they are academically or behaviorally the same, and as if academic and behavioral characteristics are unrelated, makes no sense from a biopsychosocial perspective. As you are well aware, academic achievement and psychosocial functioning are intimately related and inseparable, and as we will discover in the remainder of this book, there are neuropsychological sequelae associated with many types of LDs. The complexity of these interactions makes both identification and intervention difficult, but worthy of examination nonetheless.

Prevalence estimates suggest that children with learning disabilities represent a large minority (7%) of the school-age population and a substantial portion (51%) of the special education population (U.S. Department of Education, 1999). Children do not fit nicely into categories, but that is exactly what is expected by some directors of special education when a primary disabling category is reported to the government. Although this is standard practice, there is considerable overlap between and within various categories. As noted earlier, previous group studies of the heterogeneous "learning disability" population did not really tell us much about learning disability subtypes. We often describe children with one or more disorders as having comorbid disorders. However, this term may be a misnomer, because there is so much overlap or co-occurrence of disorders that finding children with only one disorder is unlikely (Kaplan, Dewey, Crawford, & Wilson, 2001). Understanding the interrelationship of disorder symptoms can provide you with diagnostic insight that leads to intervention efficacy—which is what this book is all about. Subtyping of learning disabilities is complex and difficult to achieve, because there is considerable overlap

IN-DEPTH 5.2. Lessons in Learning: The Teacher's World

In the beginning, I (Hale) was a teacher—a good starting place for a psychologist practicing in the schools. I became a teacher because I wanted to help children with special needs experience academic and psychosocial success. When I began my student teaching experience, I thought I had a good understanding of the knowledge base and the tools necessary to teach children with and without disabilities. I had just finished a dual-certification preparation program in learning disabilities and behavior disorders—one that had given me the confidence to teach in my cross-categorical seventh- and eighth-grade classroom. My strong belief in operant techniques had been codified by my professors. I also began my experience with a good understanding of classroom management strategies, as well as of direct instruction (e.g., advanced organizer, demonstration, modeling, guided practice, independent practice), learning strategies (e.g., self-monitoring, evaluation), and social skills (e.g., conversation skills, problem solving) curricula.

As is the case for many children with LDs, reading was a major problem in my classroom. I decided that I would collect baseline data on word recognition and reading rate with my informal reading inventory (IRI), and would complete some curriculum-based probes of comprehension skills. I determined appropriate goals based on each child's current level of functioning, developed a reinforcement menu for each one, and then set out to improve reading skills. My interventions included direct instruction with flashcards to increase word recognition/semantic knowledge (definitions on backs of cards). When students reached instructional level for these words (90% accuracy), each child read a passage that included the practiced words. Word recognition and reading speed were measured, and the students charted their own progress. However, in the months to come, I noticed that some children had trendlines well above their aimlines, while others had the opposite pattern. I also noticed that some children comprehended the passages quite well, but others had considerable difficulty, and that these patterns did not appear to be consistently related to word knowledge (semantic meaning), word recognition (accuracy), or reading speed (fluency). I had to find out why. I tried systematically manipulating schedules of reinforcement, instructional design, and measurement systems, one at a time, and still came up with different results for different children.

I remembered a lecture from graduate school about the "process–product paradigm" in teaching. The professor asked, "Is the learning process or the learning outcome more important?" Because my program was largely behavioral, I believed that outcomes or products should be my focus. Process was nebulous and intangible, and couldn't be measured effectively. But then it dawned on me: Could the process be influencing the product in my classroom? That was what my professor had concluded during her lecture. This teaching experience, combined with many others, led me to two questions I have pursued ever since:

- Why don't all children learn the same way?
- If they don't learn the same way, how do I teach them differently so they can all be successful?

When I started my doctoral program in psychology, I knew that behaviorism was an essential component of successful learning experiences. I still espouse this belief today, but I have also discovered that behaviorism is not the panacea some of my professors made it out to be. Now I am a reformed radical behaviorist—one who believes that process *and* product are important. People often ask me, "What made you change?", and my reply is always the same: "Children did." They taught me that no two children with LDs are alike. There is no "one size fits all" when it comes to serving this diverse population.

between different types of learning disabilities, with many children experiencing academic deficits in one or more areas (Keogh, 1994). Language disorders and RDs often occur in children with attention-deficit/hyperactivity disorder (ADHD) (Elbert, 1993; Pliszka, Carlson, & Swanson, 1999). Motor problems are likely to occur in children with various disorders (Dewey & Kaplan, 1994), and children with ADHD, RDs, or both also have high rates of developmental coordination disorder (Fawcett & Nicholson, 1995; Hellgren, Gillberg, & Gillberg, 1994; Kaplan et al., 2001; Wilson & McKenzie, 1998). These children are also at greater risk for deficits in social skills and socioemotional adjustment (Kavale & Forness, 1996), but there is some disagreement as to whether all children with LDs experience psychosocial deficits (Rourke, 1994). In their study of school-age children, Kaplan and colleagues (2001) found that only 48% of their sample had "pure" RDs (i.e., they did not meet criteria for another disorder). A majority of their comorbid sample also met criteria for ADHD, which is consistent with the finding that 30%–40% of children with ADHD also have RDs (Shaywitz, Fletcher, & Shaywitz, 1994; Willcutt & Pennington, 2000). However, compared to children with ADHD, those with RDs perform worse on measures of receptive and expressive language (Pisecco, Baker, Silva, & Brooke, 2001), suggesting that this distinction may be useful in differential diagnosis. Still, even children with "pure" RDs can have RDs for different causes, and comorbid symptoms are more likely with some subtypes than with others. Application 5.1 gives you an idea of why the subtype issue is important in identification and intervention of disorders.

Prevalence of RDs

Approximately 5% of school-age children have RDs (Ramus, 2001). A substantial majority of children with LDs have RDs (Kavale & Reece, 1992; Lyon & Moats, 1997); however, overall prevalence rates may vary, because discrepancy criteria do not accurately identify children with RDs (S. E. Shaywitz, Escobar, Shaywitz, Fletcher, & Makuch, 1992). This could account for early findings that children with RDs simply represent the lower tail of the normal distribution of reading

---

APPLICATION 5.1. Differential Diagnosis and Comorbidity

Why is differential diagnosis important to you as a practitioner? You certainly can recognize the danger of categorizing and stereotyping children, and we have all learned that children can develop a self-fulfilling prophecy as a result of being labeled. So why not just say that they need help? This might work if all children learned the same way. However, because they do not, labels and diagnoses help us understand the types of help children need. We can't ignore the facts that children have different learning and behavior patterns, and that different disorders and subtypes of disorders exist. Since we firmly believe that differential diagnosis of educational and psychopathological disorders is a critical component of developing effective interventions, you must remain ever vigilant in your exploration of individual differences. But at the same time, every child is ultimately a single-case study. You must not attempt to make children "fit" the category to which they "should" belong; you must see them as individuals, with unique strengths and needs. This is true even if they meet the criteria for only one particular disorder. In this and the remaining chapters of this book, this comorbidity of disorders is highlighted, and some information will be redundant because of the shared neuropsychological characteristics of many disorders. Recall that the gradiental approach (Goldberg, 2001) applies to neuropsychological functions, and as we have argued here, it applies to academic achievement and psychosocial functioning as well.

skills (S. E. Shaywitz et al., 1992). Although there is convincing evidence that RDs have a genetic basis (Compton, Davis, DeFries, Gaycen, & Olson, 2001; Pennington, 1991; Rumsey et al., 1992), genetic risk factors for RDs are associated with multiple chromosomes (Wood & Grigorenko, 2001), and the phonological subtype of RD may be more heritable (Olson, Forsberg, Wise, & Rack, 1994). There may be differences between those with congenital and acquired RDs (Rayner & Pollatsek, 1989), suggesting that some RDs may be due to biological causes, while others are primarily environmentally determined. Researchers have found that good readers read more outside of school in 2 days than poor readers do in an entire year (Cunningham & Stanovich, 1998), and that disadvantaged children enter school with lower levels of letter knowledge and phonemic awareness (Byrnes, 2001), which could lead to lower reading skills. It is likely that biological predispositions interact with environmental influences to produce RDs; in other words, RD symptoms may be the end *products* rather than the *causes* of RDs (Rumsey et al., 1999). As we have noted earlier, differentiation of "garden-variety poor readers" from those with brain-based reading disabilities is difficult, but necessary for intervention purposes.

RDS AND BRAIN FUNCTIONS

The Word Recognition Emphasis

Most of the research cited below focuses on word reading, because reading decoding or word recognition skills are often cited as a major factor in reading comprehension (Lerner, 2000). As a result, the majority of RD research has focused on single-word reading—to such an extent that the term "dyslexia" has become synonymous with word recognition deficits and RDs. This is bothersome to us. Although it is true that word recognition skills are a prerequisite to reading comprehension, the assumption that good word recognition skills and reading fluency automatically lead to comprehension does not fit well with our understanding of how the brain works, or in the types of reading problems you will encounter in your practice. Therefore, as in all academic domains, a comprehensive analysis of error patterns will be essential for making differential diagnoses and conducting individualized interventions.

Early brain researchers focused on abnormal lateralization patterns; they found that individuals with RDs were less lateralized for receptive language (Bryden, 1988) and showed smaller left planum temporale regions than is typical (Galaburda, 1985). The Geschwind and Galaburda (1987) model suggested that the path for reading begins in the occipital lobe, then proceeds to the angular gyrus and Wernicke's area for interpretation, and then moves to Broca's area via the arcuate fasciculus for expression. This certainly makes sense, given what we know about the structure and function of these areas, and it isn't far off from the actual structures implicated in reading, but subsequent research has revealed that reading competency is far more complex. For instance, this model has only an indirect relationship with language processes—specifically, phonological processing, which we know today is highly related to reading competence. There's fairly clear evidence that children with RDs can have phonological (i.e., temporal lobe), orthographic (i.e., occipital lobe), and/or naming speed (i.e., frontal lobe) deficits (Badian, 1997). In their recent review of brain imaging studies, Joseph, Noble, and Eden (2001) report that several areas are involved in reading competency. Table 5.1 highlights these regions, but it is important to recognize that Joseph and colleagues provide no discussion about hemispheric differences in reading, which we will discuss later. In addition to these areas, other "lower-level" areas implicated include the primary, premotor, and supplementary motor areas, the cerebellum, and the cingulate (Fiez & Petersen, 1998).

TABLE 5.1. Cortical Areas Implicated in Reading

- Striate and extrastriate cortex for word processing
- Perisylvian areas for phonological processing
- Angular gyrus and supramarginal gyrus in deciphering written words
- Wernicke's area for comprehension
- Broca's area for articulation, production of language, and syntax
- Dorsolateral prefrontal cortex for executive planning, organization, production, and evaluation of language output

Basic Components of Word Reading

There are several components to successful word reading. At the word recognition level, it is important to realize that words are just symbols representing our own personal reality; therefore, the development of symbolic thought is critical to developing both oral and written language. Oral language requires processing of phonemes (sounds), whereas written language requires recognition of graphemes (symbols), and children must learn to associate the two for successful reading (Stanovich, 1994). Readers must learn structural analysis to recognize morphemes, which are the smallest meaningful units in words. Some words have one morpheme (e.g., "ball"), while others have several (e.g., "mean-ing-ful"). Children can read some words by using phonetic analysis or word attack skills (e.g., "pragmatic"), while others are sight words (e.g., "taught"). Syllabication is breaking a word into its component parts, whereas phonological assembly is important for putting word parts together into a whole word. These can occur at a phonemic or morphemic level. Using both standardized and curriculum-based text to examine error patterns during oral reading can help shed light on the nature of a child's reading problems. A good way to determine the types of errors observed during a child's oral reading is to perform an error analysis. Your job is to determine the error pattern(s) observed, and to link these patterns with cognitive functioning. These patterns (with abbreviations that you can use when taking notes) include the following:

- Pause/repetition (PR)—Child delays or repeats words, suggesting limited automaticity.
- Omission (OM)—Child leaves out words, skips words, or asks for help.
- Insertion/addition (IA)—Child adds letters or words.
- Semantic substitution (SS) or paraphasia—Child substitutes whole words.
- Phonemic substitution (PS) or paraphasia—Child substitutes letters within words.
- Configuration substitution (CS)—Child uses initial letters or whole-word configuration to provide meaningful substitution (which can violate context of sentence).
- Sequencing/reversal (SR)—Child reverses word order or parts of words.
- Syntax error (SE)—Child ignores or adds punctuation by pausing or changing inflection.
- Metacognitive (executive) correction (MC)—Child automatically corrects word, either immediately or after reading additional text.

What parts of the brain are responsible for these components of word recognition? Views of the neuropsychological basis of word recognition and related RDs have undergone several speculative phases—from early beliefs that word recognition is largely visual, to more recent beliefs that it is largely phonological, to current beliefs that many areas of the brain are responsible for accurate word recognition. One of the more recent explanations for word recognition RDs is the "double-deficit" hypothesis (Wolf & Bowers, 1999). This position suggests that children with both phonological deficits and naming speed deficits are at greater risk for RDs, and that these deficits are separable sources of reading dysfunction (Wolf & Bowers, 1999). Much of the recent research reported below suggests that children with double deficits are at greater risk for reading failure (Lovett, Steinbach, & Frijters, 2000). There appear to be fairly equal numbers of children with phonological and naming speed RDs, but children with double deficits make up a majority of the samples; estimates range from 49% to 79% of the population with RDs (Goldberg, Wolf, Cirino, Morris, & Lovett, 1998; Lovett et al., 2000). Although the three-subtype model has been confirmed with cluster-analytic techniques (Morris et al., 1998), some argue that a purely orthographic RD subtype can exist, and that some children with RD can then have triple deficits (phonological, orthographic, and rapid naming) (Badian, 1997). In your examination of the underlying processes associated with reading, recognize that children with RDs can have deficits in one or more of these areas, and that differential interventions may be necessary for each.

The Neuropsychology of Word Recognition

Phonological Processes

There is a strong relationship among auditory processing, phonemic awareness, language competency, and word-reading skills (Foorman, Francis, Shaywitz, Shaywitz, & Fletcher, 1997; Hynd, Marshall, & Semrud-Clikeman, 1991; Lyon, 1995; Shaywitz, Fletcher, & Shaywitz, 1995; Shaywitz et al., 2002; Torgesen, Wagner, & Rashotte, 1994; Vellutino, Scanlon, & Tanzman, 1994). For many years, auditory processing deficits were considered to be the core deficit in RDs (Felton, 1993). In their review of phonological processes in RDs, Stanovich and Siegel (1994) found that a majority of children with dyslexia have difficulty on phonological and pseudoword tasks— possibly because they have difficulty with rapid processing of auditory information and speech (Tallal, Sainburg, & Jernigan, 1991; Tallal, Miller, & Fitch, 1993)—and a relative strength in orthographic processing. Phonological analysis relies heavily on detecting changes in sound frequency and amplitude (Stein, 2001). Critical for developing good phonological skills, sound frequency modulation accounts for a substantial amount of variance in nonword reading (Talcott, Witton, et al., 2000); thus it is not surprising that frequency modulation is difficult for many children with RDs (Stein & McAnally, 1996), and that poor frequency modulation combined with poor amplitude modulation is likely to lead to significant phonological deficits and RDs (Witton, Stein, Stoodley, Rosner, & Talcott, 2001).

This RD subtype, caused by auditory processing deficits that lead to poor phonological awareness, is often called phonological dyslexia. A child with this subtype may have a normal audiological examination, but may have a history of ear infections that result in poor phonological processing skills; however, recall also that this subtype is more likely to have a genetic basis (Olson et al., 1994). Not only do these children have problems with auditory processing and, as a result, with receptive language, but they have difficulty with basic word attack skills and perform poorly on pseudoword tasks (e.g., reading "hesrid"). This is largely because they do not have good sound–symbol awareness, which is caused by poor metalinguistic understanding that words can be broken into their phonological parts (Fletcher et al., 1994). These children tend to rely on compensatory processes for reading (Pugh et al., 2000), using a sight word approach and guessing at words based on their general configuration. This would account for the greater occipital–temporal lobe activity found in children with phonological dyslexia, who may use memory-based strategies for word recognition (Shaywitz et al., 2003). For instance, they may say "loud" for the stimulus word "lost."

Because they make many decoding errors, and may have both receptive and expressive language deficits, these children are likely to be recognized by parents and teachers as having a learning problem. Interestingly, those with phoneme–grapheme correspondence problems (i.e., superior temporal–parietal problems) may use the occipital–temporal area differently, depending on whether they successfully compensate for their deficits. Several cortical areas have been implicated in this type of RD, particularly the perisylvian temporal regions (primary and association auditory cortex), middle temporal gyrus, Wernicke's area, angular and supramarginal parietal gyri, striate and extrastriate cortex, and frontal lobe, especially in the left hemisphere (Eliez et al., 2000; Horwitz, Rumsey, & Donohue, 1998; Joseph et al., 2001; Shaywitz et al., 1995, 2002; Stein, 2001). Recent research suggests that reductions in left temporal lobe gray matter in children with phonological dyslexia are not specific to the perisylvian region (Eliez et al., 2000); this could account for the strong relationship among reading, receptive language, and crystallized/convergent/concordant processing deficits. As noted in Chapter 2, the left angular gyrus has been implicated in RDs, as this multimodal convergence zone serves to connect visual (occipital) and auditory (superior temporal gyrus) language processes (Horwitz et al., 1998; Poldrack, 2001). It is not surprising that children with this type of RD show decreased functional magnetic resonance imaging (fMRI) or positron emission tomography (PET) activation in response to phonological tasks in the left temporal and parietal regions (Demb, Poldrack, & Gabrieli, 1999). Interestingly, these children show decreased resting blood flow in the parietal region, and angular gyrus blood flow has been found to be related to reading performance in typical readers, but inversely related for children with phonological RD (Rumsey et al., 1994, 1999). These findings suggest that the left angular gyrus is the most probable site of the functional lesion in this RD type (Rumsey et al., 1999).

Researchers have found that individuals with phonological RD, as compared to controls, showed lower levels of activation in the left-hemisphere areas associated with competent reading (Shaywitz et al., 2002). They also showed lower activity during phonological assembly tasks in the superior temporal gyrus, angular gyrus, and striate and extrastriate visual cortex (Shaywitz et al., 1998). A comparison of correlations between these regions of interest showed that they were highly connected (correlated) for the typical group, but functionally disconnected for the group with phonological RD (Pugh et al., 2000). This replicates work by Horwitz and colleagues (1998), who found strong functional connectivity between angular gyrus and occipital–temporal visual areas, auditory cortex, Wernicke's area, and Broca's area in controls, but no such connections in children with phonological RD. This disconnection problem could be the result of problems with the white matter in the arcuate fasciculus and superior longitudinal fasciculus (Makris et al., 1999)—a possibility consistent with white matter deficits in this type of RD (Klingberg et al., 2000).

Could children with phonological RD be attempting to use a different pathway (i.e., the ventral stream) for word recognition? Certainly they could rely on a more ventral stream (i.e., sight word) path for word recognition (Farah, 1990), and this could possibly explain superior temporal–parietal underactivation and disconnection during word recognition tasks. However, as we will see later, fMRI studies of typical children also fail to show angular gyrus activation on some reading tasks, so this is not a clear-cut picture. As these findings suggest, the left posterior brain structures are functionally different in children with this type of RD. Therefore, determining whether it is an auditory (superior temporal), visual (ventral occipital–temporal), or integration (angular and supramarginal gyrus) problem is an important distinction to make during your evaluation, as suggested by Case Study 5.1.

CASE STUDY 5.1. Paul's Phonological Processing Deficit

Paul was an 8-year-old boy who had difficulty learning the alphabet and could not read even basic sight words, despite 2 years of remedial support. Paul was pleasant, compliant, and hard-working during the evaluation. However, some expressive language issues, including articulation problems, were noted. A review of the history revealed several instances of otitis media (ear infections), but his audiological examination was fine. For word reading, Paul read a few words correctly (e.g., "as," "then") but he had many letter reversals (e.g., reading "b" for "d"). Paul did not pass any pseudoword-decoding items. It seemed as if Paul had the classic signs of a phonological processing disorder; surprisingly, however, he had no difficulty on visual or auditory processing tasks, so further hypothesis testing was necessary. Paul made several block design orientation errors (i.e., reversals and rotations). He also had left–right confusion, as well as poor handwriting notable for uneven pencil pressure. An examination of spatial and motor skills found few problems in these areas, so what was Paul's problem? Paul apparently had difficulty with sound–symbol association, somatosensory feedback, and directional orientation—all characteristic of left parietal lobe dysfunction. Providing Paul with phonological awareness instruction wasn't the key to helping him, since he heard phonemes and saw letters just fine; he needed help with *integrating* sounds and symbols.

Grapheme/Morpheme/Orthographic Processes

We can now recognize how auditory processing skills affect phonological awareness and the acquisition of sound–symbol associations, but shouldn't visual deficits also lead to RDs? Intuitively, you know that RDs can't always be the result of auditory processing deficits, because reading is a visual task. However, after early research suggested that phonological processing deficits lead to RDs, the role of vision in reading was neglected for some time (Stein, 2001). Visual processing of words at the cortical level has been touched on briefly in the preceding section. Not only are these cortical areas implicated in this type of RD, but so are frontal and subcortical structures. Research has confirmed that orthographic skills are related to reading speed independently of phonological skills (Barker, Torgesen, & Wagner 1992), and that these skills are strong predictors of reading competency by the middle elementary grades (Torgesen, Wagner, Rashotte, Burgess, & Hecht, 1997).

The RD subtype that involves difficulty with grapheme/morpheme problems due to impaired orthography is often called orthographic dyslexia. Children with orthographic dyslexia have little difficulty with words that make phonemic sense, but they often read in a slow, laborious manner. These children tend to have problems with reading sight words; for instance, they can read the word "grand" quite well, but have problems with "right," probably saying "rig-hut." These children have also been found to have difficulty in the striate, extrastriate, and inferior parietal lobe areas. Neuroimaging studies have shown that the left ventral stream (primarily the striate, extrastriate, lingual, and fusiform areas) is important in orthography, whereas morpheme recognition and fluency are related to posterior temporal–parietal areas and Broca's area (Joseph et al., 2001).

Although these cortical areas have been implicated in reading, children with this type of RD could have deficits that result from dysfunction of early visual processes. In his review of these processes, Stein (2001) notes that children with orthographic RD appear to have impaired magnocellular functioning (see the discussion of the M pathway in Chapter 2), directly affecting the dorsal visual pathway from the occipital lobe to the parietal lobe. Consistent with this argument, children with this type of RD show reduced brain activity in the primary visual cortex and extrastriate areas (Demb, Boynton, & Heeger, 1998) and fail to activate some visual areas in response to moving dots (Eden, Van Meter, Rumsey, Maison, & Zeffiro, 1996). This would be consistent with findings that such children have poor motion sensitivity (Talcott, Hansen, Elikem, & Stein, 2000). As elaborated on in In-Depth 5.3, deficits in motion sensitivity could explain why many of these children complain that letters and words move, why they misidentify and transpose letters, and why they tend to miss middle letters when reading (Cornelissen, Hansen, Hutton, Evangelinou, & Stein, 1997; Ehri & Saltmarsh, 1995).

Fluency, Timing, and Retrieval Speed Processes

The study of fluency, timing, and retrieval speed has been a relatively recent area of inquiry into the deficits associated with RDs. Fluent reading is rapid, smooth, and automatic, without attention paid to reading mechanics such as decoding (Meyer & Felton, 1999). Reading fluency is directly related to naming speed—a skill needed for making the transition from slow, laborious reading to quick, efficient, accurate reading (Fawcett & Nicholson, 2001). Because articulation speed, naming speed, and processing speed are related to reading accuracy and speed (Kail & Hall, 1994; Scarborough & Domgaard, 1998), it is important to look for expressive speech and language characteristics, retrieval difficulties, and/or slow psychomotor or processing speed in the children you test. Children with RDs who have good phonemic and poor rapid automatized naming (RAN) skills are likely to be better at decoding, but they tend to read slowly and to make more spelling errors on tests of orthographic accuracy (Bowers, 2001; Manis, Doi, & Bhadha, 2000).

According to Torgesen, Rashotte, and Alexander (2001), the factors affecting reading fluency include the following:

- Proportion of words recognized as morphemes or orthographic units
- Speed variations in sight word processing
- Processing speed during novel word identification
- Use of context clues to facilitate word identification
- Speed of semantic access of word meanings

IN-DEPTH 5.3. The Moving Target

How could motion sensitivity be related to RDs, given that the eyes are what move, not the words? Recall that the dorsal stream is responsible for spatial and motion processing, and for self-direction of movement. Although the problem could be related to the coordination of the receptive system with the frontal eye fields (which guide and control eye movements) and the cranial nerves, as discussed in Chapter 2, much of the focus has been on the difficulties with motion processing. Tracking of visual stimuli works both ways: As the eyes move across the page, the letters must be instantly encoded and at the same time integrated, with poorly coordinated eye movements related to "movement" of the letters in working memory. Consistent with these arguments, motion sensitivity predicts orthographic skills better than phonemic skills, and accounts for 25% of the variance in reading (Stein, 2001). Although visual and motion processes are certainly important in the reading process, some researchers have suggested that phonological and orthographic deficits could reflect the same underlying pathology—a hypothesis we explore later in this chapter.

Notice how phonology is *not* one of the factors associated with RAN and reading fluency. Obviously, if you can't read a word, you can't read quickly; this is self-evident. However, studies have shown little to no correlation among auditory processing, phonological awareness, and rapid naming (Felton & Brown, 1990; Wolf & Bowers, 1999).

What brain areas could affect reading speed and fluency? Thinking back to Chapter 2, we would predict the subcortical areas associated with cortical tone; the frontal lobes, for regulation of attention, sequencing, retrieval, and temporal relationships; the cingulate, with its anterior–posterior pathway; and the cerebellum, because of its involvement in timing and skill routinization. Indeed, with the exception of the cortical tone areas, all these areas have been implicated. These areas include the thalamus and M pathway (as described in the preceding section), the cerebellum, Broca's area, and the dorsolateral prefrontal cortex. Noting that those with RDs show signs of inattention, neglect, and slower right-hemisphere processing, as well as the consequences of M-pathway deficits affecting right parietal lobe functioning, some have suggested this may be the cause of temporal information-processing deficits in RDs (Hari, Renvall, & Tanskanen, 2001). The M-pathway hypothesis could have even broader-reaching consequences, if the pathway is disturbed at the level of the thalamus, as has been suggested by postmortem studies of the brains of individuals with RDs (Galaburda & Livingstone, 1993). Recall that the lateral and medial geniculate bodies of the thalamus are the relays for visual and auditory sensory information. According to Stein (2001), the postmortem studies provide evidence that both the auditory and visual pathways could be disturbed in RDs, which could account for the phonological *and* orthographic/fluency deficits seen in many children with RDs.

However, when you think of timing, you should think of the frontal–basal ganglia–cerebellar circuit as well. Indeed, children with RDs have difficulty with selective and sustained attention, inhibition, set maintenance, flexibility, and phonemic production (Kelly, Best, & Kirk, 1989), suggesting that this functional system could account for the difficulties with sequencing and temporal relationships seen in such children (Lovegrove, 1993; Nicholson, Fawcett, & Dean, 1995; Stein, 2001; Waber et al., 2001). Although dysfunctional cross-modal temporal relationships have been found in children with various types of RDs (Waber et al., 2001), they are most likely in individuals with phonological dyslexia (Cestnick, 2001). Is this a manifestation of the frontal lobes or the left hemisphere, or is it a left–frontal combination?

If the frontal lobes are important for understanding temporal relationships, and the left hemisphere is the detailed/local/parts hemisphere, then the left–frontal combination makes good sense. Poor temporal–sequential relationships can lead to problems with auditory–sequential processing, which is important in receptive language, and even with orthography, as the visual word-processing areas (fusiform and lingual gyri) appear to be rate-dependent (Price, Wise, & Frackowiak, 1996). This explanation makes good neuropsychological sense, as executive processes are responsible for the sequential organization of responding, which occurs within a temporal framework (Berninger, Abbott, Billingsley, & Nagy, 2001). This could also explain why the brain areas associated with articulation during silent reading are used by readers with dyslexia during word attack (Shaywitz et al., 2003). Frontal processes even extend beyond this framework, as highlighted in In-Depth 5.4.

Although frontal lobe and executive problems seem to be part of the picture, it is important to consider that supporting structures, such as the cingulate and cerebellum, may also play a role in reading fluency. Researchers have recently found greater support for the cingulate's role in executive functions (especially the online monitoring of performance), and apathy is common following damage to the cingulate (Lichter & Cummings, 2001), suggesting that this could be a cause for

IN-DEPTH 5.4. The Executive Reader

How are executive functions related to RDs? Many authors have found that working memory is important in effective word reading (Breznitz, 2001), and that children with RDs have deficient executive function skills. As discussed earlier, there is considerable overlap between RDs and ADHD, possibly because frontal dysfunction may be involved in a subset of children with RDs. Studies have shown high overlap between the conditions, but children with the inattentive type of ADHD would appear to be more at risk for RDs than children with the hyperactive–impulsive type (Willcutt & Pennington, 2000). Consistent with these findings, symptoms of inattention appear to predict rapid automatic naming and orthographic processing, but hyperactivity has no significant relationship to either phonological or orthographic processes (Berninger et al., 2001). However, it is unclear whether these ADHD-like symptoms suggest comorbidity, or are primarily the result of one disorder or the other (Pennington, Groisser, & Welsh, 1993; Swanson, Mink, & Bocian, 1999).

fluency problems in RDs; however, further examination of this plausible relationship is necessary. The cerebellum seems to be the brain's main internal timepiece, as it is involved in timing, learning, and skilled performance (Ivry, Justus, & Middleton, 2001). It has reciprocal relationships with the magnocellular system (Stein, 2001), so difficulty with processing oral speech and reading could be related to poor timing secondary to cerebellar dysfunction. The cerebellum is involved in automatization of motor skills and implicit learning (Nicholson & Fawcett, 2001; Vicari, Marotta, Menghini, Molinari, & Petrosini, 2003).

Given these findings, it is not surprising that the cerebellum has been linked to reading processes (Fulbright et al., 1999), and that 80% of children with RDs show cerebellar impairment (Nicholson, Fawcett, & Dean, 2001). As noted earlier, the cerebellum is linked to frontal structures, including Broca's area, so it is essential for fluency or "verbal dexterity" (Leiner, Leiner, & Dow, 1993). In fact, cerebellar dysarthria, characterized by irregular rate and stress in speech, could be due to a timing problem (Ivry et al., 2001). Several has suggested that cerebellar dysfunction could account for the labored reading of many children with RDs. The cerebellum also affects memory retrieval and articulation rehearsal (Fiez & Raichle, 1997; Ivry et al., 2001), which is consistent with activation of Broca's area during oral reading (Stein, 2001). In the Shaywitz and colleagues (1998) RD study, recall that underactivation was found in the posterior areas, but overactivation was found for Broca's area. Overactivation is not equivalent with competence, however, as children with RDs have poor articulation speed (Avons & Hanna, 1995) and naming speed (Manis & Freedman, 2001).

Left- and Right-Hemisphere Processes

Before we discuss word-reading interventions, you will note that most of the information discussed earlier has primarily focused on the left-hemisphere and subcortical areas involved in reading. Does this mean that word reading is a left-hemisphere task and has little to do with the right hemisphere? Well, the answer is, of course, yes and no. Many of the fMRI and PET studies reported above showed activation primarily in left-hemisphere areas; however, unlike patient studies, these neuroimaging studies have provided convincing evidence of bilateral processing during reading in dyslexia, even at the word recognition level (Shaywitz et al., 2002). Since reading is a visual task, shouldn't it be a right-hemisphere activity? The assumption most researchers have made is that there are two interconnected routes: the faster, automatic *semantic route*, which relies on the visual system to retrieve whole words (i.e., sight words), and the slower *phonological route*, which depends on auditory mediation to process words (i.e., word attack skills) (Castles & Coltheart, 1993).

Based on the old left/verbal–right/nonverbal dichotomy, you would guess that the semantic route is a right-hemisphere route and the phonological route is a left-hemisphere route. This model would even fit well with the global (whole-word)–local (individual-letters) dichotomy. However, this is not quite as simple as it seems. Visual half field studies suggest that during initial stages of word processing, words are compared to phonemic and orthographic representations in memory. Similar words are likely to be processed by the left hemisphere, but dissimilar words are likely to be processed by the right in an attempt to resolve semantic ambiguity (Crossman & Polich, 1988). Recall our novel (right-hemisphere)–routinized (left-hemisphere) distinction discussed in Chapter 2; this model again explains why word recognition skills are primarily lateralized to the left hemisphere, even when they are retrieved as sight words.

As we have seen in Chapter 2, right-hemisphere processes are required during ambiguous and novel problem-solving situations, so it is not surprising that when children are first learning sound–symbol associations, right-hemisphere activity is relatively high. When infants initially process language, we have seen that the right hemisphere is important during language acquisition (Molfese & Molfese, 1997), and sure enough, these right-hemisphere processes do predict reading skills at age 8 (Molfese, Molfese, & Modgline, 2001). But as we have seen, the left hemisphere is responsible for categorizing information and developing routinized codes. Since reading fluency is related to forming new associations between phonological and orthographic representations, children with RDs could have difficulty forming these associations (Manis, Seidenburg, & Doi, 1999). Children with RDs do have difficulty with response categorization, even for nonlinguistic stimuli; this suggests that their deficit lies in categorization, not perception, of stimuli (Fawcett & Nicholson, 2001).

This difficulty with forming sound–symbol associations could account for findings that individuals with phonological dyslexia tend to use right-hemisphere global/holistic orthographic and semantic processes when reading (Coltheart, 2000; Michel, Henaff, & Intrilligator, 1996; Patterson, Varga-Khadem, & Polkey, 1989; Shaywitz et al., 2002; Weekes, Coltheart, & Gordon, 1997). They also tend to use the right frontal lobe, possibly to retrieve sight words from long-term memory (Shaywitz et al., 2003). Consistent with the works of Grabowski and Nowicka (1996), children with RDs are likely to have difficulty with high spatial frequencies or word details, and as a result are likely to rely on low spatial frequencies or global percepts to read words based on configuration. This could explain why children with RDs require more time to recognize two distinct images than a single image (Chase, 1996). Coltheart (2000) indicates that those with phonological dyslexia rely on the right inferior occipital region for letter and word recognition; this leads to right temporal and then left temporal lobe semantic activation, and finally to phonological output in Broca's area. Since these children may be less automatized in their reading performance, we would expect them to have considerable difficulty when they cannot recognize a word by using visual memory skills. This could account for their tendency to use Broca's area more in processing words, as they attempt to compensate for poor sound–symbol association skills by sounding out the words they cannot recall by sight. Because they can't access visual–verbal connections quickly (Denckla & Cutting, 1999), children with RDs are likely to require more effort when reading, and to be less efficient readers than their nondisabled peers (Fawcett & Nicholson, 2001). These arguments are consistent with electroencephalographic findings showing increased frontal lobe activity in children with RDs during word reading, suggesting more effortful processing (i.e., working memory) than automatic processing, and the use of frontal articulation areas to compensate for dysfunctional posterior systems (Rippon & Brunswick, 2000; Shaywitz et al., 2002).

Finally, it is important to evaluate the neuroimaging data suggesting differences in the use of the angular gyrus and supramarginal gyrus during reading in some studies, but not in others. Is this an artifact of the reading task, or are differences in studies meaningful? Studies that show no activation in these areas during word reading typically show activation in the occipital–temporal lobe, primarily in the lingual, fusiform, or temporal–occipital boundary areas. In their review of imaging studies, Fiez and Petersen (1998) note orthographic processing in left occipital and occipital–temporal regions (i.e., the ventral stream), near the border between the middle and superior temporal gyrus, which is involved in semantic analysis. These findings suggest two paths for word recognition (Logan, 1997): a sound–symbol association path processed through the angular and supramarginal gyri, and a more automatic path involving the left extrastriate cortex and occipital–temporal ventral stream (L. Cohen, Dehaene, Chochon, Lehericy, & Naccache, 2000; Dehaene et al., 2001; Horwitz et al., 1998; Samuelsson, 2000; Shaywitz et al., 2002, 2003). This important distinction is made evident in Case Study 5.2.

CASE STUDY 5.2. Pam's Compensatory Approach

Pam was a 12-year-old girl who was referred for an evaluation because she was having difficulty keeping up with her reading assignments, and her comprehension skills had dropped dramatically. According to parent and teacher report, Pam had had no problem with reading until recently. The teacher also noted that Pam had always been a good writer, but her handwriting was always "sloppy." The mother felt that there must be some psychosocial component to Pam's deteriorating performance, because she was also having difficulty with peer relationships. When I (Hale) asked Pam to read a passage from her text, I noticed that she read clearly, but that she skipped over some words and guessed at other words based on their initial consonant–vowel cluster. The assessment results revealed inconsistent yet average-range single-word reading, and low average comprehension, but extremely poor auditory processing, phonological awareness, phonological segmentation, sound–symbol association, and phonological assembly skills. She could barely complete any of the pseudoword-decoding items. These and other findings suggested that Pam had difficulty with superior temporal–inferior parietal regions, particularly in the left hemisphere. Interestingly, she also showed signs of poor spatial and holistic processing, directional confusion, and limited self-awareness. On a positive note, Pam had no difficulty with bimanual or right-hand motor skills, and her facial and object–word memory skills were above average.

It became clear that this was a bilateral parietal issue, not just a left parietal one. So how had Pam learned to read words successfully, and why was she having problems now? Pam had apparently memorized many high-frequency words by sight—making the association between visual and auditory words in the intact ventral stream, where the words were automatically retrieved. It wasn't until the upper elementary grades, when low-frequency words in text became more common, that Pam's compensatory approach was no longer adequate. Pam's grades began to fall because the higher-level passages included many low-frequency words, and she began to miss too many words to comprehend the passages. Had we noticed Pam's compensatory strategy earlier, we could have helped remediate her deficient word attack skills, which might have made a difference in her reading and psychosocial functioning as well. Through systematic remediation of her sound–symbol association deficits, and use of her intact sequencing skills and knowledge of morphemes, we helped Pam keep up with her reading assignments and improve her comprehension. We also helped her with spatial feedback to the motor system through occupational therapy support, and helped her improve her peer relationships through a social skills counseling group intervention.

From a neuropsychological perspective, this conceptualization of word reading makes perfect sense. We know that the ventral stream is important for object recognition, and that damage to the temporal lobe can lead to object agnosia, word agnosia, and prosopagnosia (Farah, 1990). When word recognition requires phonemic and orthographic processing at the letter or morpheme level, the dorsal stream and angular gyrus and supramarginal gyrus would be needed (as would the M pathway, described earlier), but automatic retrieval of known words would require accessing the long-term memory of words through ventral stream processes. If the left-hemisphere dorsal stream is impaired (i.e., dysfunctional angular gyrus or supramarginal gyrus), and the left ventral stream is intact (i.e., good occipital–inferior temporal lobe), we would expect a child to respond correctly on word recognition tasks by using his or her good sight vocabulary. However, if both the left dorsal and ventral streams are impaired, the child would have to rely on the right ventral stream. The child might use the right hemisphere to attempt to guess at words by morpheme knowledge or initial configuration, but this could lead to many wrong guesses based on word configuration, or to delayed word attack skills characterized by many phonemic paraphasias (sound substitutions). This hypothesis is certainly plausible, since children with RDs show increased right parietal–occipital activity, suggesting that they rely on holistic visual processing for word recognition (Flynn, Deering, Goldstein, & Rahbar, 1992); this would be consistent with Coltheart's (2000) arguments regarding phonological RD. This growing body of evidence is consistent with Logan's (1997) hypothesis about word attack and automatic word recognition routes, with the former related to the integrity of the temporal–parietal areas, and the latter associated with the occipital–ventral region (Shaywitz et al., 2002). However, one study of adults with phoneme–grapheme deficits suggests that they rely on the left-hemisphere occipital–temporal ventral stream for word reading (Shaywitz et al., 2003), with more successful compensators using it for a grapheme word attack strategy and less successful readers using it for sight word recognition. Given our understanding of the neuropsychological processes involved in word reading, you can begin to formulate ideas about a child's processing strengths and weaknesses in preparation for developing an individualized intervention designed to meet the child's needs. Several possible interventions are presented at the end of this chapter.

The Neuropsychology of Reading Comprehension

Components of Reading Comprehension

Marcus reads well in class, so why doesn't he understand what he's reading? Reading comprehension is much less studied than word recognition, because it is assumed that accurate, fluent reading leads to good comprehension, although the path may be more complex and indirect (Wolf & Bowers, 1999). A majority of research indicates that semantic processes are not as impaired as phonological processes in children with RDs (Siegel, 1993); this suggests that the problem lies at the word level, not the text level, of processing (Lyon, 1995). This may be true for some poor readers, but for average readers, listening comprehension predicts comprehension (Vellutino et al., 1994). Could it be that poor readers are limited by lower-level processes, and we never really get to higher-level instruction to determine whether comprehension is a problem? And what about children who show no lower-level problems, only higher-level comprehension problems—such as children with right-hemisphere disorders (Rourke, 1994)?

Certainly, higher-level reading skills such as word and text comprehension require accuracy and proficiency in the lower-level processes (Logan, 1997), but they also require integration of prior knowledge, suggesting that personal experience interacts with text information to create a unique interpretation of the text (Beach, 1993). Comprehension also requires much more working memory and many other executive skills, to enable the reader to interpret text meaning and draw conclusions about passages. Also, while we see little evidence of right-hemisphere activity in explicit text comprehension, interpretation of implicit, nonliteral inferences—metaphor, humor, idiom, sarcasm, and double meanings—is likely to require right-hemisphere skills (see Bryan & Hale, 2001). Children with right-hemisphere dysfunction are less likely to show comprehension problems in the early grades, as traditional elementary instruction has focused primarily on interpretation of concrete narrative plots (Williams et al., 2002). Similar to Pam's case described in Case Study 5.2, you will see children who read words and comprehend quite well until the late elementary or middle school years—but who do so for totally different reasons than nondisabled readers do, as suggested by Case Study 5.3.

At a basic level are the word recognition processes described earlier. Moving beyond these lower-level constructs, we find that word meaning, which is derived from semantic knowledge of morpheme root words, prefixes, and suffixes, is quite important. Understanding word relationships requires examination of objects, of actions, and of interactions among objects, actions, and events (Lahey, 1988). Semantics is related to both individual words (vocabulary knowledge) and sentence structure. Indeed, word knowledge and use are intimately related to syntax or grammar; syntax is the system of rules for word order and combinations and for sentence organization. Good semantic and syntactic knowledge is likely to lead to comprehension competency. However, the relationships among words and structuring of text may be explicit (requiring literal comprehension) or implicit (requiring inferential comprehension). "Pragmatics" is the final aspect of reading

CASE STUDY 5.3. "William Just Doesn't Get It"

William was referred to us for psychoeducational instruction in reading, even though his reading had been "fine" throughout elementary school. The teacher reported that his reading seemed "fine" even now, but that "William just doesn't get it." Using an informal reading inventory and his text for a curriculum-based probe of word reading and speed, William was found to be reading at the instructional level for his grade, and though his reading rate or fluency was somewhat slow, he was within grade-level expectations. However, William only answered 20% of the comprehension questions correctly. He just didn't seem to understand what he read. Few clues about his comprehension failure could be gained from the probes administered, other than that an anecdotal examination of his performance revealed little adherence to syntax. Further investigation indicated good word knowledge and language comprehension, so what could be wrong with his comprehension?

Although oral reading fluency correlates strongly with reading comprehension (Markell & Deno, 1997), the old belief that teaching William to read words would result in William's understanding everything isn't quite accurate. We have worked with numerous children who have good word recognition and fluency skills, but still don't comprehend what they read. A key to William's reading comprehension problems was found in neither his standardized test scores nor his CBM results, but in the types of answers he made. William's error responses were often phrases taken directly from the text, but only tangentially related to the question asked. In other words, he searched his semantic memory for answers and came up with "reasonable" responses. Such children often go unrecognized by teachers, because early instruction is often focused on "breaking the code," or sound–symbol association. Thinking that phonological awareness would be the key to understanding William's reading problems would ignore every other brain area except the primary auditory cortex—an area that was impaired in Pam's case (see Case Study 5.2), but just fine in William's case.

comprehension, and it is difficult to define and measure. It is best described as the function of the message conveyed, and is often used to describe communicative competence or social discourse in oral language. It is by its very nature based on personal experience and values, so in reading comprehension this area is often referred to as "evaluation" or "critical reading."

Compared to research on word reading, research into the neuropsychological basis of comprehension has been quite limited. A summary of major studies linking comprehension and brain regions can be found in Table 5.2. Although the results of these studies vary, depending on the tasks administered and subtraction tasks used, some general findings emerge. Most neuroimaging studies of semantic processing of categorical and semantic information have implicated the left temporal lobe (Daselaar, Veltman, Rombouts, Raaijmakers, & Jeroen, 2002; Shaywitz et al., 1995), both inferior and anterior to the sections described in connection with phonological processing (Joseph et al., 2001). This is consistent with our earlier arguments that the left temporal lobe serves as a warehouse of long-term memory for explicit information (Binder et al., 1997; Petersen, Fox, Snyder, & Raichle, 1990). Not surprisingly, frontal lobe activity is also required for semantic judgment and comprehension of text, although some studies show bilateral activity, and others show primarily left-hemisphere involvement during comprehension tasks. A number of researchers have shown that children with RDs have problems with executive functions (or, in cognitive–educational parlance, "metacognition"), which result in difficulty with monitoring, adjusting, and regulating cognitions (Wong, 1991). It has been suggested that for reading comprehension, executive functions such as working memory and metacognitive skills are more likely to differentiate children with RDs from controls than lower-level processes, such as phonology and morphology, which are automatic in typical readers (Swanson & Alexander, 1997). As suggested in the previous discussion, comprehension deficits due to executive dysfunction appear to be independent of the phonological/articulatory functions subserving word recognition (Swanson & Ashbaker, 2000). In a direct comparison of prefrontal and posterior measures, Kelly and colleagues (1989) found that children with RDs had greater executive deficits, including problems with selective and sustained attention, inhibition, set maintenance, flexibility, and phonemic production.

TABLE 5.2. Brain Regions Associated with Reading Comprehension and Semantic Processes

Study	IF	MF	ST/MT	IP	IO
Beauregard et al. (1997)	•	•		•	
Bookheimer et al. (1995)	•			•	•
Damasio et al. (1996)	•				•
Herbster et al. (1997)					•
Howard et al. (1992)			•		•
Kapur et al. (1994)	•				
Petersen et al. (1989)	•	•			
Price et al. (1994)			•	•	•
Pugh et al. (1997)			•	•	
Vandenberghe et al. (1996)	•		•	•	•

Note. I, inferior; M, middle; S, superior; F, frontal; T, temporal; P, parietal; O, occipital.

Neuroimaging studies have identified several key areas associated with reading comprehension. Obviously, the word recognition areas described previously play a role in reading comprehension—but possibly to a lesser extent than one would think, possibly due to other factors affecting comprehension versus simple word recognition. Many studies implicate strong bilateral activation in the occipital lobe fusiform and lingual cortices (ventral stream) in both word recognition and semantic processing (e.g., Bookheimer, Zeffiro, Blaxton, Gaillard, & Theodore, 1995; Nobre, Allison, & McCarthy, 1998). The classic left lateral superior cortex and Wernicke's areas are often activated (Just, Carpenter, Keller, Eddy, & Thulborn, 1996). Whereas superior temporal lobe activity during comprehension is often noted, mostly in the posterior Wernicke's area, the middle temporal gyrus and surrounding areas are also often active during reading comprehension. Not seen in word-reading studies, activation in the lateral and medial temporal region has been associated with semantic and episodic memory (Menon, Boyette-Anderson, Schatzberg, & Reiss, 2002). Unlike several word-reading studies, research in reading comprehension has found little or no activity in angular or supramarginal gyri (Gaillard et al., 2001). This fits nicely with our hypothesis about these areas' being involved in lower-level processes of sound–symbol association, which may not be as necessary during silent reading comprehension. Children may skip over unknown words or use context to guess at them rather than delay fluency, which could impede comprehension. They either gain access through the direct visual semantic route through the ventral visual stream associated with the left fusiform/lingual gyri (Hinojosa et al., 2001), or decide to skip or guess at the word, because the indirect phoneme–grapheme route is too slow and costly.

Frontal lobe activity also tends to be more widespread during reading comprehension than during word reading, and tends to be more bilateral (Fletcher et al., 1995; Just et al., 1996). As with word reading, Broca's area is found to be involved in some aspects of reading comprehension—specifically, in subvocal word articulation (Paulesu, Frith, & Frackowiak, 1993; Rueckert et al., 1994; Rumsey et al., 1997), understanding of temporal relationships (Keller, Carpenter, & Just, 2001), and interpretation of syntax (Stromswold, Caplan, Alpert, & Rauch, 1996). Many suggest that Broca's area is critical for understanding syntactic relationships, which the left hemisphere uses for sentence structure analysis and interpretation (Faust, 1998). Other frontal areas involved during reading comprehension include the middle frontal gyrus, which has been associated with conditional reasoning (Fletcher et al., 1995), and the dorsolateral prefrontal cortex (Fiez, 1997), which has been linked to semantic categorization, decision making, and syntax (Gaillard et al., 2001). Comparisons of word reading and sentence reading have consistently shown that sentences require more brain activity than words, and syntactic complexity requires more dorsolateral prefrontal cortex activity (Gaillard et al., 2001), presumably because of higher demands on working memory.

Left- and Right-Hemisphere Reading Comprehension Processes

The role of the right hemisphere in reading comprehension has become quite clear in recent years. Neuroimaging studies have shown that the right hemisphere is involved in many reading comprehension tasks, but that the extent of involvement varies depending on the task. The right-hemisphere counterparts to the left-hemisphere areas (i.e., fusiform/lingual gyri; angular and supramarginal gyri, superior and middle temporal gyri, Wernicke's and Broca's areas, prefrontal cortex) often become involved during complex tasks, which has led some to conclude that these regions are recruited during times of high demand (Galliard et al., 2001; Just et al., 1996). Sentence or story complexity often leads to homologous right-hemisphere activation (Galliard et al.,

2001; Just et al., 1996), but some have suggested that comparable increased cortical activation occurs regardless of the nature of the stimuli (auditory or visual). This suggests that higher-level comprehension processes operate independently of input modality (Michael, Keller, Carpenter, & Just, 2001). It is not surprising that the left hemisphere is responsible for syntax, because syntax is a highly structured and rule-governed skill; however, the right hemisphere is also likely to be involved in long, complex syntactic structures (Cooke et al., 2001).

When a reader is approaching a comprehension problem, it is likely that the left hemisphere attempts to access stored word knowledge, while the right hemisphere searches for a broader range of meanings (Beeman & Chiarello, 1998). Bryan and Hale (2001) argue that the hemispheres work simultaneously during interpretation: The right hemisphere seeks discordant information through divergent processing, while the left hemisphere attempts to find information that is consistent or concordant with existing thoughts (i.e., it tries to find the "correct" answer through convergent processing). Chiarello (1998) argues that the right hemisphere is specialized for distant semantic relations (multiple meanings of ambiguous words), whereas the left hemisphere prefers closely related meanings and single interpretation. This fits well with the finding that the left frontal lobe is important for encoding new information, as it attempts to categorize and place information in long-term storage, but that the right frontal lobe is important for searching for previously learned memories, or the process of long-term memory retrieval (Tulving, Kapur, Craik, Moscovitch, & Houle, 1994). As in most of the processes we discuss in this book, both the right and left frontal areas are involved in encoding and retrieval (Menon, Boyette-Anderson, et al., 2002); it is just the division of labor that varies.

One interesting study of right-hemisphere processes in ambiguity resolution provides convincing evidence of the right hemisphere's contribution to reading comprehension. St. George, Kutas, Martinez, and Sereno (1999) used ambiguous paragraphs and provided paragraph titles for some participants (e.g., "Horseback Riding") and no titles for others. Each passage was "clearly" about a pleasurable experience that required effort and daily activity, but it was difficult to deduce the exact activity from the passage without the title. The researchers found that both titled and untitled passages resulted in activity in the inferior frontal and temporal regions, but that right-hemisphere homologues showed greater activity in the untitled or ambiguous condition. In addition, more activity in the middle temporal area was found in the right hemisphere, but the reverse was true on the left, suggesting that this area was important for the interpretive processes necessary to achieve global story coherence (St. George et al., 1999). These findings are consistent with those of other studies that show a similar bilateral activation pattern, typically in the middle temporal area, during reading of random sentences, metaphors, and fables (Bottini et al., 1994; Fletcher et al., 1995; Nichelli et al., 1995).

The right hemisphere keeps the proverbial doors open in interpretation, until the left hemisphere can help draw the appropriate conclusions about the passage. Whereas we would expect the left hemisphere to select the most probable or literal interpretation for text, children with right-hemisphere dysfunction are more likely to miss the "gist" of implicit messages. As the metaphor goes, they live in the "land of the literal." It is not surprising, then, that children with right-hemisphere dysfunction have little difficulty in elementary school, because the "correct" answer to an explicit/literal comprehension question is often provided in the text. In the story presented in Application 2.4 of Chapter 2, for example, the left hemisphere quickly picks up that the store manager's name was Ms. Smith; this is just the kind of detail the left hemisphere is looking for when a child is reading. It is likely that increased text ambiguity or complexity requires coordination between the left and right hemispheres—coordination carried out by the prefrontal cortex.

While the left hemisphere analyzes the text for syntactic structure and details, the right hemisphere explores multiple semantic relationships between words and phrases (Beeman & Chiarello, 1998). This comparing and contrasting of information can only be carried out by the brain's manager, the prefrontal cortex, with the right hemisphere developing predictive inferences and the left making connective inferences (Beeman & Chiarello, 1998).

Given our understanding of the importance of executive and novel problem-solving abilities, we are not surprised that ambiguous lexical–semantic relationships and syntactic complexity result in higher right-hemisphere and frontal activity. As the complexity of sentences increases, bilateral dorsolateral prefrontal activation is more likely (Just et al., 1996), and diffuse activity is more likely on the right than on the left side (St. George et al., 1999), consistent with our presumptions of greater association cortex in the right hemisphere (Goldberg, 2001). Some have suggested that the right frontal areas may be necessary to sustain attention, maintain contextual elements in working memory, and use implicit reasoning skills to interpret story themes (Michael et al., 2001; Price et al., 1996). These right-hemisphere skills may be essential to integrate new information into existing interpretations, or to reinterpret existing information when new information is presented (Beeman & Chiarello, 1998). However, let's not forget another important component of this left–right involvement in comprehension: Information is transferred between the hemispheres via the corpus callosum. This supports the "callosal relay model" of semantic category processing (Khateb et al., 2001). Possible differences in the anterior or posterior areas of the corpus callosum could affect the rapid transfer of information between the left and right hemispheres (Hynd et al., 1995), leading to comprehension breakdown.

You can see that multiple brain areas and neuropsychological processes are involved in reading comprehension. Not only are the basic psychological processes of word recognition included in reading comprehension, but several other higher-level skills associated with left- and right-hemisphere tertiary areas are required as well. As has been proposed by some researchers, adequate word recognition and fluency skills are important, but not sufficient, for adequate reading comprehension.

INSTRUCTIONAL STRATEGIES FOR CHILDREN WITH RDs

Individual Differences and Intervention

Now that we have a basic understanding of the neuropsychological bases of word recognition and reading comprehension, let us turn briefly to intervention. As stated in the previous chapters, we feel that a majority of children can be helped by using prereferral strategies, and for those who cannot be, comprehensive evaluation and individualized interventions may be in order. With the information on the neuropsychological bases of RDs described above, you can develop an assessment protocol designed to examine each child's unique characteristics, develop and test hypotheses about his or her strengths and weaknesses, and provide recommendations for intervention that are uniquely tailored to the child's needs. As stated in previous chapters, this is merely the *beginning* of linking assessment to intervention. Building upon your shared knowledge with the teacher, you can work collaboratively with him or her to brainstorm instructional strategies, develop data-based interventions, and evaluate the efficacy of your intervention. The continuation of the CHT model beyond the initial "diagnosis" is what allows you to be sure that interventions are effective for each child, and that your assessment results have true treatment validity.

As a result, we do not offer you a "diagnostic–prescriptive" model in this or the remaining chapters. The early attempts to find ATIs largely failed because researchers had poorly constructed measures of cognitive processes, little understanding of how the brain really worked, and interventions that were not designed to meet the unique needs of individual children (Hale & Fiorello, 2002; Hale, Fiorello, Kavanagh, Hoeppner, & Gaither, 2001). If you develop large-group ATI designs, and put heterogeneous children in each group, it is not surprising that the overall results will be insignificant. As Braden and Kratochwill (1997) appropriately argue, we cannot accept the null hypothesis about ATI—that there is no relationship between neuropsychological functioning and educational and psychosocial outcomes. We must instead continue to explore individual ATIs at the single-subject level, but this cannot happen if we fail to recognize each child's unique pattern of neuropsychological performance (Hale, Fiorello, et al., 2001). We have given you a model of neuropsychological functioning, and reliable and valid measures to tap those constructs. It is now up to you to establish concurrent, ecological, and treatment validity for each individual child.

Interventions for Word Reading and Reading Comprehension

Given the caveat above, let's explore the major interventions for word reading and reading comprehension. In addition to the ideas presented here, you may wish to purchase one or more general texts on special education or specific reading interventions. Listed in Appendix 5.2 are several of the recommended interventions for word recognition cited in the literature, and Appendix 5.3 offers ideas for reading comprehension. We make no claims as to the efficacy of these interventions, and further consultation with the sources will be necessary before you undertake any one intervention. These interventions should be beneficial for addressing many of the reading deficits described in this chapter, but programs must be tailored to the child's individual needs. In addition, recall that the use of compensation, remediation, or both is dependent on the child's age and the severity of his or her problems, as noted in Chapter 3.

READING CASE STUDY: LINKING ASSESSMENT TO INTERVENTION

The complexity of these issues is highlighted in Case Study 5.4, where we take you from assessment to intervention with a boy who appeared to have attention problems, but who was found to have a different cause for his attention and reading difficulties. As you can see from John's unique pattern of performance, he did seem at first to fit well into a category. If we are to serve the real needs of children like John, however, we must not make recommendations based on initial teacher referral questions or even preliminary test data. Instead, we can only make recommendations for such children after we understand the complexities of their cognitive profiles, and this information can be gathered through the systematic CHT approach.

John was a boy with a history of reading and attention difficulties. At the time of referral, John's teacher reported that she thought he had ADHD, inattentive type, and speculated that he might "need to be on medicine." She added, "He can't pay attention long enough to know what he's reading." A review of the history indicated that John was born a month prematurely and had a low birth weight. He had several ear infections as a young child, but was otherwise healthy. Vision and hearing were within normal limits. Prereferral and functional analysis data indicated that time on task was a significant problem, especially during reading and language arts instruction. John typically ignored the teacher during these times; he played with his materials in or on his desk, or talked quietly with a peer. The prereferral interventions decreased his off-task performance, but his reading performance was still quite poor. An analysis of his error patterns indicated a tendency to guess at words by configuration, labored oral reading with many phonemic paraphasias (letter sound errors), and a tendency to skip over unknown words. During an interview with John, he said that reading was hard, math was his favorite subject, and he preferred watching television or playing video games with his friends. Although reportedly somewhat withdrawn, John appeared to have adequate relationships with peers and family members. Other than attention problems, no aberrant behavior was reported.

On the basis of this history, what hypotheses could you generate? Although it is important to keep an open mind while developing your theory, you should be concerned about attention, executive functions, auditory processing, receptive and expressive language, and possible withdrawal/anxiety (less likely) affecting reading skills. Let's see what happened when we tested a theory.

CHT: INITIAL DATA COLLECTION

During initial testing, the teacher's ratings suggested clinical-range attention problems and elevated withdrawal, but the parents' ratings were in the typical range. This could be a difference in environments or expectations, so we shouldn't rule out ADHD yet. Direct observation, sentence completion, and clinical interview results suggested that John had some preference for being alone, but that he was generally well liked by his peers, and his family relationships were reportedly strong. John presented as a somewhat quiet child, but he was generally pleasant, engaged, related, and relaxed during the evaluation. He did, however, begin to fidget during the reading subtests. The following initial cognitive and achievement (limited to reading) testing results were obtained.

WECHSLER INTELLIGENCE SCALE FOR CHILDREN—THIRD EDITION (WISC-III)

IQ/Index scores	SS	%ile	95% confidence interval
Full Scale IQ (FSIQ)	92	30	87–98
Verbal IQ (VIQ)	89	23	83–96
Verbal Comprehension (VC)	91	27	85–98
Freedom from Distractibility (FD)/Working Memory (WM)	81	10	74–93
Performance IQ (PIQ)	98	45	90–106
Perceptual Organization (PO)	102	55	93–110
Processing Speed (PS)	99	47	89–109

Verbal subtests	SS	Performance subtests	SS
Information	8	Picture Completion	12
Similarities	6	Coding	7
Arithmetic	7	Picture Arrangement	9
Vocabulary	10	Block Design	10
Comprehension	9	Object Assembly	10
Digit Span (6F, 3B)	6	Symbol Search	12

(continued)

WECHSLER INDIVIDUAL ACHIEVEMENT TEST—SECOND EDITION (WIAT-II)

Subtest	SS	Supplemental scores	Quartile
Word Reading	68	Target Words	1
Reading Comprehension	79	Reading Speed	1
Pseudoword Decoding	65		

First, let's look at the WISC-III results. Can you tell which global scores should be used if you were asked to calculate concordance and discordance statistics? The FSIQ at first glance seems valid, because there is no significant difference between the VIQ and PIQ SSs. Moving top-down, however, we see that Vocabulary is significantly higher than Similarities, so the VIQ SS is invalid, and this would also rule out VC. So, from the bottom up, VC, VIQ, and FSIQ cannot be interpreted. Moving top-down for the PIQ SS, there is a significant difference between Picture Completion and Coding, resulting in PIQ invalidity (you could substitute Symbol Search, however; see Reynolds, Sanchez, & Wilson, 1996). However, the PO SS of 102 is valid, because there are no significant differences between the subtests that compose it. With this as our "processing strength" measure, we find that John's PO is discordant in all areas of reading, with Word Reading and Pseudoword Decoding being the most impaired. So now we need a "processing weakness" measure for the concordance analysis. What cognitive processes are most associated with reading? We (Hale, Fiorello, et al., 2001) found the VC and FD/WM factors to be most closely related to word recognition and reading comprehension. Since we found that VC is not valid, we are left with FD, which is valid. The concordance analysis found no difference between FD and Reading Comprehension, but there almost was a difference found with Word Reading—with this subtest even lower than expected, given the cognitive weakness. This tells us that there might be some other cognitive processing weaknesses not accounted for by the FD/WM.

In terms of subtest performance, John certainly was better at Performance tasks, suggesting good visual discrimination, perceptual analysis, visual memory, and holistic/global processes. With the scores fairly comparable, you should not interpret slight subtest differences. However, John's Coding SS was low, compared to the SSs for other measures. Examining this and other measures suggests that low psychomotor speed could have affected his score, but it could also be a problem with number–symbol association, visual working memory, graphomotor skills, or attention/executive function. John's Verbal subtest scores were also comparatively low, but (surprisingly) his Vocabulary score was adequate, suggesting good word knowledge and semantic information. Verbal retrieval could be a problem, however, as it is generally easier to use expressive language skills to compensate on Vocabulary and Comprehension. Sure enough, John did fairly well on these subtests, because he was able to use lengthy, circumlocutious speech to respond successfully. Certainly the Arithmetic and Digit Span scores were low, but not that much different from those for the other Verbal subtests. The 6 Forward and 3 Backward scores on Digit Span could suggest attention or executive problems, so we need to look further into this performance profile.

Take a minute to think of the measures you would use for hypothesis testing in this case. What brain areas do you think could be involved for John? Why were his Coding results different from those for the other Performance subtests? These initial findings might lead you to be concerned about attention, auditory–verbal, and reading skills, but not visual–spatial/holistic processes.

(continued)

CHT: CONFIRMING OR REFUTING HYPOTHESES

Several measures were used to test hypotheses about John's cognitive strengths and weaknesses, including the NEPSY, CTOPP, the WJ-III, and others.

Visual–motor	SS	Verbal/phonemic	SS
NEPSY		CTOPP	
Arrows	95	Elision	65
Visuomotor Precision	84	WJ-III	
Developmental Test of VMI	88	Sound Blending	70
Halstead–Reitan		Incomplete Words	78
Finger Tapping	105		
		Verbal/orthographic/fluency	
Attention/executive function		CTOPP	
Conners Continuous Performance Test II		Rapid Letter Naming	86
Omissions	115	Rapid Digit Naming	83
Commissions	105	NEPSY	
Reaction Time	98	Speeded Naming	92
Reaction Time Block Change	100		
Reaction Time Interstimulus	97	Verbal long-term memory retrieval/fluency	
Interval Change		WISC-III Processing Instrument	
Cognitive Assessment System		Information	95
Planned Directions	105	NEPSY	
Expressive Attention	96	Verbal Fluency	90
NEPSY			
Tower	112		
WJ-III			
Numbers Reversed	98		
Planning	105		

In addition to testing these hypotheses, I (Hale) administered the WJ-III Reading Fluency subtest because I was worried about fluency problems, and found John's score to be in the low average range. What do these results suggest? Remember what we said about conclusions in Chapter 3: The strength of the data determines what we conclude and how we report the findings.

Let's begin with what areas appeared to be adequate. This is a good strategy in interpretation and report writing. When we look at the results of the attention and executive function measures, we see that John appeared to have good attention and executive functions (including working memory), suggesting that at least the orbital and dorsolateral areas were adequate. We need to find an alternative explanation for the attention problems, and the history and observations suggested that it could be a problem with auditory processing/phonological awareness/language. However, let's look at visual–motor skills first. These skills appeared to be specifically affected by the use of a pencil, so graphomotor skills rather than simple motor speed was affected. Because John's visual–spatial skills appeared to be strong, and the Planning subtest did not appear to be affected, we should be more concerned with the left somatosensory or motor primary or secondary premotor or supplementary motor cortex. So this leaves us concerned with auditory and verbal fluency skills, because John would appear to have a classic "double deficit" RD. It seems clear that he had difficulty with phonemic awareness. Although he did seem to have some difficulty with rapid naming, his verbal fluency and long-term memory retrieval appeared to

(continued)

be pretty good, and processing speed on other measures was adequate. So we have good support suggesting that John's problems were due to auditory processing, the most common type of RD, which is typically associated with problems in the superior temporal region in the primary and association auditory cortex. We have some support for a rapid naming/fluency problem, but the data were inconsistent, so our conclusions must be tentative at best.

Could any other data shed light on our findings? What about the WISC-III Similarities and Coding scores? First, John's semantic knowledge appeared to be adequate in general, and his Information and Similarities scores could be partially related to performance anxiety or retrieval. But the Similarities subtest was quite hard for him, despite his adequate word knowledge. Remember that his speech was characterized by circumlocutions, articulation errors, and limited verbal fluency. Could another area beyond the prefrontal cortex be causing these difficulties? This is a hard one. Could it be the cingulate, corpus callosum, or arcuate fasciculus, which connect the different regions? The cingulate is associated with memory retrieval, and we might postulate that John's attention and retrieval issues were not prefrontal, but secondary to difficulties with efficient cingulate activity. But processing speed is again adequate for nonverbal material, so we are again pointed toward a more posterior focus, with cingulate/anterior problems secondary. So although we cannot say that John definitely had a "classic" double-deficit RD, he had enough of a problem that he might benefit from instructional support to improve oral/reading fluency and flexibility in word choice, and possibly from extended testing time for auditory/linguistic information. Finally, the Coding problem has not been resolved. John's visual–spatial skills seemed fine, his basic motor skills were adequate, and his executive motor control seemed intact—so he should be able to draw well, right? Well, these could be signs of the frontal–basal ganglia–cerebellar problem discussed in connection with fluency in the text. This makes sense, as articulation and other fine motor problems were evident. However, recall that the left parietal cortex is needed to provide somatosensory feedback to the motor system in the right hand. Also, recall that the left inferior parietal cortex is also responsible for integrating sound–symbol relationships, so this could possibly fit with our data. Interestingly, although John's Block Design score was adequate, he had three block reversal errors. This is another situation when going beyond the summative score to understand the underlying psychological processes can help us understand a child's unique pattern of performance. (Of course, it might also have helped if his numerous letter reversals had been mentioned.)

CHT: LINKING ASSESSMENT TO INTERVENTION

Although these hypotheses regarding John's pattern of performance provide us with insight into possible areas of strength and need, they remain somewhat speculative. They do, however, give us important starting points for intervention. Remember that understanding a child's strengths and needs from a neuropsychological perspective merely helps us develop strategies that might be effective for a child. In John's case, I worked collaboratively with John's teacher, and we developed a phonemic awareness and sound–symbol association intervention. John listened to and read words in graded passages, charting his own accuracy and time. Error responses were used as stimuli for phonemes/graphemes/morphemes practice sessions, in which John used note cards. He made steady progress in these areas. When I retested his processing speed, rapid naming skills, and reading speed and comprehension, I found that John had improved somewhat in these areas, scoring within the average range; this suggested that these issues had interfered with reading fluency and comprehension. In addition, we continued the prereferral program to increase John's on-task performance, and his attention problems began to decline across academic subjects. Had only the initial test results, and the teacher's complaints about attention, been used to make diagnostic and intervention decisions, John might have been referred to his pediatrician for an ADHD assessment. Obviously, based on the data we present here, John would not have benefited from medication treatment.

APPENDIX 5.1. Significant Instructional Components in Swanson and Colleagues' Meta-Analysis of LD Treatment

	WR	P	RC (all)	RC (ex DV)	GR	S	W	M	SE
Sequencing—Breaking down the task, fading of prompts or cues, matching the difficulty level of the task to the child, sequencing short activities and/or using step-by-step prompts.		*				**			0.89 Lg
Drill/repetition and practice/review—Mastery criteria, distributed review and practice, use of redundant materials or text, repeated practice, sequenced reviews, daily feedback, and/or weekly reviews.	*					*			0.96 Lg
Anticipatory or preparatory responses—Asking the child to look over material prior to instruction, directing the child to focus on material or concepts prior to instruction, providing information to prepare the child for discussion, and/or stating the learning objectives for the lesson prior to instruction.							**		
Strategy modeling + attribution training—Processing components or multisteps related to modeling from the teacher; simplified demonstrations modeled by the teacher to solve a problem or complete a task successfully; teacher modeling; teacher providing child with reminders to use certain strategies, steps, and/or procedures; use of think-aloud models; and/or the teacher presenting the benefits of taught strategies.	*								0.89 Lg
Probing reinforcement—Intermittent or consistent use of probes, daily feedback, fading of prompts and cues, and/or overt administration of rewards and reinforcers.							*		
Segmentation—Breaking down the targeted skill into smaller units, breaking it into component parts, or segmenting and/or synthesizing component parts.						**			0.85 Lg
Technology—Use of formal curricula, newly developed pictorial representations, specific material or computers, and/or other media to facilitate presentation and feedback.						*			0.88 Lg
Modeling by teacher of steps—Modeling from the teacher in terms of demonstration of processes and/or steps the children are to follow.					*				
Small-group instruction—Instruction in a small group, and/or verbal interaction occurring in a small group with children and/or teacher.								*	0.93 Lg
One-on-one instruction—Independent practice, tutoring, individually paced or tailored instruction.									0.86 Lg
A supplement to teacher involvement besides peers—Homework, parents' help in reinforcing instruction, and the like.							*		2.00 Lg
Control of difficulty—Short activities, level of difficulty controlled, task analysis, tasks sequenced from easy to difficult, teacher providing necessary assistance or simplified demonstration.									1.10 Lg
Strategy cues without attribution training—Reminders to use strategies or multisteps, teacher verbalizing steps or procedures to solve problems, use of think-aloud models, and/or teacher presenting the benefits of strategy use or procedures.		*							0.74 Md
Weighted mean effect sizes for interventions in each academic area	0.61 Md	0.64 Md	0.82 Lg	0.90 Lg	0.42 Sm	0.46 Sm	0.66 Md	0.45 Sm	

Note. Definitions taken from Swanson, Hoskyn, and Lee (1999, pp. 30–32). exp DV, Experimental Dependent Variable; WR, word recognition; P, phonology; RC, reading comprehension; GR, general reading; S, spelling; W, writing; M, math; SE, significant effect; Lg, large; Md, medium; Sm, small.
*Significant at $p < .05$. **Significant at $p < .01$.

APPENDIX 5.2. Word Recognition Interventions

Reference	Intervention description
Berninger (1998)	"Talking letters," pseudoword instruction for phonemic awareness and processing
Berninger et al. (2001)	Teaching phonemic, orthographic, and fluency components within a temporal framework, including repeated reading, precision teaching, and/or metacognitive instruction (including self-monitoring/evaluation)
Bowers (1993)	Repeated reading for word recognition automaticity and reading fluency
Breznitz (1997)	Improving fluency by increasing rate over self-paced reading
Browder & Lalli (1991)	Sight word instruction using antecedent stimulus control (errorless learning) and fading of added stimuli (prompt elimination/stimulus fading); presenting easy-to-hard discrimination
Carnine et al. (1997)	Synthetic phonics approach or phonological assembly
Cunningham (1979)	Phonemic awareness training incorporated in regular reading lessons
Engelmann et al. (1999)	Corrective reading program featuring synthetic phonics, sound–symbol association, sequencing, blending, and comprehension, through demonstration, modeling, frequent student response, feedback
Fawcett & Nicholson (2001)	Automaticity instruction using direct instruction, task analysis, and mastery
Fernald (1988); Fry et al. (1984)	Popular multisensory "VAKT" (visual–auditory–kinesthetic–tactile) strategy Sight word list of most commonly used words in English ordered by frequency of occurrence, covering 90% of all written material
Folk & Campbell (1978)	Instruction in functional or survival reading of sight words
Glass & Glass (1978)	"Glass analysis" for teaching letter clusters or morphemes
Iversen & Tunmer (1993)	Focus and phoneme–grapheme correspondence in related words, and on phonological coding
Kirk et al. (1985)	Focus on duration and sequence of sounds in words
Lenz & Hughes (1990)	"DISSECT"; Discovering content, isolating prefix, separating suffix, saying stem, examining stem, checking with someone, trying a dictionary for unknown words
Levy (2001)	Segmentation training, leading to rapid acquisition of words and orthographic patterns
Levy et al. (1997)	Word-reading practice followed by story reading
Lovett et al. (1994)	Systematic phonological analysis and blending program
Lovett et al. (2000)	Metacognitive phonics program to improve word recognition skills
Meyer & Felton (1999)	Repeated reading technique for improved fluency
Orton-Gillingham & Stillman (1973)	Highly structured multisensory approach, focusing on 48 English phonemes and rules for consonant and vowel combinations
Read Naturally (1997)	Rereading of high-interest passages at instructional level, self-charting time, answering questions, and summarizing
Simmons, Gunn, et al. (1994)	Phonological awareness training, including auditory analysis, explicit to implicit, word properties, scaffolding of blending/segmenting, integration of sound–symbol associations
Stewart & Cegelka (1995)	Systematic phonics approach modeling, letter hierarchy, pacing, blending, digraphs, irregular words, connected text reading
Torgesen et al. (2001)	Systematic instruction in phonemic and orthographic skills for accuracy, repeated reading with peer, feedback regarding accuracy and fluency
Williams (1980)	"ABDs of reading": Focus on phonemic analysis and sound blending

APPENDIX 5.3. Reading Comprehension Interventions

Reference	Intervention description
Adams (1990)	Systematic phonics instruction with reading connected text; repeated readings for word recognition, fluency, and comprehension
Beck & McKeown (1981)	Story-mapping procedure for determining plot, theme, and question format
Bos & Van Reusen (1991)	Interactive learning, linking prior knowledge with text and prediction
Carnine & Kinder (1985)	Identifying text characters, goal, action, and outcome
Carnine et al. (1997)	Vocabulary definition, providing positive and negative examples, reviewing new and old words
Chan & Cole (1986)	Metacognitive training, including student-made questions, underlining words of interest, and self-questioning
Chan et al. (1987)	Monitoring narrative text for inconsistent sentences
Clark et al. (1984)	"RIDER": Read, image, describe, evaluate, repeat
Eeds & Cockrum (1985)	Teacher interaction method: Activating common experiences, recording individual experiences, recording nonexample, and translating into own words
Englert & Mariage (1991)	"POSSE": Predict, organize, search, summarize, evaluate (in reciprocal teaching format)
Fuchs et al. (1997)	"PALS": Peer tutoring program of partner reading, paragraph summary, prediction
Grant (1993)	"SCROLL": Surveying, connecting, reading, outlining, looking for comprehension
Heckelman (1986)	Presenting method with three phases: Auditory, paraphrasing, echoing
Gurney et al. (1990)	Story grammar technique for identifying conflict, characters, resolution, theme
Idol & Croll (1987)	Story mapping graphic organizer for setting, problem, goal, action, outcome
Idol-Maestas (1985)	"TELLS" advanced organizer: Studying story titles, examining pages for clues, looking for key words, looking for difficult words, evaluating setting for fact–fiction decision
Jenkins et al. (1987)	Restatement procedure for story retelling in own words and in writing
Johnson & Pearson (1984)	Semantic mapping technique: Brainstorming multiple words associated with stimulus word (teaches semantic categorization and fluency)
Mercer & Mercer (2001)	High-interest/low-vocabulary technique for older children; use of Fry readability formula to foster motivation
Palinscar & Brown (1988)	Reciprocal teaching; comprehension monitoring through predicting, questioning, summarizing, clarifying
Robinson (1961)	"SQ3R": Surveying, questioning, reading, reciting, reviewing
Rye (1982)	Cloze/maze technique: Fill-in-blank strategy (free-recall or multiple-choice)
Sachs (1983)	"DRA": Directed reading activity (solicits student interest through own experience)
Samuels (1979)	Repeated readings of same text until read fluently
Schumaker et al. (1982)	"MULTIPASS," "Survey Pass," "Size-Up Pass," "Sort-Out Pass"; also strategies for word identification, visual imagery, self-questioning, paraphrasing
Simmons, Chard, et al. (1994)	Directed reading of basal readers with supplemental modeling and phonological awareness instruction
Simmonds (1992)	"QAR": Question–answer relationships; identification of "Right There" (text explicit), "Think and Search" (text implicit), and "On My Own" (script implicit) comprehension questions
Sinatra et al. (1985)	Semantic mapping, providing graphic outline of story and linking parts together (can be used before, during, or after reading)
Williams et al. (2002)	Direct instruction approach of explanation, modeling, guided practice, and independent practice to teach story themes
Wolf, Miller, et al. (2000)	"RAVE-O": Retrieval, automaticity, vocabulary elaboration, and orthography (addresses automaticity at lower-process and higher-concept levels)
Wong & Jones (1982)	Self-questioning to identify purpose, main idea, reading to answer question
Wood et al. (2001)	Prediction used for anticipatory fluency and goal-directedness in reading

CHAPTER 6

The Neuropsychology of Mathematics Disorders

CHARACTERISTICS OF CHILDREN WITH MATHEMATICS DISORDERS

Is Math Different?

As we have noted in Chapter 5, much more is known about reading disorders (RDs) than about mathematics disorders (MDs) and other types of learning disorders (LDs). Because there is so much emphasis on reading in teacher-training programs, teachers find themselves struggling with mathematics computation and word problem instruction, especially when children have difficulty in these areas. Many children with math problems also have problems in reading and written language, and in these cases there may be similar neuropsychological reasons for their difficulties. Some children with MDs have significant psychosocial concerns, while others seem to be well adjusted. The reasons for their differential presentation can be environmental, biological, or (most likely) some combination of both. Some children are quite anxious when it comes to math skills; others take great pleasure in learning math concepts and computation skills. Recognizing how children with MDs solve math problems, and what types of errors they commit, can provide us with an understanding of how to remediate or compensate for their deficient performance. As we have stressed throughout this book, each child's MD is unique in some way, and a thorough investigation may reveal different underlying causes for his or her difficulties, as can be seen in Case Study 6.1.

Basic Components of Math Competency

To understand the underlying neurospsychological processes required for math competency, it is important to recognize how math skills develop. What do children need in order to learn math skills? In his discussion of concrete operations, Piaget (1965) taught us about several important underlying concepts critical for math competency, including one-to-one correspondence, classification, seriation, and conservation. When children are learning about quantity and operations (es-

CASE STUDY 6.1. Lessons in Learning: Making Math Count for Mary

I (Hale) had Mary, an 8-year-old girl, referred to me for a comprehensive evaluation because of her persistent difficulty with math computation and word problems (the latter was especially problematic). When I met with the teacher, Jane, to discuss the case, she said that no matter how hard Mary tried, "she just didn't get it." Although Jane was hard pressed to provide details, she said that Mary's homework wasn't too bad, but that she couldn't remember how to do the work during board time (when children did problems at the board) or on tests. Jane suspected that Mary's concerned mother was helping her complete her homework, which took "hours" every night. I looked at Mary's file and permanent products, always finding the same pattern: fairly good homework performance and abysmal test scores. When I conducted the initial evaluation, I found some signs of retrieval and processing speed difficulties, but these findings were inconsistent. My CHT did not sufficiently support these deficits, and again findings were inconsistent. I noticed that Mary did much better on multiple-choice than on free-recall tasks, consistent with retrieval problems; however, her language skills and verbal fluency were intact. In addition, Mary did fine with math computation, had greater difficulty with word problems, and performed quite poorly on a math fluency subtest. Mary's math problems were a neuropsychological mystery.

When there appears to be no consistent pattern of performance borne out during CHT, it may be because there are no real neuropsychological deficits, and you should look for psychosocial explanations. The personality/behavioral evaluation results revealed signs of anxiety, withdrawal, depression, and isolation. Mary also had low self-esteem and unresolved attachment issues. In addition, Mary said during the interview that she had always hated math, became nervous when she had to work at the board, and froze during the math tests. She felt "stupid" when it came to doing math, and "sick" when it came time to take tests. As you will see in Chapter 8, there is a strong interrelationship between psychosocial and neuropsychological functioning, and Mary's case seemed to be a prime example of this. After the evaluation was completed, it became clear that Mary's problems were largely related to psychosocial issues. I subsequently worked with the teacher to develop an intervention to increase Mary's sense of math self-efficacy, enhance her test-taking skills, and improve her peer relationships. This was combined with anxiety management strategies (systematic desensitization, relaxing breaths, and progressive muscle relaxation). We also suggested strategies to improve the mother–daughter relationship and decrease homework completion time. Mary's performance began to improve over the following months, and eventually she gained confidence in her math skills. Soon thereafter, Mary began to do just as well in class and on tests as she had during her homework sessions, and her homework only took a half hour every night.

pecially addition), teachers often use concrete objects at first, then move on to semiabstract symbols, and finally use numbers. From these basic skills, students learn addition, subtraction, multiplication, division, and fractions in a hierarchical fashion. Most researchers recommend introduction of word problems early during this sequence, if not at the very beginning. More advanced areas, such as geometry and algebra, are not always taught in the same order or in the same grade. Although math instruction is fairly predictable, it is important to examine each child's curriculum and exposure to different math concepts before determining whether the child has a math deficit on the basis of standardized tests. As many children will tell you, one reason they can't do a particular math operation is "We haven't done that yet."

There has been some debate about the core cognitive features associated with math competency, because visual–spatial, linguistic, and working memory skills are needed for math computation (Dehaene, Spelke, Pinel, Stanescu, & Tsivkin, 1999; Keogh, 1994; McLean & Hitch, 1999). Semantic or declarative knowledge of math facts and quantitative relationships is an important component of math computation skills (Byrnes, 2001). In addition to facts, one needs to have procedural knowledge of how to carry out operations, which also requires an understanding of math syntax (Hiebert & LeFevre, 1987) and visual-perceptual–motor skills for mechanical arithmetic computation (Rourke, 1994). McCloskey, Aliminosa, and Sokol (1991) suggest that adequate computation skills require both a number-processing system for understanding quantity and a calculation system for retrieving information and carrying out algorithmic procedures.

These findings suggest that there are several possible types of MDs. As noted in Chapter 5, part of linking assessment to intervention requires an examination of the types of cognitive and achievement errors a child displays during testing. As is the case with reading error patterns, it is important for you to identify the child's math error patterns during your comprehensive cognitive hypothesis-testing (CHT) evaluation. This cannot always be ascertained by looking at the child's final answers, so if error types are found, it is often helpful to have the child verbalize the algorithm steps as he or she completes the problem. Take, for example, the following verbalization from a child named Lucy as she solved a problem:

64	*"First I look and see if it is addition or subtraction. OK, addition, so you always*
+ 13	*go top to bottom and left to right. So I add 6 + 4, and that equals 10, and then*
14	*1 + 3 equals 4, and then I add them together, top to bottom, 10 + 4 equals 14."*

As you can see, what at first seems to be a random response, or a poor attempt at subtraction, becomes clear from Lucy's commentary. Her simple addition is OK, but she has little concept of place value or of the algorithm she needs to respond successfully to such two-digit problems. Look for these and other error patterns when you are conducting CHT evaluations for children with MDs. The following error patterns (with abbreviations that you can use in making notes) are frequently found in children with various types of MDs:

- Math fact error (FE)—Child has not learned math fact, or does not automatically retrieve it from long-term memory.
- Operand error (OE)—Child performs one operation instead of another (e.g., performs 6 + 3 for 6 – 3 problem).
- Algorithm error (AE)—Child performs steps out of sequence, or follows idiosyncratic algorithm or pattern of solving problem (e.g., subtracting larger from smaller number, regardless of position: 123 – 87 = 164).
- Place value error (PE)—Child carries out the steps in order, but makes a place value error (which could be due to visual–spatial processes, but also to algorithm problems).
- Regrouping errors (RE)—Child regroups when not required, forgets to subtract from regrouped column during subtraction, or adds regrouped number before multiplication.

Prevalence of MDs

There has been considerably more research on reading and RDs than on math and MDs. This is somewhat surprising, since prevalence rates indicate that RDs and MDs are each found in about 6% of the population (Fleischner, 1994; Geary, Hamson, & Hoard, 2000; Mazzocco, 2001). There is some debate as to the nature of MDs in relation to RDs and other LDs. Whereas some have suggested that MDs can be unique LDs (Rourke, 1993), others suggest that MDs are due to more generalized LDs, they frequently co-occur with other LDs (Fleischner, 1994). MDs and RDs may share some of the same underlying processing difficulties, as they often co-occur, with comorbidity estimates reaching as high as 40% (Geary, 1993; Light & DeFries, 1995). Although this could suggest a common underlying deficit associated with MDs and RDs, others are quick to point out that poor instructional techniques and textbooks could take the blame for some math problems (Engelmann, Carnine, & Steely, 1991). Because math instruction is sequential and hierarchical, students with learning problems quickly fall behind (Cawley & Miller, 1989); without intervention, most fail to benefit from instruction beyond the seventh grade (Warner, Alley, Schumaker, Deshler, & Clark, 1980).

MDs AND BRAIN FUNCTIONS

Subtypes of MDs

How can you tell whether a child has an MD or not? You may be thinking that we will provide you with a "red flag" test predictor, but actually longitudinal studies show that the best predictor to date is repeated math failure in multiple areas across grades (Geary et al., 2000). Some think that MD is synonymous with the neuropsychological term "dyscalculia," a specific impairment in math computation or concepts (Fleischner, 1994); as we have discussed earlier, however, the likelihood of a "pure" MD in the children you see is unlikely. Instead, you should become familiar with the subtypes of MDs and the ways they are likely to affect academic achievement across the domains. Consistent with the cognitive skills needed for math as described above, researchers have found several types of MDs. Although there is variability between and within subtypes, there is a growing consensus that at least three types of MD exist: the *semantic memory, procedural,* and *visual–spatial* subtypes (Mazzocco, 2001). The *semantic-memory subtype* is characterized by poor number–symbol association and math fact automaticity. This subtype often has comorbid RDs and language disorders. The *procedural subtype* often involves poor strategy or algorithm use, and has been associated with attention-deficit/hyperactivity disorder (ADHD). Finally, the visual–spatial subtype includes problems with column alignment, place values, and operand adherence. This is the subtype most often associated with Rourke's (1994) nonverbal learning disabilities.

The semantic-memory subtype commonly co-occurs with the other LDs, so problems with oral and/or written language are common. Similar to the symbolic relationships discussed in connection with word recognition, number processing requires translation of verbal to Arabic numbers (Seron & Fayol, 1994), so sound–symbol (number) association is important in math as well. Quantitative concepts are similar to other semantic knowledge, and the number–symbol association is similar to the letter–symbol association found for reading. Children gradually learn to associate concrete, semiconcrete, and then abstract representations of this quantitative–symbolic relationship, as highlighted in In-Depth 6.1.

Not surprisingly, children with the semantic-memory subtype of MD have difficulty with learning and/or retrieving basic math facts from memory. They take longer amounts of time to retrieve facts, and their retrieval accuracy is typically poor (Geary, 1993). Because these children are likely to have comorbid RDs, they are at risk for poorer math performance, especially in the areas of number comprehension and production (Geary, Hoard, & Hamson, 1999). As the name of this MD subtype suggests, cognitive assessment indicates that these children have problems with phonological and/or semantic memory, not the working memory problems found for children with the procedural subtype (Geary, 1993; Geary et al., 1999). Drawing upon their extensive research

IN-DEPTH 6.1. Developmental Progression of Basic Arithmetic

Most children learn initial quantitative relationships by simply counting, using a one-to-one correspondence. As the developmental progression advances, a typical sequence of quantitative knowledge and computation skills is observed. As Geary and colleagues (2000) describe, children gradually shift from counting on fingers, to verbal counting, and then to using what these authors call the MIN (counting on), MAX, or SUM (counting all) procedures until memory-based strategies are used. For the MIN procedure, children usually take the larger addend as a starting point, and then count the quantity necessary to reach the smaller number total (e.g., 7 + 3 = 7, 8-9-10). In the SUM procedure, the child starts at 1 and counts both numbers (e.g., 1-2-3-4-5-6-7, 8-9-10). The MAX procedure starts with the smaller addend, and then counts up from there (e.g., 3, 4-5-6-7-8-9-10). Developmentally, after finger and verbal counting, SUM and MAX are typically used, but MIN is the last procedure to emerge prior to obtaining math fact automaticity. Not only are children with MDs (especially those with comorbid RDs) more likely to use SUM and MAX procedures, but they continue to use these strategies when their peers have attained automaticity of basic math facts (Geary et al., 2000).

findings, Geary and colleagues (1999) concluded that both children with comorbid MDs/RDs and those with only RDs have difficulty encoding and retrieving information from long-term memory; this difficulty affects quantitative knowledge, number concepts, counting, arithmetic skills, and cognitive functions beyond the influence of global intelligence.

Children with the procedural subtype of MD demonstrate adequate quantitative knowledge and quantity–symbol relationships, but their computation and strategy use are characterized by slow processing speed, and they make many calculation errors (Geary, 1993). As a result, they tend to rely on immature strategies such as SUM or MIN (see In-Depth 6.1) to solve problems (Geary, 1993), possibly because they have difficulty with retrieval of quantitative information from long-term memory. A major difference between the semantic memory and procedural subtypes is related to attention and executive function, with cognitive assessments demonstrating that children with the procedural subtype have considerable difficulty manipulating information in working memory (Geary et al., 1999; Hitch & McAuley, 1991). Irrelevant associations in working memory could lead to the increased error rates and delayed reaction times seen in some children with MDs (Conway & Engle, 1994), as well as their overreliance on immature counting strategies. Consistent with findings suggesting that Digits Backward performance is related to attention and executive functions (Hale, Fiorello, & Hoeppner, 2001), children with this subtype perform worse on Digits Backward than do those with comorbid MDs/RDs or the semantic-memory subtype (Geary et al., 1999). It is likely that the procedural subtype involves executive deficits, which lead to limited flexibility, sequencing errors, and difficulty with maintaining information in working memory.

Given this evidence suggesting that children with the procedural subtype of MD are more likely to experience attention and executive function deficits, you should not be surprised to find that MDs have been associated with the inattentive type, but not the hyperactive–impulsive type, of ADHD (Marshall, Schafer, O'Donnell, Elliott, & Handwerk, 1999). However, some researchers have noted that children with MDs and ADHD have problems with fact retrieval (Zentall, 1990), which has been associated with activity level (Zentall, Smith, Yung-bin, & Wieczorek, 1994). Although it makes neuropsychological sense that the inattentive type of ADHD is more likely to be accompanied by characteristics of procedural MD than the hyperactive–impulsive type, the Zentall and colleagues (1994) study seems to contradict this assumption. Perhaps the overactivity and impulsivity symptoms interact with online monitoring of retrieval strategies and status (see the discussion of orbital and cingulate functions in Chapter 2), so the semantic memory problems are qualitatively different in children with ADHD. However, it is important to remember that there is a high degree of comorbidity among these conditions, and that finding "pure" samples is rare. In fact, the Zentall and colleagues study's sample with ADHD had problems in reading and understanding math concepts, not in math problem solving per se, which would suggest that they really had a procedural and/or semantic memory subtype of MD.

The third subtype of MD, the visual–spatial subtype, has been researched and described extensively by Byron Rourke at the University of Windsor. Using Goldberg and Costa's (1981) model (see Chapter 2), Rourke (1988) has suggested that right-hemisphere dysfunction is largely due to a white matter syndrome affecting the right hemisphere. Recall that the right hemisphere has more association cortex, as well as more white than gray matter to allow for intersensory integration. In his studies of hundreds of children with LDs, Rourke (1994) has provided convincing evidence that children with this subtype of MD have poor visual–spatial–organizational, psychomotor, tactile-perceptual, and concept formation skills, but adequate rote, automatic, verbal skills; this combination leads to pedantic speech, social isolation, low self-esteem, depression, anxiety, and of course MDs. They also show semantic problems when verbal information is complex or novel, which can lead to comprehension deficits. As you can see, children with this MD subtype have numerous nonverbal and verbal problems, but for some reason, the primary focus of researchers and clinicians has been on their visual and spatial deficits.

Support for Rourke's findings can be found in multiple studies of children with MDs and attention problems (Semrud-Clikeman & Hynd, 1990). In a comparison of children with RDs, MDs, and both, White, Moffitt, and Silva (1992) found that only children with MDs had a nonverbal learning disability neuropsychological profile, but socioemotional problems were found for all groups. Moreover, they found that 18% of the variance in math performance was accounted for by visual–spatial skills, 3% was accounted for by verbal skills, and 8% was accounted for by visual–motor integration. This pattern has also been found in psychiatric populations, where children with symptoms of right-hemisphere white matter dysfunction had arithmetic difficulties and showed significant levels of depression (Cleaver & Whitman, 1998). In another study of those with right-hemisphere dysfunction, two-thirds had poor math computation skills due to visual–spatial column alignment and poor math fact automatization (Gross-Tsur, Shalev, Manor, & Amir, 1995). Interestingly, some children with MDs show slow counting speed and difficulty with retaining numbers in working memory during counting (Hitch & McAuley, 1991), which are somewhat similar to the orthographic/fluency problems experienced in children with RDs. In the Marshall and colleagues (1999) ADHD study described earlier, the calculation errors and higher WISC Verbal than Performance scores for children with the inattentive type of ADHD led the researchers to suggest that this type could be similar to nonverbal learning disabilities. Although these findings certainly support the substantial database from the University of Windsor, they do not answer an important diagnostic question: Are the problems associated with this subtype right frontal (difficulties with novel problem solving), right posterior (visual–spatial–holistic problems), or both? Could there be two separate "nonverbal learning disability" subtypes, related to right anterior and posterior deficits? This certainly makes sense, as highlighted in Case Study 6.2. More importantly, if these different subtypes exist, do children with each subtype require instruction that is more carefully tailored to their particular needs?

CASE STUDY 6.2. Jerry's Nonverbal Learning Disorder

I (Hale) was asked to do a reevaluation of Jerry, a child with a "nonverbal learning disorder," who had been diagnosed with Asperger syndrome and a MD by a clinical psychologist 3 years prior to my evaluation. He was currently in a resource room setting for math and written language instruction, and was receiving social skills instruction and counseling. The special education teacher, Lisa, told me that Jerry was doing well with his math calculations, but he was having difficulty with word problems and still had difficulty with peer and adult interactions. She said that drawing lines to ensure column alignment had worked well, but he had never really had a problem with writing his numbers or letters, and his written language problems involved ideas and organization rather than handwriting. For word problems, Jerry couldn't seem to sort the relevant from the irrelevant information, or to turn the verbal information into written equations. I asked the school psychologist, Fred, about the social skills instruction, and Fred said that he was teaching Jerry to recognize facial and verbal affect by labeling different pictures and voices with emotions. Jerry reportedly had done so well with this affect recognition intervention that Fred was thinking about discontinuing the service, until he talked with Lisa about Jerry's continuing social problems. Fred thought that maybe Jerry just needed additional instruction, so that he could generalize the skills he had learned to the classroom environment.

Reviewing the previous psychological evaluation, I found the telltale WISC-III Verbal–Performance split, which was 22 points. Jerry also had relative difficulty with Arithmetic and Comprehension compared to his other Verbal subtests, but these scores were well above his Performance subtest scores, and Digit Span (both Digits Forward and Digits Backward) was fine. Surprisingly, his score on the Developmental Test of Visual–Motor Integration was pretty good and in the low average range. Rating scale data generally showed social and attention problems. I conducted a CHT evaluation with the Woodcock–Johnson III (WJ-III) as my screening intellectual/cognitive instrument. I found that Jerry's *Gv* (visual–spatial) and *Gs* scores were just fine. He had some relative difficulty with the *Gsm* subtests (measures of attention, working memory and executive function), but these processes did not appear to be impaired. Where were Jerry's nonverbal deficits that were seen on the WISC-III? They were there all the time, but assuming they were related to visual-perceptual difficulties had led the special education teacher and the school psychologist down the wrong intervention path. It was the *Gf* (fluid reasoning) subtests that were impaired on the WJ-III, and this was confirmed with the Differential Ability Scales (DAS) Nonverbal Reasoning subtests. What Jerry needed help with were anterior right-hemisphere functions (novel problem-solving skills), not the posterior ones the teacher and school psychologist were addressing with their generic "nonverbal LD" interventions. Although these would be excellent interventions for children with posterior right-hemisphere problems, they would not meet Jerry's needs.

The Neuropsychology of Mathematics

Although "dyscalculia" has traditionally been associated with Gerstmann syndrome and damage to the left parietal region (Mayer et al., 1999), it is not surprising to find that several areas of the brain are associated with math competency, and that disruption to one or more of these regions can lead to MDs. It is not uncommon for people to claim that language and reading are "left-brain" functions, but this is clearly not the case for math (Shalev, Manor, Amir, Wertman-Elad, & Gross-Tsur, 1995). In fact, excellent math skills are associated with bilateral, not lateral, strengths (Benbow & Lubinski, 1997), and MDs can result from both left- and right-hemisphere damage (Grafman, Passafiume, & Faglioni, & Boller, 1982). Most neuroimaging studies have confirmed bilateral activation in most homologous areas. It has been suggested that the right hemisphere may preferentially determine numerical magnitude, while the left hemisphere preferentially caries out arithmetic (Rickard et al., 2000). Some have suggested that the difference is between "exact" and "approximate" arithmetic, with the former drawing upon language processes and the latter relying on numerical magnitudes and visual–spatial processes (Dehaene et al., 1999). However, notice how this exact–approximate distinction fits well with our reconceptualization of hemispheric processes in Chapter 2.

Patient Studies and Left-Hemisphere Math Processes

Patient studies have found that damage to the left frontal region, perisylvian region, inferior parietal lobe, and basal ganglia are all associated with deficient math skills and MDs (Butterworth, 1999; L. Cohen, Dehaene, Chochon, Lehericy, & Naccache, 2000; Hittair-Delazer, Semenza, & Denes, 1994; Kahn & Whitaker, 1991; Lucchelli & DeRenzi, 1993; Whalon, McCloskey, Lesser, & Gordon, 1997). Although bilateral parietal lobe functions appear to be necessary for math skills, patient studies suggest that left parietal dysfunction alone may lead to MDs (Isaacs, Edmonds, Lucas, & Gadian, 2001). In fact, Isaacs and colleagues (2001) found that calculation deficits were associated with less gray matter in the left parietal lobe. Left-hemisphere damage to the perisylvian areas can selectively impair retrieval of math facts, but if the left inferior parietal region is unaffected, calculation skills may be spared (L. Cohen et al., 2000). Given these findings regarding the left-hemisphere processes associated with math computation, we would likely conclude that the structures associated with reading competency are same ones involved in math calculation.

Patient Studies and Right-Hemisphere Math Processes

As would be expected from the research cited earlier, several studies have noted that individuals with right-hemisphere damage also have problems with calculation. Individuals with MDs due to right-hemisphere damage often have incorrect spatial alignment of columns or neglect of stimuli in the left visual field (Basso, Burgio, & Caporali, 2000; Langdon & Warrington, 1997; Rosselli & Ardila, 1989). Math problems are typically presented in a vertical format, and, not surprisingly, these individuals often ignore or "misread" the operands for problems. Neglect, most often due to right parietal lobe dysfunction, would also be consistent with the high rate of constructional apraxia in individuals with MDs who have right-brain damage (Basso et al., 2000). Fleischner (1994) has argued that recalling numbers, writing numbers by hand, and performing calculations are all right-hemisphere skills.

Right Hemisphere, Left Hemisphere, or Both?

Although many have endorsed the idea that right-hemisphere damage is the cause for MDs (see Rourke, 2000, for a review), recall that McCloskey and colleagues (1991) found that a majority of subjects with MDs had frank left-hemisphere damage, and that Branch, Cohen, and Hynd (1995) found little support for the right-hemisphere theory of math deficits. Our recent study (Hale, Fiorello, Bertin, & Sherman, 2003) showed that visual–graphomotor skills and processing speed predict math achievement, but a majority of the variance was accounted for by semantic memory and working memory/executive function factors. These conflicting views and findings lead us to believe that math is a bilateral task, requiring both the right and left hemispheres. In contrasting the left and right hemispheres' roles in computation, Isaacs and colleagues (2001) suggest that the visual–spatial areas are necessary for approximation, but that exact calculation is language-based. It may be the nature of the math task that detects hemispheric differences, as patients with left-hemisphere damage have difficulty with calculation, but those with right-hemisphere damage only have difficulty with math reasoning (Langdon & Warrington, 1997). These two studies fit nicely with our notion of the right hemisphere as important for processing novel, coarse, and global information, and of the left hemisphere as important for fine, detail-oriented, and rule-governed processing.

Neuroimaging of Math Competency

The debate over left-brain versus right-brain functions in math competency is far from over, but recent neuroimaging studies have shed new light on the mental processes involved in math. Most of these studies suggest that the prefrontal and inferior parietal areas (including the angular and supramarginal gyri) are most involved in math computation skills (Burbaud et al., 1995; Chochon, Cohen, van de Moortele, & Dehaene, 1999; Cowell, Egan, Code, Harasty, & Watson, 2000; Gruber, Indefrey, Steinmetz, & Kleinschmidt, 2001; Menon et al., 2000; Roland & Friberg, 1985; Rueckert et al., 1996). However, other studies have failed to find activation in the angular or supramarginal gyri during math calculation (Deheane et al., 1996). As we have noted in previous chapters, this difference could be related to the math and control tasks used during neuroimaging. However, think about these findings for a minute. Recall from Chapter 5 that we have posited a direct route and an indirect route for word recognition. Could the same be true for math computation, as suggested in In-Depth 6.2? If children use different routes for similar problems, then differential diagnosis beyond the nomothetic total correct score is essential.

IN-DEPTH 6.2. Different Math Routes for Similar Problems

As is the case in reading, it is likely that different areas of the brain are differentially active in math, depending on the child's level of math competency. Recall that the angular gyrus is active when sound–symbol association is required, but that when words are retrieved automatically, this area is silent. Could it be that the inferior parietal math functions (particularly the supramarginal and angular gyri) are needed when rote retrieval of math facts fails (Dehaene & Cohen, 1997)? Consistent with this hypothesis, it is not surprising that the Deheane and colleagues (1996) study found activation in the striate and extrastriate areas, particularly the left fusiform and lingual gyri, but not the inferior parietal regions—maybe because the math was easy and automatic for their subjects. This suggests that their subjects used the ventral stream and temporal lobe for retrieval of rote, automatic math facts (Rickard et al., 2000). Menon and colleagues (2000) found that perfect performers had less activation in the left angular gyrus—a finding generally associated with skill accuracy and proficiency. Rickard and colleagues (2000) found bilateral activity both posterior and superior to the angular and supramarginal gyri on a verification task, suggesting that the angular gyrus is only necessary for complex calculations requiring borrowing and carrying.

These findings have dramatic implications for your assessment and intervention practices. Not only do they suggest that different brain areas carry out different functions during math calculation, but they also suggest that not every child will solve the same math problem in the same way. For instance, think of the problem 8 × 7, and you easily rely on your ventral stream/temporal lobe to come up with 56. Now think of 16 × 7. Most of us do not know the multiplication tables beyond the 12 or 13 level, so this now becomes a computation task—one that will require both parietal and frontal lobe functioning to carry it out. If different brain areas are used for different problems, and children have different levels of competency, then children in the same classroom may arrive at their answers via different methods, and these methods will take different amounts of time to complete. In addition, consistent with this line of reasoning, different types of error patterns may emerge for each child, requiring thorough examination to ensure understanding of each child's math competency and needs.

As noted earlier, several studies have found frontal activation during math tasks. Activation has been found in Broca's area and the premotor region—areas that have been associated with syntactic requirements, oral expression, and motor control (Gruber et al., 2001; Menon et al., 2000; Prabhakaran, Rypma, & Gabrieli, 2001; Rickard et al., 2000), as has been found for reading. Considering their purported role in executive functions, we would expect prefrontal areas to be highly involved in math calculation. The prefrontal cortex is likely to be needed for working memory and retrieval of math facts (Menon et al., 2000), as well as for the sequential solving of multistep problems (Gruber et al., 2001). Whereas simple calculation problems require more parietal than frontal activity, complex computations require bilateral frontal activation (Prabhakaran et al., 2001). Stanescu-Cosson and colleagues (2000) found bilateral prefrontal activation during a math approximation task, but only left inferior frontal activation during a calculation task. As you would expect, they found bilateral angular gyrus activity to be greater during calculation than during approximation. Making judgments about math equations also requires prefrontal involvement. In a study that asked participants to determine whether equations were correct or not, dorsolateral prefrontal activation was common in processing of all equations, but this area and the ventrolateral prefrontal area were both active during processing of incorrect equations, suggesting that interference and working memory demands were higher (Menon, Mackenzie, Rivera, & Reiss, 2002).

The findings reported above clearly show that bilateral and frontal activity is important for solving math problems. Consistent with our discussion of brain functioning in Chapter 2, we find that as complexity or ambiguity increases, frontal and right-hemisphere skills are required. The prefrontal cortex is important for problem solving, whereas the inferior region is likely to be involved in vocal output and syntax or algorithm rules, which makes this aspect of math lateralize to the left-hemisphere frontal region. In addition, we find that the striate is important for visual perception, and that the inferior and sometimes medial parietal cortices are much more important for math calculation than they are for reading. However, like reading well-known words, retrieving simple math facts may not require either the prefrontal or parietal areas; this automatic retrieval of facts may necessitate ventral stream involvement. However, as retrieval demands increase, the role of the frontal cortex increases as well (as with verbal fluency tasks). This generalization would also be true for multistep problems, which require greater working memory, as well as the executive skills of planning, organization, sequencing, flexibility, monitoring, and evaluating performance.

Given our understanding of the neuropsychological processes involved in math computation, you can begin to formulate ideas about a child's processing strengths and weaknesses, and to determine which brain areas are involved during math performance. However, recall that different brain areas may be involved as a child ascends some computational hierarchy, and that children with MDs may use different problem-solving routes when completing their math assignments and exams. This can help you develop individualized interventions designed to meet the needs of children with MDs, several of which are presented at the end of this chapter.

INSTRUCTIONAL STRATEGIES FOR CHILDREN WITH MDs

Now that you have a basic understanding of the cognitive and neuropsychological characteristics of children with MDs, we must now move to intervention. Interventions for math problems have received a great deal of attention by investigators, but as you will see in Appendix 6.1, most programs are not tailored for individual strengths and weaknesses. Recognizing the reason why a child is struggling with mathematics is an important first step.

Using the information described in the preceding section, you should be able to recognize the cognitive pattern associated with the math deficit, but it is also important to do an error analysis of failed responses and to compare these to correct responses. First, look for types of error responses in permanent products from the classroom. In addition, it may be important to conduct a process assessment (Rivera & Bryant, 1992) so that you can see the pattern of errors. Having a child talk out loud or use the think-aloud technique (Ginsburg, 1987) to tell you the steps he or she uses during computation is often extremely helpful. This additional information cannot be obtained from standardized measures, which should really be considered as math screening measures (Vaughn & Wilson, 1994), so it might be helpful to ask the child's teacher for some math computation worksheets to further examine the pattern of performance.

After you have conducted these initial steps, you will have a better understanding of the reason why the child is having problems in math. In preparation for your consultation meeting with Billy's teacher, for example, ask yourself the following questions. Is the problem related to prior learning and/or difficulty with retention/retrieval of math facts? Does Billy find math difficult because it is boring and too abstract for him? Billy seems to have difficulty with algorithm understanding or use; is this because he has difficulty following the sequence of steps? Does he show attentional concerns, failing to recognize the operands at times? Does he have difficulty with the spatial characteristics of multistep math problems and show poor handwriting? Or is the solving of novel problems, especially word problems, difficult for him? Is the severity great enough that you should suggest a compensatory technique, or is remediation sufficient? Has Billy tried these techniques without success for too long, or is he still young enough to make good progress through systematic intervention designed to reduce error responding? These questions must be asked as you begin to work collaboratively with the teacher to brainstorm appropriate intervention strategies and formulate a plan to evaluate the efficacy of your intervention.

MATH CASE STUDY: LINKING ASSESSMENT TO INTERVENTION

The complexity of these assessment and intervention issues in highlighted in Case Study 6.3, where we take you from assessment to intervention with a boy who appeared to his teacher to have problems with math secondary to a nonverbal LD or ADHD. As you can see from Matt's unique pattern of performance, he did immediately seem to fit well into a "category" of MD; however, even though he did seem to show characteristics of the procedural subtype of MD, assuming that this pattern would automatically be associated with ADHD would have been problematic. As we emphasize throughout this book, if we are to truly serve the needs of children like Matt, we must not make recommendations based on initial teacher referral questions or even preliminary test data. Instead, we can only make recommendations for such children after we understand the complexities of their cognitive profiles, and the ways they use those cognitive processes to solve math problems.

CASE STUDY 6.3. Matt and Math

I (Hale) was called into a local school to consult with a fourth-grade teacher, Rita, who was perplexed about Matt's poor math performance. Matt had a history of fairly adequate math performance until last year, when his math grades started to deteriorate. In addition, although his reading skills were excellent, his comprehension began to fail as well. Rita described Matt as a "good kid" who was never disruptive, but he seemed somewhat inattentive and withdrawn. His mother wanted to put Matt on medication for what she called "ADD," but the school-based support team suggested that he should have a psychological evaluation first. At the team meeting, the school psychologist concluded that Matt had test anxiety, particularly in the areas of math and comprehension. This hypothesis was also invoked to explain his attention problems in the classroom. Matt did not qualify for special education services because the team adhered strictly to the discrepancy model, and his WISC-III Full Scale IQ was in the average range and his KeyMath scores were only low average. The team recommended Americans with Disabilities Act/Rehabilitation Act counseling accommodations for Matt's anxiety problem.

Rita agreed that Matt would tense up at times, but she didn't really see Matt as an anxious child. She remembered reading something about nonverbal LD and math disabilities, so she decided to do some research. She read several learning disability subtype studies from the Windsor Taxonomic Laboratory (see Rourke, 1994). In these studies, children with math problems were found to have good reading/spelling skills and poor mechanical arithmetic performance. They also tended to have a characteristic WISC-III Verbal > Performance IQ split, suggesting possible right-hemisphere dysfunction. Because Rita had some knowledge of brain–behavior relationships, she easily understood the assumption that children with math disabilities must have deficient visual–spatial, nonverbal, and graphomotor skills. These perceptual deficits would lead to problems with spatial processes and column alignment in math calculation. She also agreed that Matt showed some of the socioemotional signs of nonverbal learning disabilities, as he was somewhat "peculiar" and socially reticent.

Returning to Matt's student file and his permanent products (e.g., worksheets, tests), Rita looked at the data for evidence of this pattern. She was surprised to find that Matt didn't have this Verbal–Performance split at all, but she noticed significant WISC-III subtest scatter. Matt did have problems with Block Design and Coding, which brought down his Performance score, but he was still in the average range. He also had a low average Arithmetic and Comprehension score, but the Digit Span subtest was average (although Digits Forward was significantly better than Digits Backward). Other than a low average Bender–Gestalt score, there were no other cognitive data available. Achievement test results revealed inattention to signs or operands, and messy, disorganized work, but little other evidence of a math deficit. Matt's classroom math papers and tests did not show any column alignment errors in multistep problems, but he did show several algorithm and apparently some math fact retrieval errors. Matt rarely completed his math assignments on time, and he missed many points on tests for the same reason. The only psychosocial evaluation data available were the Bender–Gestalt score interpreted from a projective approach (we do not recommend this!) and a score on a Conners rating scale, which was significant for attention problems. When we sat down to discuss the case, we first explored changes in home or classroom that could have accounted for Matt's deteriorating performance. There seemed to be nothing out of the ordinary going on in the home, but Rita commented that she wasn't sure whether Matt's mom was a reliable informant. When questioned about this comment, Rita said, "Sometimes it seems like she's not all there"—that is, as if the mother were distracted by something.

Our initial hypothesis was that an attention problem could explain the computation errors, and that Matt might have ADHD, inattentive type (consistent with executive dysfunction), with comorbid anxiety. However, the history obtained from the mother and Rita revealed other interesting facts, including a possible birth trauma and a family history of psychiatric problems. When I began my assessment, I decided that I would collect more information on Matt's personality and behavior, including mother, teacher, and self-report forms. I began my evaluation by using the DAS as my screening tool, to see whether Matt indeed had "adequate" nonverbal skills, and to compare nonverbal reasoning to visual–spatial skills. The following data were obtained (the General Cognitive Ability [GCA] and clusters are in standard scores [SSs], subtests are in T scores):

(continued)

$$\text{GCA} = 95$$

Verbal Ability = 87	Nonverbal Reasoning Ability = 93	Spatial Ability = 106
Word Definitions = 45	Matrices = 48	Recall of Designs = 52
Similarities = 40	Sequential and Quantitative Reasoning = 45	Pattern Construction=56

Consistent with the WISC-III results, Matt's scores on measures of visual-perceptual skills were adequate, and nonverbal reasoning skills, while in the lower end of the average range, were not impaired. Matt was often perseverative and inflexible on these measures, but never disinhibited or impulsive. So far, the results appeared to be consistent with ADHD, inattentive type. However, after the CHT theory was developed, we had to test our hypothesis that attention and executive problems were the source of Matt's problems. We decided to use our repeatable ADHD drug trial battery in preparation for a possible drug trial (recall that Matt's mother wanted medication for "ADD"), supplemented by additional executive function measures (most results are converted to SSs, with higher scores = better performance).

Task	Variable	SS	Raw score
Hale Cancellation Task	Correct	95	
	Time	82	
Selective Reminding Test	Long-Term Storage	85	
	Consistent Retrieval	80	
Go–No Go Test	Correct		29/30
Conners Continuous Performance Test II	Omissions	90	
	Commissions	110	
	Reaction Time	65	
	Reaction Time Block Change	88	
	Reaction Time ISI Change	80	
Stroop Color–Word Test	Interference	78	
	Errors		8
Trail Making Test, Part B	Correct	95	
	Time	79	
Test of Memory and Learning	Digits Backward	85	
Wisconsin Card Sorting Test	Errors	88	
	Perseverative Responses	80	
	Perseverative Errors	86	
	Categories		5
	Failure to Maintain Set		0
	Trials to First Category		18
Controlled Oral Word Association Test (COWAT)	Letters (F/A/S)	96	
	Category	68	
WJ-III	Planning	87	
Developmental Neuropsychological Assessment (NEPSY)	Tower	75	
	Design Fluency	92	

(continued)

Certainly the test results and environmental data pointed to ADHD, inattentive type. The test data were all suggesting that Matt's dorsolateral prefrontal cortex and/or cingulate circuits were impaired, but something didn't quite fit. Was it just psychometric "noise"—a very real possibility, given the number of measures and different norm groups? Why the low Comprehension score on the WISC-III? Why was his COWAT Category score so low, and the Letters score so high? Why did he have such slow psychomotor speed on some tasks but not others? Why were his graphomotor skills adequate, but his drawings disorganized and perseverative? Why were his nonverbal skills adequate when these skills are often difficult for children with ADHD? The reported classroom behaviors and family psychiatric history made me consider an additional possibility: thought disorder. Sure enough, through further examination of the behavior ratings and of Matt's self-report, I felt comfortable suggesting that Matt's math and comprehension problems were probably due to executive and attention problems. But I didn't stop there; I added that I thought these problems did not constitute a "primary" attention deficit (one that would benefit from stimulant treatment), but were "secondary" to his "internal distraction" and "unique way of thinking about and solving problems." In other words, it seemed that evidence was emerging that Matt had a thought disorder. During the feedback, I discussed these concerns with the teacher and mother. Both confirmed that Matt displayed idiosyncratic and "peculiar" (both actually used this word!) behaviors in the classroom and at home. He also had a rich fantasy life that he claimed was "real" at times. In addition, the family history of psychiatric problems included an incarcerated uncle who had "lost it" and was "on lots of medication."

Why was this differentiation important? First, we discovered that the apparent reasons for Matt's math and comprehension problems were attentional and executive in nature, not due to anxiety or nonverbal LD. Systematic desensitization would not really help Matt, but metacognitive instruction designed to foster self-structure and evaluation during academic tasks could help him. He was taught to use a checklist to ensure that he double-checked the operand and his math facts after completing each problem. He was also given extended time for math and other language-based subjects. Furthermore, we wouldn't waste time trying to teach spatial skills, column alignment, or graphomotor skills in an attempt to overcome a nonverbal LD. Finally, it is true that all of these decisions could have been made with our finding of attention and executive function deficits, regardless of the underlying pathology—but we might not have recognized the psychosocial issues as such, because Rita reported that Matt was a "good kid" (as we will note in Chapter 8, internalizers are always seen as "good kids"). In addition, if a pediatrician or psychiatrist were to read our report and conclude that Matt had ADHD, he or she might have treated Matt with a dopamine *agonist* (e.g., Ritalin), which could have a *detrimental* effect on a child with a thought disorder. What he needed was counseling, social skills training, help with peer interactions, and careful psychiatric monitoring to ensure that a dopamine *antagonist* wasn't needed.

APPENDIX 6.1. Mathematics Interventions

Reference	Intervention description
Ashlock (1998)	Estimation: Adding or subtracting to round to nearest whole number, then carrying out operation using tens, hundreds, etc.
Bley & Thornton (1995)	A problem-solving approach that includes decision making; understanding vocabulary; using information; and identifying patterns/sequences, strategies, and solutions
Bullock & Walentas (1989)	Touch Math Technique: Counting aloud and touching dots on numbers, with direction determining addition and subtraction
Cawley et al. (1976)	Project MATH: Interactive model that provides students with variable teacher presentation and student response formats
Dunlap & Brennan (1979)	Concrete–semiconcrete–abstract progression: Manipulatives, mental images, 1:1 correspondence of manipulatives and paper/pencil, object movement
Engelmann & Carmine (1981)	Corrective Mathematics: Module strands for remediation, including facts, operations, story problems
Fitzmaurice-Hayes (1984)	Left-to-right subtraction algorithm requiring regrouping in the answer
Fleischner et al. (1987)	Reading, rereading, thinking, solving, checking word problems
Friebel & Gingrich (1972)	Math Applications Kit: Applications of math materials in real-life situations
Hayes (1985)	Improving math fact automaticity by teaching a few facts at a time; ensuring mastery; regular drill, repetition, and review; providing accommodations
Hutchings (1975, 1976)	Low-Stress Method for subtraction and multiplication algorithms
Hutchinson (1993)	Teacher modeling, scripts, prompts, self-questions, feedback, guided practice, independent practice, and graphing progress
Lombardo & Drabman (1985)	Write–Say Technique: Students write/talk selves through problem, evaluate selves, make corrections through repetition of problem
McTighe & Lyman (1988)	Think–Pair–Share: Cooperative learning technique in which students think about problem, pair in twos, share results of discussions in whole group
Mercer & Mercer (2001)	Teaching steps, modeling, teacher–student interaction, concrete–semiconcrete–abstract, concepts, rules, monitoring, providing feedback
Mercer & Miller (1991–1993)	Strategic Math Series: Pretest, concrete level, representation, abstract level (guided practice), posttest (independent practice), fluency instruction, and problem solving
Miller et al. (1998)	Goal setting, strategy instruction, direct instruction, self-regulation, manipulatives, drawing, timing, and lecture/pause
Montague (1992)	Reading word problem, paraphrasing, visualizing, hypothesizing, estimating, computing, checking
Montague & Bos (1986)	Metacognitive approach for problem solving and accuracy evaluation
Pearson (1986)	Left-to-right addition algorithm for understanding regrouping
Reisman (1977)	Division algorithm shortcut using multiples of 10
Rourke (1989)	Sequential problem solving with feedback and verbal mediation
Ruais (1978)	Ray multiplication algorithm for addition and subtraction of fractions
Silbert et al. (1990)	Direct Instruction Mathematics: Objectives, problem-solving strategies, prerequisite skills, sequence of new skills, procedure, format, examples, guided practice, independent practice
Sosniak & Ethington (1994)	Cognitively Demanding Instructional Model: Problem-solving approach, difficult problems, use of teacher materials, encouragement of students, address teacher beliefs
Thornton & Toohley (1985)	MATHFACT program: Prerequisite skills, ongoing assessment, modifying sequences, strategy instruction, modifying presentation for individuals, controlling pacing, promoting generalization, using prompts, self-monitoring, overlearning
Underhill et al. (1980)	Understanding at concrete, semiconcrete, abstract levels; memorization of basic facts; emphasis on place value, structures, regrouping (carrying/borrowing)
Watanabe (1991)	SIGNS: Surveying question, identifying key words, graphically drawing problem, noting operations needed, solving and checking answer
Zawaiza & Gerber (1993)	Strategy instruction of modeling, sufficient exemplar problems, practice with feedback, student discussion, and application

CHAPTER 7

|_|_|_|_|_|_|_|_|_|_|_|_|

The Neuropsychology
of Written Language Disorders

CHARACTERISTICS OF CHILDREN WITH WRITTEN LANGUAGE DISORDERS

Complexity of Written Language Disorders

From a neuropsychological perspective, written language is by far the most difficult academic skill (Lerner, 2000); yet it has probably received less empirical examination than any other domain (Hooper et al., 1994). Why has written language received so little attention? The old belief that writing is a natural extension of language may have something to do with it. This belief, long held by the educational establishment, is that if you provide children with handwriting instruction, they will be able to convey their thoughts on paper as easily as they do when speaking. If a child can speak, and can use a pencil, then he or she will have no difficulty with written language. As empirical evidence emerges that oral and written language are dissociable, the basis of this belief is slowly being eroded. We now know that there are many cognitive processes associated with written language achievement, and that dysfunction in one or more of those areas can lead to a written language disorder (WLD).

Unlike the other academic domains discussed so far, written language is the only academic skill that is primarily an output task. Written language depends on the input system for memory and feedback to the output system, but it is more of a "frontal" skill than the others, because it requires formulating ideas, organizing the ideas into paragraphs and sentences, using words to convey meaning and link ideas, using graphomotor skills to write and spell words, evaluating the accuracy of the product, and editing as necessary. In fact, the executive or critical analysis of the written language product may be the single most important determinant of success (Harris & Graham, 1997), but the executive skills of planning and revising written language products are seldom used by children with WLDs (Graham, Harris, MacArthur, & Schwartz, 1991).

Written language is by no means *solely* a frontal task, however, because the posterior regions are required at every step. Writing requires some comprehension of the writing problem prior to ideation, prior knowledge and experiences to develop the written material, visualization of word spellings, and somatosensory and spatial feedback to direct the hand during writing. Spelling and handwriting are important parts of written language, and both are covered in this chapter; however, these prerequisite skills are subsumed under the broader, more complex skill of written language. WLDs can occur because of problems in any of these areas, and while difficulties with spelling and handwriting can be overcome with the use of a computer-based compensatory technique, the other types of WLDs require additional individualized interventions. It is the complexity of the written language process that has probably dissuaded researchers and practitioners from allotting the necessary time and resources to examine this important academic domain thoroughly.

Prevalence and Comorbidity of WLD

Given the paucity of research into the nature and causes of WLDs, it is not surprising to find limited information about their prevalence and comorbidity with other disorders. Because writing skills require many of the cognitive processes required for other academic domains, it is not surprising that WLDs are likely to co-occur with other disorders. WLDs rarely occur in isolation, and are typically comorbid with many other language disorders and language-based learning disabilities (Hooper et al., 1994). This is not surprising given that children with receptive and expressive language disorders should also have difficulty with written expression. Children with WLDs tend to write fewer words and sentences (Houck & Billingsley, 1989), thereby limiting analysis of their writing strengths and weaknesses. Difficulty with determining prevalence and comorbidity rates is also confounded by difficulty with task definition and measurement problems (Hooper et al., 1994). Because there are numerous complex skills required for written language, and these skills interact with other processes and each other, defining and measuring WLDs are difficult—and this difficulty precludes accurate classification of WLDs.

Epidemiological studies using absolute criteria cutoffs have revealed prevalence rates for WLDs to be quite high, with 4% showing absolute-criteria handwriting problems, and as many as 17% showing problems with syntactic skills (Hooper et al., 1994). These high rates are not surprising when one considers that auditory–verbal, visual–spatial, and executive function processes are all required for successful written expression (Gregg, 1992). As basic literacy skills and writing affect one another in a reciprocal manner (Richek, Caldwell, Jennings, & Lerner, 1996), it must also be determined whether a WLD is primary or secondary to a language disorder. Instead of classifying children on the basis of the discrepancy model, some have suggested that identification of children with WLDs should be based on their specific processing deficits (Roeltgen, 1985); this is consistent with the instructional emphasis on the process instead of the product of written language (Graves, 1994). Careful analysis of the processing requirements of written expression can help you determine whether a breakdown in the writing process is occurring at one or more levels of cognitive processing. This deficit-based subtyping of WLDs could lead to more accurate prevalence and comorbidity estimates in future research.

WLDs AND BRAIN FUNCTIONS

Spelling

Spelling is an integral part of written language, but it is a seldom-studied academic domain, especially when it comes to brain–behavior research. Perhaps few studies have been done because English spelling is fraught with exceptions to the rules, or because the advent of spell checking in computer programs has diminished the importance of this skill for some educators. However, we briefly examine spelling issues here, as we feel that everyone will need to spell at least occasionally throughout life. Spelling disorders (SDs) are often associated with problems with phonological awareness (Torgesen, 1996), but they are also seen in children with certain executive disorders (e.g., attention-deficit/hyperactivity disorder [ADHD]), and children with nonverbal LDs also display spelling errors, dysgraphia, and graphomotor problems (Gross-Tsur, Shalev, Manor, & Amir, 1995). As is the case with other LDs, we must identify the types of spelling problems displayed, link them to cognitive processes, and offer appropriate remediation and/or compensation to help children overcome their SDs. In addition, we believe that early writing activities prepare students for future computer writing. As is the case with oral language, we all communicate with others through our writing, and failure to prepare students for this eventuality will limit their potential.

Development of Spelling Skills

As with other academic skills, students move through developmental stages in acquiring spelling competency. Recognizing the developmental progression of spelling stages can help you determine whether a child's spelling errors are developmentally appropriate. Gentry (1982) has indicated that children go through five stages when learning to spell. In the first stage, preschool-age children produce letter-like forms, but show little understanding of phoneme–grapheme correspondence. The next stage is characterized by the use of letter abbreviations, such as "CT" for "cat." Upon entering first grade, children begin to spell words that make phonemic sense, such as "brot" for "brought." A couple of years later, children enter a stage where they spell conventionally, but continue to have some difficulty with exception or sight words. By about the age of 8 or 9, most children spell according to orthographic rules and recognize exception words, providing alternative spellings for words and checking the accuracy of their spellings.

Although this is the typical pattern of spelling development, this stage approach may not be entirely accurate, because children consider both phonetics and orthography as they learn to spell (Treiman, Cassar, & Zukowski, 1994). Directly related to spelling competency, morphology skills tend to increase throughout the late elementary to middle school period, but children with SDs tend to lag behind their peers (Carlisle, 1987). As is the case with other academic domains, it is important to look for error patterns within the developmental context. For instance, young children may frequently use invented spellings or show letter reversals, but this is uncommon in older children. Polloway and Smith (1999) have identified the most common error patterns in children with SDs as follows:

- Letter additions
- Letter omissions
- Letter reversals
- Sequencing errors
- Consonant substitutions
- Vowel substitutions

In addition to examining a child's error patterns and phoneme–grapheme correspondence skills, it is important to recognize that graphomotor skills are developing during this period and can affect spelling competency. Your job is to determine whether poor graphomotor skills are interfering with the writing process or with accurate letter reproduction. Children with SDs tend to show poorer letter formation, spacing, and size, and their overall spelling and written language output is lower than that of their same-age peers (Johnson & Carlisle, 1996). Are the graphomotor skill problems inherent in SDs, or are they comorbid? They certainly would seem to require different brain areas, so we would expect to see a dissociation between SDs and graphomotor problems. However, as you might expect, the notion that poor graphomotor skills interfere with spelling and writing competency has been hotly contested, with researchers arguing both for and against the dissociation of letter representations and sensory–motor processes, as can be seen in In-Depth 7.1.

Given that phonological awareness is an important prerequisite for both reading and spelling (Torgesen, 1996), it is not surprising that children with reading problems tend to have spelling problems as well (Shanker & Ekwall, 1998). In many ways spelling is more difficult than reading, because it requires many of the skills that word recognition does, but also requires visual–motor coordination and graphomotor skills to produce written words. Another substantial difference between spelling and reading is that the former requires orthographic retrieval, whereas the latter requires only recognition of graphemes. There are only 26 letters in the alphabet, but over 500 spellings used in representing the 44 phonemes in the English language (Tompkins, 1998). To cover that much ground, we must think of unique ways to order the letters to produce the desired product. Add on top of this the irregular sight words—those words that do not follow standard orthographic–phonemic rules—and it is easy to see why so many children have difficulties with spelling that persist even after their reading decoding skills have improved (Bruck, 1987).

IN-DEPTH 7.1. The Sensory–Motor Controversy

Written spelling is by definition a visual–motor integration task. Spelling requires encoding and retrieval of the visual shape of letters, uppercase and lowercase formats, and print and cursive styles (Shuren, Maher, & Heilman, 1996). As grapheme retrieval is necessary for spelling, it would seem as though this orthographic code, because of its very nature, must be represented in a visual format (Margolin & Goodman-Shulman, 1992). The orthographic or graphemic representation is important for developing a letter image, which in turn provides spatial information feedback for sensory–motor integration (Crary & Heilman, 1988). Others have suggested that visualization is not always necessary for spelling if the lexical–semantic route is used (Shuren et al., 1996). If spelling can occur independently of the phoneme–grapheme route, then representations of letters and words must be independent of motor functions, yet individual letter strokes will still require involvement of motor areas (Wright & Lindemann, 1993).

Rapp and Caramazza (1997) suggest that the semantic and graphemic representations of words and letters are amodal; in other words, they aren't related to visual, auditory, somatosensory, or motor processes. According to this model, the semantic representation of the spelling is transferred to a graphemic representation area that is amodal. The grapheme's position and organization are then sent to the motor areas for processing and output (either writing, typing, or speaking). Consistent with the assumption that language, whether oral or written, requires the same neuropsychological processes, this model suggests that phoneme perception (i.e., superior temporal lobe) and oral–motor skills (i.e., Broca's area) lead to oral language competency, which then allows for development of written language skills (Lindamood, 1994). According to this perspective, visual graphemic representations are not necessary for spelling; however, they may subserve spelling when written language is required.

The Neuropsychology of Spelling

It is not surprising that neuropsychological studies of spelling suggest that it depends on a network of relatively independent, albeit interconnected, cognitive processes and several different brain areas (Hillis et al., 2002). As is the case with other academic areas, most of the research points to the importance of left-hemisphere functions in spelling (Baxter & Warrington, 1994; Hillis et al., 2002; Hodges & Marshall, 1992). Development of the left-hemisphere lexical–semantic and phonemic awareness skills affects both reading and spelling, so it is not surprising that children who have deficits in these areas experience impaired reading and spelling (Ogden, 1996).

Several cases of impaired written spelling in the presence of adequate oral spelling have been used to suggest that spelling knowledge and skills actually exist beyond the sensory–motor areas responsible for carrying out the physical act of spelling (Rapp & Caramazza, 1997). Consistent with these findings, it has been found that written language fluency is more closely related to spelling than to handwriting (Johnson & Carlisle, 1996), and that visual imagery is not necessary for spelling orally or for recognizing orally spelled words (Shuren, Maher, & Heilman, 1996). It has been suggested that phonemic awareness serves as a foundation for morphemes, syllables, and words of written language (Lindamood, 1994), which would be consistent with the finding that oral and written spelling share the same cognitive processes (Shuren et al., 1996).

Others contend that oral and written spelling can be dissociated, because the latter is dependent on graphemic representations (Cipolotti & Warrington, 1996). Letter substitutions, reversals, and transpositions can occur within well-written sentences, suggesting that no one area is associated with all written language deficits (Caramazza, Miceli, Villa, & Romani, 1987). Damage to the left superior temporal–parietal lobe can lead to grapheme impairment for letters and words; this indicates that the parietal lobe mediates visual input and is the possible source of the visual–kinesthetic or graphic letter representation (Katanoda, Yoshikawa, & Sugishita, 2001; Moretti, Torre, Antonello, Ukmar, & Cazzato, 2001). Graphemic–orthographic impairments have been found to lead to phonological-equivalent spelling errors (Cameron, Cubelli, & Della Sala, 2002). In fact, phoneme–grapheme skills might be used for word stems, but morphemes such as prefixes or suffixes could be processed in lexical or automatic fashion (Badecker, Rapp, & Caramazza, 1996).

Could these positions be reconciled with what we know about reading, and about how the temporal and parietal lobes work? We have evidence of a lexical–semantic route (ventral stream) and a phoneme–grapheme route (dorsal stream) in reading. As we recognize that whole words or parts of words can be represented in the different visual streams, we must consider whether this applies to spelling as well. Although there are subtle differences between the language and writing systems, they interact in predictable ways (Berninger, Abbott, Abbott, Graham, & Richards, 2002). Some have suggested that a common cause of both semantic and graphemic deficits in writing can be linked to the frontal–subcortical pathways responsible for self-regulation and ordering/sequencing of information. As we can see, many of the brain areas and cognitive processes involved in reading and math contribute to spelling competency. However, the addition of graphomotor skills, and the fact that it is a production rather than a recognition task, make spelling different: It requires additional frontal lobe functions, as well as left sensory–motor areas to carry out the act of handwriting.

Given our understanding of brain–behavior relationships, it is not surprising that multiple cognitive processes are necessary for successful oral and/or written spelling (Rapp, 2001). In a model that provides us with a conceptualization of these processes, Hillis and colleagues (2002) contrast different paths for familiar and unfamiliar words and for oral and written spelling. Figure 7.1 depicts the separate paths for familiar and unfamiliar words, with familiar words being channeled through the lexical route to the graphemic buffer, which then can be transferred into oral and written spelling output. Hillis and colleagues found support for this model in a large sample of patients with either hypoperfusion or infarcts in several brain areas associated with these constructs. For lexical–semantic processes, Wernicke's area was impaired in a majority of these patients. For written word form for output, Broca's area was implicated. Support was also found for the hypotheses that the angular gyrus is responsible for phonemic–graphemic skills, and that the graphemic buffer is associated with the occipital cortex. Finally, in regard to the allographic conversion area (the premotor or "Exner's" area; see below), strong support was found for a relationship between hypoperfusion/damage and the motoric production of letters.

As is the case with reading disorders (RDs), several possible areas could be affected in SDs, including the ventral route, dorsal route, dorsal and medial frontal areas, and the sensory–motor regions. Clinically, it is important to recognize how children's spelling skills relate to their word attack skills. Is there a tendency to use sight word approaches and spell from memory (ventral stream)? Do children use sound–symbol association skills to spell words phonetically (temporal–parietal)? Do they make the same or different type of errors, and when they make errors, do they recognize and change them (frontal)? Do they have problems with letter order (frontal) or reversals (parietal)? Recognizing these error patterns will provide you with a better understanding of each child's spelling and word recognition skills, leading to more effective interventions as a result.

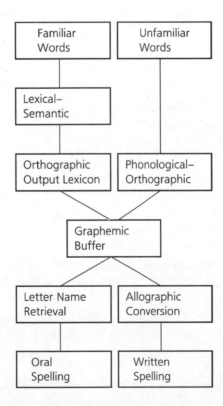

FIGURE 7.1. Schematic of cognitive spelling processes. Adapted from Hillis et al. (2002). Copyright 2002 by Psychology Press Ltd. Adapted by permission of Psychology Press Ltd., Hove, East Sussex, UK.

Interventions for Children with SDs

Appendix 7.1 lists some of the major teaching strategies for spelling instruction. Although many of the techniques for developing sound (phoneme)–symbol (grapheme) association listed in Chapter 5 (see Appendix 5.2) apply to spelling instruction, the additional importance of visual memory retrieval in spelling is worth recognizing. As we have noted above, spelling by its very nature is an output or production task, whereas reading is a recognition task. In reading, individuals have the correct word in front of them, but having the auditory representation (e.g., "I want you to spell the word 'comprehensive' ") requires a systematic search (frontal executive) for visual word images (ventral stream). In addition, this information must be translated into a sequential representation of the motor plan for writing the word (frontal and supplementary motor cortex), then sensory–motor integration for handwriting (left somatosensory–motor cortices), and finally evaluation of response and modification as necessary (frontal). We can't just assume that because Barbara can read well, she can also spell, because there are many more processes involved in the latter.

As we can see from Appendix 7.1, several interventions require multiple steps and recommend a multisensory approach. The belief regarding most interventions in special education has been "Let's put together all the strategies we know are effective, and something will work." We believe that this will change in the years to come as researchers begin to establish that interventions are not uniformly equally effective for all children with special needs. However, an examination of the spelling interventions described in Appendix 7.1 offers you some idea of what has been effective in the literature. Again, the combination of your knowledge about cognitive patterns of performance, your familiarity with successful strategies reported in the literature, and your effective collaborative consultation meetings with teachers will help you to develop, implement, and evaluate interventions for children with SDs.

Handwriting

Handwriting is often a problem for children with LDs, and this can certainly affect written language. If Joey doesn't like to write because it hurts his hand, because it takes too much time, or because his writing is illegible, Joey is less likely to write, even though he may have good ideas. Joey may readily discuss his ideas and provide you with a coherent oral narrative, easily telling you about the people, actions, and outcome of his story. However, when Joey sits down to write about the same topic, he struggles and becomes frustrated. His writing sample lacks fluency and clarity; he produces only three sentences, and these are disconnected and flat. How could this be? Although there are several possibilities—one that we have already discussed (spelling), and another that we will discuss later (written language)—many children with LDs have difficulty with writing tasks because of their poor handwriting. Some observers have questioned the use of handwriting at all, suggesting that keyboarding has become the skill to learn. However, as Greenland and Polloway (1994) note, people form impressions about others on the basis of their handwriting skills. In addition, as is the case with spelling, determining whether handwriting is interfering with written language, math computation, or other skills requiring visual–somatosensory–motor integration (e.g., art) is a critical part of your comprehensive cognitive hypothesis-testing (CHT) approach to serving children with LDs.

Several areas of written language should be considered during your evaluation of a child with an LD, handwriting problems, and poor visual–motor integration skills (Hagborg & Aiello-Coulter, 1994). In addition to looking for signs of constructional (apraxia) problems and poor psychomotor speed, it is important to look directly at the quality of handwriting either produced by the child during testing or gathered informally. This can help you determine whether the difficulty is a visual–spatial (dorsal stream), somatosensory (tactile and kinesthetic feedback to motor system), motor (primary or secondary motor areas), or integration (corpus callosum) problem. According to Mercer and Mercer (2001), the following attributes should be examined in your handwriting assessment:

- Letter shape (letter slant/changes)
- Letter size (large, small, not uniform)
- Letter spacing (crowding, too much)
- Letter alignment (not on line)
- Line quality (slant/directional issues)

There is some debate about the print (manuscript)–cursive (script) distinction in handwriting: Printing is easier to produce and read, but cursive is less likely to produce reversals or interfere with the flow of thought. Certainly there are similar neuropsychological processes associated with both, so let's briefly explore them before we move on to written language.

The Neuropsychology of Handwriting

More neuroimaging studies of hand movements and handwriting have been completed than studies of spelling and written language. Before we review them, let's review the processes we think should be involved in visual–somatosensory–motor integration for handwriting—specifically, copying notes from the board. Recall that constructional abilities typically require bilateral visual perception, so the frontal eye fields coordinate eye movement with the cranial nerves to receive the image in the retina. This is transferred to the subcortical thalamus and the superior colliculi structures en route to the striate or primary visual cortex. From there, the dorsal stream is probably needed, as this area is important for part–whole relationships and spatial processing.

This receptive information must be translated to the left premotor and/or supplementary motor area, which then directs the left primary motor cortex (in right-handed people) to carry out the motor act, with somatosensory (tactile and kinesthetic) feedback provided by the left superior parietal cortex. Let's not forget that the corpus callosum may be needed if new learning or holistic perceptual and/or motor processes require right-hemisphere involvement. This seems simple enough, but let's see whether this generalizes to handwriting, and also whether this varies based on whether the task is novel or routinized.

For handwriting competency, most researchers have identified two areas associated with writing deficits from the clinical literature: the posterior end of the left middle frontal gyrus, or "Exner's" area; and the left anterior superior parietal region, associated with Gerstmann syndrome (Menon & Desmond, 2001). Frontal lobe activity during writing has been mostly limited to the lateral premotor area, the medial supplementary motor area, and in some cases the prefrontal cortex, depending on the task (Haslinger et al., 2002; Katanoda et al., 2001; Muller, Kleinhans, Pierce, Kemmotsu, & Courchesne, 2002). The association motor areas responsible for writing are often referred to as "Exner's" area; it is both anterior and superior to the primary motor cortex hand area (Menon & Desmond, 2001).

As you will recall from Chapter 2, these secondary motor areas are needed for providing directions to the primary motor cortex. Although some have suggested the premotor cortex is responsible for motor actions in response to the environment, and the supplementary motor cortex is responsible for internally driven motor behavior (Petersen, van Mier, Fiez, & Raichle, 1998; van Mier, Tempel,

Perlmutter, Raichle, & Petersen, 1998), others have argued that the premotor–supplementary motor distinction is more complex (Haslinger et al., 2002). This is consistent with the findings that supplementary motor cortex activity is found during both early and later stages of learning, with no significant difference between the two periods (Muller et al., 2002). These findings lead some to suggest that the distinction is one of skill complexity, with the premotor area designed for intricate movements and modulation during movement execution (Siebner et al., 2001).

Consistent with our novel–automatic distinction, studies demonstrating prefrontal effects often examine new motor learning, with the right frontal region activated during initial stages, and later learning associated with left superior frontal activation (Muller et al., 2002; Shadmehr & Holcomb, 1997). Prefrontal activity also seems to be most prevalent during new learning, and as tasks become routinized, more posterior activity is likely (Staines, Padilla, & Knight, 2002). Not surprisingly, handwriting and motor program studies have implicated the frontal–subcortical circuits, and the subcortical structures receiving attention have included the hippocampus, thalamus, basal ganglia, and cerebellum (Haslinger et al., 2002; Katanoda et al., 2001; Muller et al., 2002; Siebner et al., 2001). However, even Broca's area has been implicated in handwriting and fine motor skills, as suggested in In-Depth 7.2.

Aside from the expected activation in the primary sensory–motor, striate, and extrastriate regions (Haslinger et al., 2002; Katanoda et al., 2001; Muller et al., 2002), many have found activation in the superior and inferior parietal regions (Haslinger et al., 2002; Katanoda et al., 2001; Menon & Desmond, 2001), including the secondary somatosensory cortex and supramarginal gyrus (Siebner et al., 2001), but not the angular gyrus. Interestingly, learning novel motor sequences requires bilateral activation, and this activation diminishes with learning (Deiber, Honda, Ibanez, Sadato, & Hallett, 1999; Muller et al., 2002; van Mier et al., 1998). In keeping with our earlier arguments about the differences between parietal and temporal activation in reading and math, we find evidence suggesting that the parietal lobe is more active during initial learning. But is there evidence to indicate that learned motor skills require more temporal lobe

IN-DEPTH 7.2. Broca's Area and Handwriting

When you think of Broca's area, you often think of nonfluent or expressive aphasia, affecting *oral* language or speech production. However, unilateral or bilateral activity in Broca's area has also been reported during handwriting and fine motor activity (Haslinger et al., 2002; Muller et al., 2002); at first glance, this is somewhat surprising, considering that this is the expressive speech area. Since Broca first described his aphasic patients, it has been a basic tenet of neuropsychology that damage to Broca's area leads to expressive aphasia. Although no one disputes this finding, some have questioned whether this area is solely responsible for expressive language. If we think back to our arguments presented in earlier chapters, could it be that the psychological *processes* are more important than the (verbal) output? Instead of thinking that Broca's area is responsible for verbal functions, many have noted that expressive language is a *motor* skill. It just so happens that Broca's area is responsible for producing detailed motor responses within time (Schubotz & von Cramon, 2001) or sequence, and so it is a likely candidate for both oral and handwritten language skills. Since this activity is sometimes bilateral during learning of motor behaviors, the right and left Broca's areas are working together to fine-tune motor movements to form a synchronized motor (verbal or nonverbal) pattern. This could account for the high comorbidity rate of aphasias and apraxias (Liepmann, 1908), with the underlying psychological processes affecting both types of output.

involvement? Indeed, Muller and colleagues (2002) found that as parietal lobe activity declined, medial temporal lobe activation was stronger in later stages of motor learning.

Finally, before we leave the topic of handwriting, we have provided important evidence that Gerstmann was correct in his assertion that the parietal lobe is a source of both agraphia (handwriting problems) and acalculia (math calculation problems). With our recognition that the angular gyrus is involved in sound–symbol associations, and our knowledge that left-hemisphere dysfunction leads to Block Design reversals, could the parietal association cortex be responsible for both the letter reversals seen in RDs and the left–right orientation problems seen in Gerstmann syndrome? Certainly the available evidence would point to this plausible explanation for why children with LDs experience so many related deficits in apparently disparate academic and linguistic areas. Recognizing these interrelationships may hold the key to effective interventions for children with handwriting problems, as is suggested in Case Study 7.1.

Interventions for Children with Handwriting Disorders

Now that you have a good idea about the brain–behavior relationships involved in handwriting, it is important to think about whether the intervention can be handled by you, the teacher, the parent, or an occupational therapist. One important decision you must make is related to whether the problem is uniquely a graphomotor problem that causes difficulty with handwriting, or a more severe developmental coordination disorder (apraxia) requiring an occupational therapy evaluation and treatment plan. As in many of the disorders we discuss, there is probably a continuum spanning adequate, delayed, and deficient psychomotor skills. Thus you will require an understanding of both fine motor development in general, and the child's unique profile of psychomotor skills.

CASE STUDY 7.1. **Nathaniel's Handwriting Problem**

Nathaniel was a 7-year-old boy who was originally evaluated and classified as having a learning disability 2 years prior to my (Hale's) consultation with his teacher. He had been receiving resource room services for reading problems and speech–language services. A review of existing records and evaluations revealed that Nathaniel had a classic "double-deficit" reading disability, and both receptive and expressive language delays. In addition to his linguistic deficits, the psychological and educational evaluations said that Nathaniel had "visual–spatial" problems, because his graphomotor skills were poor. Test results confirmed difficulty with graphomotor skills, processing speed, and visual–motor integration, but nonmotor visual–perceptual skills appeared to be adequate. The resource room teacher reported that Nathaniel had made much progress in the visual–spatial area, as he easily discriminated simple and complex visual stimuli, recognized spatial relationships, and identified part–whole relationships. But Nathaniel still had difficulty with his handwriting. An examination of his handwriting confirmed that he had difficulty in this area. Although I did not give Nathaniel a full CHT evaluation, I used the hypothesis-testing approach to look at his visual–motor functioning. Sure enough, Nathaniel's visual–motor integration skills were poor; however, I found his visual processes to be intact, whereas motor skills were significantly delayed. He also had particular difficulty with learning and replicating motor sequences. In other words, Nathaniel showed classic signs of apraxia secondary to left-hemisphere dysfunction, consistent with his aphasic symptoms, and no amount of visual training would remediate his apparent motor problems. With this information, the teacher began helping Nathaniel sequence motor actions and coordinate graphomotor skills, using templates and tracing guidelines to improve his handwriting. But the focus was now on the motor action, not on the nonexistent visual–spatial problems thought to be present during his evaluation.

As is the case with deficit types in reading, it may be important to determine whether a child has a single, double, or triple fine motor deficit (i.e., sensory, motor, and/or frontal–subcortical); the more severe conditions will definitely necessitate occupational therapy. However, the distinction is dependent on many factors, including how severely affected the child is in each area, how old he or she is, and whether remediation has been successful in the past. That being said, we offer a number of handwriting recommendations in Appendix 7.2 for you and/or the teacher to help children with handwriting deficits. Although these are offered for manuscript, many of the same ideas apply to cursive writing as well. It is important to recognize that these are not prescriptions; rather, they are suggestions to help you through the process of brainstorming for interventions during CHT consultation.

Written Language

In the preceding two sections, we have developed an understanding of how two technical skills, spelling and handwriting, can contribute to written language problems. When you also consider the cognitive demands of expressive language and executive skills required in written language, it is easy to see why some children have difficulty developing, writing, and editing their writing assignments. Although prevalence rates vary, some studies have suggested that as many as 10%–18% of school-age children have a significant writing problem in one of these areas (Hooper et al., 1994). Some children readily enjoy putting their ideas on paper: They easily develop their ideas before writing, write flexibly and with ease, and then revise their prose. Other children may struggle with the writing process—planning little before starting, writing very little in an attempt just to get something on the paper, and then failing to check the paper for understanding, grammar, or legibility (Englert, Raphael, Fear, & Anderson, 1988).

Given that many children experience written language problems, it is somewhat surprising that the study of written expression has lagged behind that of other academic domains, as noted earlier (Hooper et al., 1994). Partly as a result of this lack of research, while children with WLDs may show improvement in language and reading skills, their written language deficits may persist into adulthood and affect their vocational skills (Johnson, 1987). Compared to peers, children with WLDs tend to write fewer long sentences; produce more fragments; use fewer advanced vocabulary words; and have higher rates of spelling, capitalization, and punctuation errors (Houck & Billingsley, 1989; Newcomer & Barenbaum, 1991; Singer, 1995). They do not develop their ideas well and organize them poorly in writing, often failing to develop a coherent theme (Smith, 1998). This may be due to limited oral language automaticity (Lahey & Bloom, 1994) or limited fluency, which results in a labored effort as they try to translate oral to written language (Singer, 1995).

What are the components of written language? In addition to the spelling and handwriting components discussed above, executive functions and semantic knowledge are required, both of which require memory processes (i.e., long-term and working memory). The same types of metacognitive processes are used in reading and written language, including self-planning, monitoring, evaluation, and modification (Wong, 1991). Expert writers tend to be goal-directed, moving from ideas to written text to planning for the next sentence or paragraph (Hooper et al., 1994). Semantic knowledge, which is so important in oral language and written language, is also critical for writing (Berninger, 1994). In a factor analysis of the writing samples of school-age children, Tindal and Parker (1991) found three factors that accounted for 81% of the variance. The Production/ Word Sequence, Conventions, and Idea/Cohesion/Organization factors they identified accounted for 37%, 26%, and 18% of the variance, respectively. Production appears to be a key element in written language, as fluency is related to most other writing skills (Isaacson, 1988).

Because WLDs are by definition complex and interrelated with other disorders, differential diagnosis of WLDs requires careful examination of multiple subcomponent processes. Your job is to examine the written language process and products beyond spelling and handwriting to determine the problematic areas for subsequent intervention. According to Mercer and Mercer (2001), it is important to examine the following written language processes during your evaluation:

- Content (accuracy/ideas/organization)
- Structure (grammatical correctness ratio/errors)
- Vocabulary (type token ratio/diversification index/unusual words)
- Syntax (sentence type variety/thought unit length)
- Fluency (average sentence length/length of sample)

WLD Subtypes

Although the description above gives us insight into the elements of written language, age serves as an important mitigating factor. Children with WLDs often experience what has been called a "developmental output disorder" (Levine, Oberklaid, & Meltzer, 1981), so that changes in the writing process with age may influence predictors of writing competency (Berninger, Mizokawa, & Bragg, 1991). Abbott and Berninger (1993) provide a neuropsychological model of the writing process that includes three major factors: Oral Language/Verbal Reasoning, Compositional Fluency, and Reading Skills. Included in their model are intellectual, achievement, processing, and writing measures. They found in one study that the Reading Skills factor was more closely related to writing for younger children, but that the Oral Language/Verbal Reasoning factor became increasingly important with age. It is important to realize that developmental influences on executive functions, visual–spatial processes, and language processes can all have an impact on written language competency (Gregg, 1992).

Most of the research has explored poor versus competent writers, but one study examined subtypes of children with WLDs. In a cluster analysis of clinic-referred children they classified as having WLDs, Sandler and colleagues (1992) found that a majority of the children had fine motor and linguistic deficits. A second group had visual–spatial deficits and poor handwriting, but good spelling and idea development. Attention and memory problems were notable in the third group, with problems noted in the areas of spelling, organization, and monitoring. A fourth group had poor letter production, legibility problems, and sequencing deficits. Executive impairments may be at the core of many written language problems, as executive and working memory deficits have been associated with poor sentence coherence, output, efficiency, and lexical cohesion (Wilson & Proctor, 2000). Although research is needed the effects of these cognitive processes on WLD, it is apparent that exploration of written language subtypes and their underlying neuropsychological characteristics may provide us with the necessary information to develop more effective interventions for children with WLDs (Hooper et al., 1994). Consistent with the arguments made throughout this book, we must move beyond levels of performance and examine intraindividual differences across domains if we are truly interested in understanding children with WLDs (Berninger & Abbott, 1992).

The Neuropsychology of WLDs

Although neuropsychological studies of WLDs are limited due to the complexity of studying these disorders, let's explore some of the neuropsychological factors that could influence written language competency. In addition to spelling and handwriting, several additional factors contribute to a child's written product. As noted earlier, attention, memory, and executive functions play an important role in written language, with the frontal lobe playing an important role in all of these. Long-term semantic memory retrieval is needed for choosing words and developing arguments, so the right prefrontal cortex would be important for accessing this prior knowledge (Cardebat et al., 1996). As noted in Chapter 2, the left temporal lobe has been found to be especially important for semantic memory (Daniele, Giustolisi, Silveri, Colosimo, & Gainotti, 1994; Gourovitch et al., 2000), with anterior regions more closely related to living things and posterior areas to objects (Damasio, Grabowski, Tranel, Hichwa, & Damasio, 1996; Strauss et al., 2000). This suggests that there could be a dissociation between writing narratives (with people included) and expository writing (especially if it is about a thing). Also recall that verbs are more likely to be represented in frontal areas (action = motor) (Daniele et al., 1994), so noun–verb agreement could be related to the interaction between the frontal and temporal lobes.

Appropriate grammar and syntax are important as well, with much research suggesting that the inferior frontal areas, particularly Broca's area, are responsible for syntax (Delazer, Girelli, Semenza, & Denes, 1999; Sirigu et al., 1998). Planning, organizing, shifting, monitoring, evaluating, and changing are all important skills during writing, so the prefrontal areas are needed to carry out working memory and other executive function demands (Chapman et al., 1992; Gershberg & Shimamura, 1995; Wilson & Proctor, 2000). Working memory would be essential to keep these processes "online" and ensure progress toward the writing objective. In addition, the prefrontal area would also be essential for establishing the story sequence or a temporally coherent narrative (Sirigu et al., 1998). Of course, the frontal–basal ganglia–cerebellar circuit would also be important during written language.

Left- and Right-Hemisphere Processes

Finally, let's examine the left- and right-hemisphere processes in written language. As noted in Chapter 2, our model of hemispheric functioning suggests that the left- and right-hemisphere processes can be characterized by local–global (Delis, Robertson, & Efron, 1986), microstructural–macrostructural (Glosser, 1993), fine–coarse (Beeman, 1993), and concordant/convergent–discordant/divergent (Bryan & Hale, 2001) distinctions. When the hemispheres are working together in a complementary rather than segregated way during writing, the left hemisphere may provide a quick, efficient, and predictable response (Coney, 1998), but homologous right-hemisphere areas may be recruited to increase the linguistic complexity of the output (Just, Carpenter, Keller, Eddy, & Thulborn, 1996). Children with left-hemisphere dysfunction may then have difficulty adhering to grammatical rules and structured responses. These are the children who may get assigned two grades on their writing assignments: an A for content and an F for grammar.

Children with right-hemisphere dysfunction may show a more subtle pattern of deficits—one that may not emerge until the late elementary or middle school years. During the early school years, these children are likely to produce grammatically correct sentences that obey conventional syntactic rules, but they are less likely to produce complex syntactic structures (Beeman & Chiarello, 1998), which are not required until later grades. For lexical–semantic use in writing, they may produce straightforward sentences using common words, but may have more difficulty thinking of alternative words to represent their ideas. Recall that the right hemisphere is essential for considering multiple possible word and sentence meanings and distant semantic relations, whereas the left hemisphere is specialized for closely related words, single interpretations, and semantic integration (Chiarello, 1998; Richards & Chiarello, 1997). Unlike the left hemisphere, which is likely to respond with highly probable, predictable, routinized, and concrete writing discourse, the right hemisphere is likely to provide rich, complex, and creative prose. As a result, children with right-hemisphere dysfunction are likely to produce serviceable, but not very interesting or complex, writing samples. They may be overly focused and literal, missing the ultimate objective of their writing assignment.

During writing, children with right-hemisphere dysfunction are likely to use left-hemisphere *convergent* processing to locate and select information that is *concordant* with their existing thoughts, but they may have difficulty maintaining the flexibility necessary to revise preliminary work to integrate a novel perspective or additional information (Bowden & Beeman, 1998; Stemmer & Joanette, 1998). This is because they are likely to have difficulty with *divergent* thinking and fail to consider *discordant* information. Not only does this affect communicative intent, but it also impairs word choice, leading to prose that may be marked by trivial, tangential, and/or unrelated information (Cherney & Canter, 1993; Myers, 1993). This may affect not only content, but sentence and paragraph structure as well. Children with right-hemisphere dysfunction may capitalize and punctuate correctly, and have all elements of a sentence in place, but they are unlikely to produce creative or interesting prose.

As you can see, multiple areas of the brain are involved in written language. Written language is by far the most difficult academic subject, requiring virtually every part of the brain to work concertedly toward a final product. Obviously, many more cognitive processes are required for written language competency than for other academic skills. It requires brainstorming, planning, and organization skills; choosing appropriate words and phrases; putting together a coherent sequence of words and sentences; adherence to grammar and syntax conventions; handwriting and spelling; and monitoring, evaluating, and changing the written product. Determining where a child is having difficulty can help you understand how to help that child, so that he or she may effectively communicate ideas in both oral and written form.

Interventions for Children with WLDs

You will find a number of techniques to assist you with written expression in Appendix 7.3. As we have discussed in regard to spelling intervention, written expression requires all of the visual memory, graphomotor skills, and executive functions that spelling does. However, the executive demands are what set written expression apart from all other achievement activities. Let's think of them. Writers need to brainstorm and retrieve ideas; develop a plan; organize their ideas into a sequence; develop a strategy for writing and integrating information; monitor their writing at the word, sentence, paragraph, and whole-product levels; remain flexible to change their ideas, words, or sentences; and evaluate the clarity of their content. Even if they do this well, they still must focus on the mechanics, such as proper spelling, punctuation, capitalization, and grammar. It is no wonder that many children with LDs have problems with written language. As with other academic areas, you must first attempt to recognize a child's cognitive pattern of performance, link this information to the written language product (both formal and informal assessment data), and then work collaboratively with the teacher to develop an effective intervention. However, because written language is so complex, there may be more than one problem area, so it is important for you and the teacher to remain flexible and open to exploring multiple strategies and interventions. Again, the key is the use of progress monitoring and recycling to ensure intervention efficacy.

It is important to recognize that few, if any, of the interventions in Appendix 7.3 were developed with the knowledge we now have about brain–behavior relationships. Therefore, even a very good strategy may be individually effective for some children, but not for others. It is essential that you design interventions for each individual child during the collaborative problem-solving meeting with the teacher(s) and/or parents. The intervention ideas presented in this chapter are merely suggestions to help you generate ideas in the problem-solving interview. Even an intervention that works for most children may need to be tailored to the child's unique characteristics so that it may be even more effective. Your ongoing intervention monitoring, evaluation, and recycling will be the key for ensuring the treatment validity of your evaluation and maximizing individualized instruction practices in written language.

WRITTEN LANGUAGE CASE STUDY

Case Study 7.2 presents an interesting case study of a child with a WLD that wasn't quite what it seemed. As is the case with oral language, written language competency is related to both the fluency and the quality of the response. As we can see in Elise's case, she didn't really seem to have good ideas at all (of course, it depends on how you define "good"). The case again highlights how referral questions, histories, and observations are limited in helping you understand written language problems. If it weren't for our CHT evaluation, there were several interventions we might have considered, but few would have been related to the actual cause for Elise's writing problems.

CASE STUDY 7.2. Elise's Ideas

Elise was an 11-year-old girl referred for a psychological evaluation because of parental concerns about her writing. She reportedly had good ideas, but couldn't seem to convey them on paper. Elise was described as a polite, cooperative, and reserved girl who was slow to warm up, but could be quite talkative with her best friend and family. Elise was hard-working and conscientious about her schoolwork, and had earned above-average grades for most of her schooling. Socially, Elise was best friends with Debbie, but she had few other friendships. She seemed to get along well with others, sometimes talking extensively about a particular book or topic she was interested in. However, Elise was somewhat isolated and teased by others, and one of Elise's teachers, Bert, couldn't seem to pinpoint why. Bert said that sometimes Elise seemed awkward in social situations. Sometimes Elise would get angry when others were joking around, and would say things that were unrelated to the conversation; other than that, however, she seemed fine. Bert said that Elise was an avid reader, preferring reading to any other activity, and often remained in the periphery during social situations.

The social studies teacher reported that Elise had no difficulty with objective exams; she just had problems with essay exams. She also had difficulty with both expository and creative writing in English, often writing little during creative writing exercises. Examining her writing, I (Hale) found that her handwriting was fairly good (she had big loops on some curved letters, though), and she had adequate capitalization and punctuation for the most part. The sentences mostly followed the same subject–verb–object pattern, however, and ideas were seldom connected. Overall, the longer samples had very limited organization, and the paragraphs didn't seem to flow well. Despite her reported reading skill, Elise tended to answer comprehension questions that asked her to retrieve facts and details from assignments.

A CHT evaluation was undertaken, using the Differential Ability Scales (DAS) as the screening tool. The following results were obtained:

General Cognitive Ability (GCA) = 94		
Verbal Ability = 108	Nonverbal Reasoning Ability = 86	Spatial Ability = 90
Word Definitions = 59	Matrices = 39	Recall of Designs = 37
Similarities = 52	Sequential and Quantitative Reasoning = 45	Pattern Construction = 52
Recall of Digits = 55		
Recall of Objects—Immediate = 41		
Recall of Objects—Delayed = 47		
Speed of Information Processing = 48		

From this evaluation, it appeared that Elise had adequate skills in many areas, and that verbal areas appeared to be a strength—an uncommon finding for children with WLDs. Her nonverbal reasoning or fluid abilities seemed to be somewhat low, and there was a large difference between the two DAS Spatial Ability subtests, with Recall of Designs much poorer than Pattern Construction. This led me to the hypothesis that something about Elise's visual–motor integration or constructional praxis could be affecting handwriting, but Recall of Designs also taps memory, so memory problems were another possibility. The diagnostic subtests were largely adequate, but Elise's memory for objects was low. Interestingly, the Immediate score on Recall of Objects was worse than the Delayed score, suggesting that once she had these word–object associations in memory, she was fine. Obviously, there was nothing in the data that would suggest a writing problem, so some detective work was necessary. Could Elise be a child with a "nonverbal" learning disorder affecting a "verbal" skill such as written language? In an attempt to examine this possibility, I looked into nonverbal or fluid reasoning, visual memory, and nonliteral language as possible causes for her difficulties. Given the history of problems with organization and flexibility, I also thought it would be important to look at executive functions as well. The following were the results of the hypothesis-testing stage (all scores are converted to standard scores):

(continued)

239

NEPSY

Tower = 95
Design Fluency = 85
Verbal Fluency = 95
Design Copy = 105
Arrows = 100
Memory for Faces = 85
Narrative Memory = 105

Test of Memory and Learning

Memory for Location = 100
Object Recall = 85

Wisconsin Card Sorting Test (WCST)

Errors = 92
Perseverative Responses = 85
Perseverative Errors = 88
Categories, Trials to First Category,
Failure to Maintain Set > 16th %ile

Cognitive Assessment System (CAS)

Nonverbal Matrices = 95
Planned Connections = 105
Expressive Attention = 100

Woodcock–Johnson III

Concept Formation = 86

Comprehensive Assessment of Spoken Language (CASL)

Antonyms = 106
Synonyms = 114
Sentence Completion = 92
Idiomatic Language = 102

Grammatical Morphemes = 104
Sentence Comprehension = 89
Grammaticality Judgment = 108

Nonliteral Language = 75
Meaning from Context = 87
Inference = 82
Ambiguous Sentences = 80
Pragmatic Judgment = 92

The hypothesis-testing results revealed that Elise did not appear to have significant difficulty with nonverbal reasoning and fluid ability, but as these tasks became less structured, she had more difficulty; she performed best when given a multiple-choice format. Similarly, her attention and executive functions appeared to be good, but she was somewhat perseverative on the WCST, an unstructured, self-directed task. She also seemed to have more difficulty on the last items of the CAS Planned Connections subtest (consistent with Trails B difficulties), making several errors. On the NEPSY, there was an apparent dissociation between her Verbal Fluency, which was fine, and her Design Fluency, which was low average; this suggested that maybe the visual nature of this task or the graphomotor skills required were causing her difficulty. However, her skill at drawing designs according to a model was intact, and other dorsal or visual–spatial–memory skills appeared to be adequate. Elise's memory for object–word associations and facial memory were limited, pointing to possible ventral stream problems. The CASL results appeared to confirm that Elise had language difficulties associated with right-hemisphere temporal lobe dysfunction. She had difficulty with nonliteral language, gaining meaning from context, drawing inferences, and deciphering ambiguous sentences. She performed adequately on the CASL Idiomatic Language subtest, which is somewhat surprising at first glance. But an examination of this subtest reveals that the idioms used are fairly straightforward and commonly used. This is why the CASL's author placed the Idiomatic Language subtest in the Lexical/Semantic category. Consistent with this assumption, Elise easily recognized these simple idioms by using her good rote memory skills, and she had no problem providing the appropriate definition of each.

The results of the CHT evaluation confirmed the hypothesis that Elise apparently had a "nonverbal" LD affecting written language. Subsequent to the CHT, I worked with the teacher to develop some written language strategies designed to increase Elise's brainstorming of ideas prior to writing, her flexibility in interpretation and production of language, her consideration of multiple word choices and meanings, and her skill at linking ideas and concepts; she was encouraged to provide details only after the concepts were developed and associated. The teacher also came up with a great strategy—namely, using poems to work on Elise's skill at interpreting multiple meanings of words. Finally, we offered counseling to help Elise read facial and vocal affect and recognize colloquial language during conversation.

APPENDIX 7.1. Spelling Interventions

Reference	Intervention description
Berninger et al. (2002)	Alphabet principle and teacher scaffolding
Dixon (1991)	Phoneme–grapheme rule-based instruction, with morphological analysis to reduce misspellings due to phonetically irregular words
Fernald (1988)	Multisensory approach: Writing, checking, tracing, repeating, writing from memory
Gillingham & Stillman (1973)	Gillingham method: Simultaneous oral spelling, written spelling, and reading in logical sequential word hierarchy
Graham & Freeman (1986)	Six steps: Saying word, writing/saying word, checking word with model, tracing model and saying word, writing word, checking word with model (steps repeated as necessary)
Graham, Harris, & Loynachan (1994)	Spelling for Writing word list: Most frequently used words in writing, including irregular words, for Grades 1–3
Graham & Voth (1990)	Test–teach–test approach: Daily practice with self-correction for accuracy and fluency; game-like format for spelling activities
Greene (1994)	Look–cover–write–check: Visual and semantic mnemonics (e.g., "principal" is your "pal")
Harp (1988)	Spelling notebook of difficult-to-spell words for use when writing
Horn (1954)	Horn method: Pronouncing, looking, saying letters in sequence, spelling from memory, checking, repeating steps if words misspelled
Kauffman et al. (1978)	Imitation of student error, then modeling of correct spelling
Kearney & Drabman (1993)	Multisensory procedure: Individual study, practice with feedback, oral and written respelling of words
Mercer & Mercer (2001)	Cover and write method: Looking and saying word, writing word while looking, covering word and writing it, and uncovering to see if correct
McGuigan (1975)	Add-a-Word Flow spelling lists (words added after mastery of previous words)
McNaughton et al. (1994)	Self-directed and peer-mediated instruction; linking of oral and written spelling; regular practice, evaluation, and review with feedback
Shanker & Ekwall (1998)	Teaching spelling of common words across curriculum and linking to effective written communication
Stein (1983)	Finger spelling and sound blending combined
Stephens (1977)	Teaching auditory discrimination, consonants, phonograms, plurals, syllabication, structural analysis, suffixes, digraphs, diphthongs, silent "e"
Templeton (1986)	Teaching spelling in context of oral reading and semantic understanding
Wirtz et al. (1996)	Hearing word, writing word, comparing to model, correcting errors with proofreading marks, writing correctly, repeating first five steps
Wong (1986)	Metacognitive self-questioning strategy ("Know word? Syllables? Syllables match? Parts I don't know? Look right?"); self-reinforcement

APPENDIX 7.2. Handwriting Interventions (for Manuscript Printing)[1]

Problem	Possible cause	Remediation
Letters slanted	Paper slanted	Straighten paper/pull strokes toward body
Shapes vary	Poor grapheme image	Write problem letters "nearpoint" (paper) to "farpoint" (chalkboard); prompt and tracing
Too large	Poor line recognition	Reteach size within line restrictions; use physical prompting and manual guidance
	Exaggerated arm movement	Reduce arm movement on circle-type letters
	Poor grapheme image	Write problem letters nearpoint (paper) to farpoint (chalkboard); prompt and tracing
Too small	Poor line recognition	Reteach size within line restriction; prompting and manual guidance
	Finger movement	Stress arm movement; check pencil grasp; check hand–pencil and arm–hand positions; write within model borders
	Poor grapheme image	Write problem letters nearpoint to farpoint; use pointing and tracing
Crowded	Spatial perception	Reteach uniform spacing using pencil tip, prompt, trace, fade
Excess space	Improper case size/shape	Review size concept; provide space model; move nearpoint to farpoint; trace and fade
Poor alignment	Improper letter formation	Review size; stress bringing strokes down to line; demonstrate, trace, prompt, fade, provide feedback
	Improper grasp/position	Check grasp; check hand and hand–arm positions
Improper letter height	Poor size concept	Provide different letter size within lines; model, trace, and fade guidance
Poor line quality	Improper pressure	Check grasp; check hand–arm position; use tissue paper/pencil in palm to relax grip; use special grip support; check darkness with model

From Mercer and Mercer (2001). Copyright 2001 by Pearson Education. Adapted by permission.

APPENDIX 7.3. Written Language Interventions

Reference	Intervention description
Bos & Vaughn (1988)	SCOPE proofreading technique: Spelling, capitalization, order/syntax, punctuation, expressing complete thoughts
Czarnecki et al. (1998)	CALL-UP for note taking: Copying from board, adding details, listening/writing teacher questions, listening/writing answers, utilizing text, putting in own words
de la Paz (1997)	STOP: Suspending judgment; telling thesis statement; organizing ideas; planning as you write, using "DARE" (different sentences, avoiding pronouns, remembering grammar, exciting and interesting)
Englert (1990)	Cognitive strategy instruction for planning, organizing, editing, revising
Englert (1992)	Modeling writing, thinking aloud during writing, student editing
Gordon & Braun (1983)	Story grammar of characters, setting, plot, problem, action, resolution
Graham (1992)	Writing objectives: Student interest, goals, multiple audiences, project format, incorporating writing in activities, pragmatic writing
Graves (1994)	Write–teach approach, emphasizing composition before mechanics
Graves & Hauge (1993)	Story grammar cue system: Setting, characters, problem, action, ending
Harris & Graham (1992)	W-W-W, What-2, How-2: Who, when, where; what (protagonist), what (environment); how (ending), how (protagonist feeling)
Harris & Graham (1997)	Self-regulated strategy development: background knowledge, discussion, modeling, memorization, position support, independent practice
Isaacson (1995)	Process approach to writing: Modeling, collaboration, prompting, self-initiation, self-monitoring
Leavell & Ioannides (1993)	Identifying character attributes, speech, actions, thoughts, and emotions in own writing
MacArthur et al. (1991)	Peer revising strategy: Listening/reading, providing feedback, rereading, making suggestions, revising and checking for errors, exchanging papers and checking for errors
Mercer (1997)	Prewriting, drafting, revising, editing, publishing stages
Mercer & Mercer (2001)	TOWER: Thinking about content, ordering topics/details, writing draft, engaging in error analysis with COPS (see below), revising/rewriting
Phelps-Terasaki & Phelps-Gunn (2000)	Modified Fitzgerald key, using "wh-" questions for ordering sentences in paragraphs according to structured sequence
Polloway et al. (1981)	Oral proofreading strategy designed to have students recognize inconsistencies in the content and sentence structure
Rico (1983)	Clustering prewriting technique for nucleus word, and free association of related ideas forming clusters; words/clusters are connected with arrows
Schumaker et al. (1985)	COPS editing strategy: capitalization, overall appearance, punctuation, spelling accuracy
Schumaker et al. (1984)	RAP: Reading paragraph, asking self about main ideas, putting main idea and details into own paragraph
Schumaker & Sheldon (1985)	PENS sentence composition: Picking sentence type/formula; exploring words for formula; noting words; searching for verbs and subjects, then checking
Stevens & Englert (1993)	PODE: Planning, organizing, drafting, editing/revising writing
Strong (1983)	Combining sentences into clusters and paragraphs
Tompkins & Friend (1985)	Semantic mapping of ideas/shapes with topic and supporting subordinate ideas, linked together with lines and/or arrows
Welch (1992)	PLEASE metacognitive strategy: Picking topic, listing information, evaluating list and planning organization, activating with topic sentence, supplying supporting sentences, ending with conclusion and evaluating mechanics
Wong et al. (1996)	Interactive-dialogue reciprocal teaching technique to plan, write, revise

CHAPTER 8

└┴┴┴┴┴┴┴┴┴┴┴┘

Neuropsychological Principles and Psychopathology

THE POLITICS OF PSYCHOPATHOLOGY

School and Mental Health Practitioners

We are all taught about personality theories and psychopathology in our training programs. We learn the different theories, study differential diagnoses, and are taught to administer objective and projective measures of behavior and personality. However, we seldom see training programs focus on the relationship between cognitive functioning and psychopathology. Just as we tend to assume that academic achievement is a teacher's responsibility, we tend to think of psychological disorders as something a psychiatrist or clinic-based mental health practitioner should handle. We feel a little uneasy about identifying psychopathological disorders, preferring to use the seemingly more benign label "behavior disorders." If "serious emotional disturbance" makes us uncomfortable, making a formal diagnosis is even less appealing. It is easier to say that a child is "sad" or "acting out" than to say that the child has depression (DE) or conduct disorder (CD). As we will discuss in the following sections, psychopathological disorders do exist in children, and recognizing the signs of such a disorder can lead to preventative early intervention, possibly limiting the impact of the condition. At the same time, we recognize that more weight can be placed on the symptoms expressed by a child rather than the underlying etiology, at least at the present time.

Unfortunately, we all have a tendency to segregate and compartmentalize the highly interrelated domains of cognition and behavior, even though categorical approaches seldom reflect the complexity of children. You may recall Bandura's (1978) model of reciprocal determinism from your training. It is important to remember the major tenet of this model: that cognition, behavior, and environment are inextricably interrelated and mutually determined, resulting in an ever-changing, dynamic individual. Therefore, assessment of child psychopathology requires a transactional interpretive framework—one that considers the interaction of biological and environmental factors in relation to brain development (Teeter & Semrud-Clikeman, 1995). When children interact with their environment, the behaviors they display in any given situation are invariably related to their previous experiences, the contingencies they have experienced, and the cognitive templates in which they perceive the world. These multiple "realities" that all children construct are what make them unique individuals. Unfortunately, these idiosyncratic manifestations of cognitive and behavior problems also make the study of the neuropsychology of childhood psychopathology extremely difficult, though intriguing.

Although neurocognitive impairments are more closely related to psychiatric symptoms displayed in school than in home settings (Szatmari, Offord, Siegel, Finlayson, & Tuff, 1990), school psychologists may be reluctant to explore the relationship between neuropsychological constructs and psychopathology for several reasons. Many claim that psychopathology is a "mental health" issue—something "clinical psychologists" deal with—and that referral to appropriate agencies is necessary unless a child has "just a behavior problem." We agree that the severity of some cases warrants referral for psychiatric and/or psychological treatment outside the schools, but it is important to realize that psychologists in the schools serve as the "front line" of mental health services for children and their families. Even children who have received mental health services in a hospital or residential setting were once in a school like yours, and will probably return to a school after treatment. With today's administrative climate in managed care clinical settings, there is an increased likelihood that you will be required to serve more children with significant mental health needs within the regular school setting. Hospital stays and residential care are quite expensive, so you and your colleagues are responsible for caring for these children. As we will discuss later, children who experience psychopathology have a greater tendency to have brain-based disorders, and recognizing the interrelationship of brain and behavior thus becomes essential for the school-based psychologist. Whether your training in personality/behavioral assessment and intervention was extensive or minimal, it is critical that you recognize the relationship among development, cognition, achievement, and personality/behavior if you are to gain a holistic understanding of a child.

Neuropsychological Principles for Child Mental Health

Many practitioners rely on interview methods and on the multiaxial system of the *Diagnostic and Statistical Manual for Mental Disorders*, fourth edition (DSM-IV; American Psychiatric Association, 1994) or the DSM-IV text revision (DSM-IV-TR; American Psychiatric Association, 2000) for differential diagnosis of childhood psychological disorders. The DSM-IV/DSM-IV-TR system provides important information regarding the prevalence rates, etiological factors, associated characteristics, and diagnostic criteria for numerous disorders. Although a careful history and evaluation corroborated by medical, developmental, historical, and informant data may reveal classic signs and symptoms of specific disorders, the presence of neuropsychological symptoms, comorbid conditions, rapid decline in academic performance or behavior, or poor response to intervention may indicate the need for a more comprehensive evaluation. As we will discuss later, the use of categorical models is helpful in understanding childhood disorders; however, the complex interplay of cognition, behavior, and environment often requires much more than a clinical interview using DSM-IV/DSM-IV-TR criteria.

Advocates of the problem-solving services delivery model argue that interview and observation methods are sufficient for appropriate problem identification and analysis. This is probably more accurate for children with emotional or behavioral disorders that are secondary to environmental issues (e.g., inappropriate reinforcement or punishment). These children have "behavior disorders." However, you can seldom say with certainty that a disorder is "brain-based" or "environmental" in practice, because these descriptors should be seen as the endpoints of an interactive continuum, not as an either–or dichotomy (Dean, 1986). Interview techniques alone may not be effective for complex cases, and as we have discussed in earlier chapters, similar symptoms can result from very disparate neuropsychological disorders. Detailing the relationships among neurological, cognitive, and behavioral characteristics of children with associated psychological disorders (Keefe, 1995) can provide practitioners with the information necessary to confirm initial diagnostic impressions, rule out confounding or conflicting data, and monitor intervention efficacy. As part of a team, you can become a key player in differential diagnosis and treatment of childhood disorders of psychopathology, as highlighted in regard to attention-deficit/hyperactivity disorder (ADHD) in In-Depth 8.1.

Your role in the assessment and treatment of child psychopathology requires a fine-grained examination of the interrelationship of cognition, achievement, and behavior. This analysis must be undertaken within an ecological and developmental framework, as the behavioral manifestations of neuropsychological impairment appear to change over time and situations (Tramontana, Hooper, & Nardolillo, 1988). Although many children present with learning problems that may mask comorbid emotional and behavior disorders (Hagin, 1997), children with neuropsychological impairment are more likely to display overt signs of psychiatric disturbance (Bornstein, Miller, & van Schoor, 1989), and neuropsychological assessment is sensitive to both cerebral dysfunction and psychopathology (Flor-Henry, 1990). For example, a child with a pervasive developmental disorder (PDD) may display concomitant intellectual deficits, speech impairment, dysphoria, and self-injurious behavior. Another child with a mathematics disorder may present with psychomotor slowing, poor abstract verbal comprehension, and both internalizing disorders (IDs) such as DE and externalizing disorders (EDs) such as CD. As is the case with cognitive and neuropsychological measures, your assessment strategy should be determined by the presenting problems and previous data acquired, because not all measures will be equally effective in addressing the wide array of childhood behavioral, social, and emotional problems (Merrell, 1999).

For a complex, multidimensional case, quantitative and qualitative analysis of neuropsychological patterns of performance can provide you with insight into the child's problems for subsequent treatment planning or modification (Milberg, Hebben, & Kaplan, 1996). This insight is also critical for providing you with the necessary information for "manifest determination" of whether the child's emotional or behavioral difficulties are related to his or her inappropriate behavior; this determination can affect subsequent disciplinary action (Melroy, 1999). When treatment adherence, compliance, and/or response are of concern, you can use neuropsychological and other measures to help physicians and other practitioners develop single-subject research designs for monitoring response over time or across conditions (Hale & Fiorello, 2002).

NEUROPSYCHOLOGICAL BASIS OF EMOTION AND BEHAVIOR

Although the famous case of Phineas Gage (the man with the iron rod accident) demonstrated the first clear association between the frontal lobes and psychopathology in the mid-1800s, the relationship among brain, emotion, and behavior has only recently begun to receive much needed attention. In your training, you probably heard of the nebulous "limbic system" as the emotional area of the brain, but it is always unclear how these and other structures interact to produce the complexity of human behavior. Not only is neuroanatomy important in this study, but neurochemistry research has been instrumental as well. We know that stimulants (e.g., Ritalin,

IN-DEPTH 8.1. ADHD and Differential Diagnosis

There are advantages and disadvantages of individual versus team diagnosis of disorders. Research on decision making suggests that individuals are quicker and more efficient at arriving at decisions, but that the *quality* of a decision is often better when it is made by a group of individuals. Nowhere is this issue more relevant than in the diagnosis of ADHD. Many administrators and school psychologists operate under the assumption that only physicians are qualified to diagnose ADHD. Not only do many school practitioners believe this; so do many physicians, as evidenced by a statement one of us recently heard a pediatrician make to a large group of teachers. It is not uncommon to hear the sentence, "I think Johnny has ADHD; send him to the doctor for medicine" echoed in school team meetings. True, physicians presently are the only professionals with prescription privileges (in most states). However, you must ask yourself several questions before making this medical referral:

- What are the other possible reasons for the child's inattention, impulsivity, or overactivity?
- What do the results of the functional analysis (i.e., antecedent → behavior → consequence) reveal?
- What are the results of the prereferral efforts undertaken by you, the teacher, and/or the parents?
- What objective measures have you administered for differential diagnosis?
- What will you do to communicate with the physician and facilitate his or her assessment of the child?
- What is your plan for monitoring medication response if medication treatment is attempted?
- What adjunctive academic and behavioral interventions will you attempt to ensure optimal care?

The point here is that you should play an integral role in diagnosing and treating children with ADHD and other disorders. The bottom line is that most physicians make ADHD diagnoses on the basis of parent interview and observation over a 10- to 20-minute evaluation, as there are no formal medical tests for ADHD. Some physicians may perform a soft sign exam (see Chapter 3), but as we have noted earlier, soft signs are often positive in many childhood disorders. Physicians sometimes use brief behavior rating scales, but these are often screening tools that include ADHD symptoms only. Psychologists have many more objective tools, including cognitive and neuropsychological tests, as well as multidimensional rating scales that can provide critical information regarding the signs and symptoms of the disorder. Including a physician's evaluation is helpful—indeed, it is important for developing treatment strategies and monitoring response—but physicians who receive objective information from teachers and psychologists are more likely to make accurate diagnoses and develop more comprehensive treatment plans. In fact, most physicians desire this information from the schools. Therefore, working with physicians and other outside professionals is an integral component of the school psychologist's role and function.

Teamwork is the key, both inside and outside the schools. In most cases, the team approach is less likely to result in error, and we have seen many diagnoses made solely by individual clinicians change when comprehensive team evaluations are undertaken. We really need to change our thinking from an emphasis on independent *multidisciplinary* evaluation and treatment to the encouragement of *interdisciplinary* collaboration and cooperation, so that we can all truly meet the needs of children (Hale & Kavanagh, 1991).

Adderall) may be the drugs of choice for ADHD, and that selective serotonin reuptake inhibitors (SSRIs) are often used to treat DE. Researchers thus have concluded that dopamine is related to ADHD symptoms and serotonin is related to DE, but we are only now beginning to understand how both of these neurotransmitters, and others, work together to produce the types of neuropsychological and behavioral patterns seen in these disorders. Unfortunately, none of the psychopathological disorders we discuss have been uniformly identified by discrete brain lesions; therefore, we must start with overt behavior and work backward to understand the underlying anomalous neural systems that produce the observed problems (Filipek, 1999).

This book largely examines cortical relationships and behavior, but this section necessarily begins with an exploration of subcortical structures associated with emotion and personality. We are more likely to have an impact on cortical areas in our interventions, of course, but understanding the basis of these disorders helps with differential diagnosis and treatment strategies. Given the complexity of human emotions and behavior, you will not be surprised to find that multiple structures and systems have been implicated. The amygdala, with its "fight-or-flight" reputation, is the structure most likely to be associated with emotional valence (Gray, 1987)—from attraction (approach) to withdrawal (avoidance). It affects not only behavior, but endocrine and autonomic activity as well (LeDoux, 1995). The amygdala also helps identify emotionally laden information, and therefore has an important function for constructing long-term memories (Krishnan, 1999). The left amygdala has been associated with positive emotions, whereas bilateral amygdala activity has been noted with negative emotions (Hamann, Ely, Hoffman, & Kilts, 2002). Interestingly, the hippocampus becomes more active as problems are solved, suggesting that learning has occurred, but frustrating, unsolvable problems lead to amygdala activation (Schneider et al., 1996). Certainly, physiological response could be the result of hypothalamic dysregulation, as the hypothalamus is the subcortical structure essential for regulating drives such as eating and sexual behavior (Capote, Flaherty, & Lichter, 2001), and hypothalamic dysfunction has been associated with intermittent explosive disorder (Krishnan, 1999). Certainly the thalamic "relay station" can have a modulating effect on emotional processing; the striatum can affect executive and emotional regulation, and motoric response to social or emotional stimuli; and the hippocampus may be involved in formulating emotional valence or memories.

Although cortical areas may be directly or indirectly related to emotional experiences, they certainly have a modulating influence. The prefrontal cortex allows individuals to think about the emotional consequences of their actions before they engage in a behavior, or mull over a behavior after they have completed it (Davidson, 2000). As a result, it is not surprising that the prefrontal–striatal–thalamic circuits have been strong candidates for many of the different psychopathological disorders, with the orbital prefrontal cortex seen as the prime culprit. Consistent with the activation hypothesis, orbital underactivation or dysfunction results in disinhibition, while overactivation results in inhibition or overcontrolled behavior. This area may be one source of what has been termed "affective information processing" (Murphy & Sahakian, 2001) or "emotion regulation"—a dynamic process that allows for examination of intrinsic factors (self) in relation to extrinsic ones (others) (Slattery, Garvey, & Swedo, 2001). Damage to the orbital area has been associated with lability, irritability, poor judgment, antisocial behavior, distractibility, and socially inappropriate behavior (Lichter & Cummings, 2001). Evidence is mounting that the orbital cortex is *underactive* in children with ADHD (Voeller, 2001), but *overactive* in children with IDs such as obsessive–compulsive disorder (OCD) (Baxter, Clark, Iqbal, & Ackerman, 2001). The orbital cortex has close connections with several subcortical structures, including the ventral anterior cingulate, which (as noted earlier) is related to online monitoring of environmental stimuli and self-control of behavior. Damage to the anterior cingulate has been associated with lethargy, apathy, and slow psychomotor speed, similar to the symptoms of DE (Mayberg, 2001). However, damage to the dorsolateral prefrontal area can also lead to these symptoms, as well as difficulty with attention, working memory, and executive function, found in DE, ADHD, and other syndromes (Lichter & Cummings, 2001). As we can see, oversimplifying the dorsolateral prefrontal cortex as the "executive function" area, and the orbital prefrontal cortex as the "emotion regulation" area, does not provide us with an accurate understanding of the complex relationship between these important areas and functions (Slattery et al., 2001). In addition, there may be left–right frontal differences that need elucidation. For instance, children with ADHD show right frontal–subcortical hypoactivity, while those with schizophrenia show underactivation in the left homologue frontal–subcortical areas (Rubia, 2002). The "frontal metaphor" has been invoked to explain many developmental psychopathologies (Pennington & Ozonoff, 1996), but we are only now beginning to recognize how these frontal–subcortical relationships affect the social and emotional functioning of children.

Although much of the emphasis on the neuropsychological causes of psychopathology has been on the frontal and temporal lobes, it is important to recognize that left- and right-hemisphere processes are probably also associated with emotion and behavior. Fitting nicely with our dichotomy between the left and right hemispheres, the left hemisphere is responsible for voluntary expressions (prior learning), but spontaneous expressions can be initiated by either hemisphere (Gazzaniga, Ivry, & Mangun, 1998). Interestingly, some research has shown left-hemisphere activation to be associated with positive affect and right-hemisphere activation with negative affect; this suggests that the left frontal area is associated with approach behavior and positive affect, whereas the right is linked to avoidant/withdrawal behavior and negative affect (Davidson, 1995). Could it be that novel, complex, and ambiguous situations cause individuals to experience negative emotions (i.e., right-hemisphere activation), while automatic, routinized, and familiar situations lead to positive emotions (i.e., left-hemisphere activation)? This possible link with our neuropsychological model discussed in Chapter 2 makes sense, given what we know about cognitive dissonance—we all like the things we know and tend to discount those ideas unfamiliar to us! Based on this left–right affect lateralization pattern, we might also suggest that if the left hemisphere is underactive or dysfunctional, then negative affect and avoidance behaviors may occur, and if the right is underactive, then positive affect and approach behaviors may occur. Consistent with this argument, crying, depressed behaviors, and catastrophic reactions have been associated with left-hemisphere lesions, while laughter, euphoria, or indifference are more likely following right-hemisphere lesions (Heilman, Bowers, & Valenstein, 1993; Sackheim, Decima, & Malitz, 1982). Extroverted individuals who are optimistic, social, and positive tend to show increased left frontal activity, whereas lower left frontal activity has been associated with negative, neurotic, introverted behavior (Canli et al., 2001).

As we have seen in previous chapters, we are not surprised to find that cortical–subcortical structures act upon emotional information in complex and multifaceted ways. When it comes to cortical–subcortical relationships and psychopathology, the top-down or bottom-up question becomes a big one. The frontal–subcortical circuits can affect an individual's interest in the environment, with overarousal resulting in a tendency toward withdrawal (e.g., "Everything is too overwhelming; I need to avoid others") and underarousal associated with approach behaviors (e.g., "Everything is boring; I need to approach others"). Examining this propensity, Gray (1987) has argued that there are two interrelated systems: the behavioral activation system (BAS), sensitive to reward and escape from punishment, and the behavioral inhibition system (BIS), sensitive to punishment and nonreward. Could psychological disorders be related to the interaction of these two systems? An accumulating body of research supports a notion first posited by Eysenck (1983) several years ago: Individuals with EDs (e.g., CD) have cortical *underarousal,* while those with IDs (e.g., anxiety [AN], DE) are likely to experience cortical *overarousal.* Beauchaine (2001) suggests that an underactive BIS is characteristic of ADHD and CD, because the BAS works without BIS balance. For anxiety and depression, the BIS is overactive, limiting the effects of the BAS. Consistent with these arguments, introverts tend to have greater cortical activity, while extroverts show lower levels of activity (Johnson et al., 1999). This extends beyond the central nervous system to the autonomic nervous system as well, with children with IDs showing high parasympathetic reactivity, and those with EDs showing low reactivity in both the sympathetic and parasympathetic systems (Boyce et al., 2001).

THE COMORBIDITY ISSUE AND CHILD PSYCHOPATHOLOGY

As we have suggested throughout this book, the cognitive hypothesis-testing (CHT) model requires a comprehensive yet flexible examination of brain–behavior relationships and their influence on a child's academic and behavioral functioning. This approach suggests that most children will not fit neatly into categories. When we think about the comorbidity of childhood psychopathological disorders, we need to think of an inherent tension between the "clumper" and "splitter" orientations (Hale & Fiorello, 2002). Clumpers tend to group children into large heterogeneous groups and adhere to a nomothetic or normative orientation. At the extreme end of the clumper continuum is the belief that all children are the same, learn the same way, and act they way they do for the same reasons. Although the number of groups in the clumper approach is fewer, these groups tend to be quite heterogeneous. The more clumping, the more heterogeneous the groups. Splitters, on the other hand, prefer to create smaller, more discrete groups by clumping only the most similar children together. Although doing this will reduce heterogeneity, it also increases the likelihood that the groups will be comorbid with each other (Sonuga-Barke, 1998). An extreme splitter will use idiographic analysis to evaluate the unique determinants of a each child's cognition and behavior. No child is identical, so each child must be treated as a single-case study. We agree with this extreme position; yet we adhere to both clumping and splitting orientations in practice, as this gives an understanding of the similarities and differences among children, of the covariation among childhood disorders that defines comorbidity (Lilienfeld, Waldman, & Israel, 1994), and of the way each child's uniqueness fits within the "big picture" of child psychopathology.

The DSM-IV/DSM-IV-TR categorical approach is thought to be an atheoretical one, but it is really a "medical model" approach to differential diagnosis. We diagnose children to determine the best treatment for them, right? Well, yes and no. In a categorical approach, a distinction is made between "normal" and "pathological" on the basis of category membership, not the degree that they differ from each other (Wilson, 1993). For instance, a child who meets only five of nine DSM-IV inattention criteria for ADHD is "normal," but a child who meets six of nine is "disordered" or has ADHD. This is one of the problems with a categorical approach for both practice and research, especially if services are only provided to children who meet the required number of criteria. However, a possibly more important issue has to do with the reliability and validity of the categorical criteria. The "S" in DSM-IV stands for *Statistical,* but there is no statistical algorithm offered for assessment tools, so that you can be "sure" a child has a particular diagnosis. To be fair, the DSM-IV-TR provides the latest information on disorders, and the criteria are often based on the results of empirical studies; however, these studies are often inconsistent in subject selection, methodology, data analysis, and interpretation, as we will see in our discussion of disorders below.

Even if we assume that the diagnostic criteria are fairly reliable and valid, we must consider the thorny issue of whether a given child meets those criteria. Diagnostic uncertainty is a major limitation in developing and utilizing effective treatment strategies for children with psychopathology (Vitiello, 2001), so it is not surprising that most of us want to use those left brains of ours to come up with a definitive decision about a child's diagnosis. We see our job as being one in which we "answer" that typical parent or teacher question: "So what is *it*? Did you find out what *the problem* is?" We often reluctantly fall for this ploy—saying definitively, "It's X," when we know that a host of diagnoses and factors are affecting the child's current status. After lengthy team discussions about a child, we are always amazed when the team looks at us in disbelief when we sheepishly say we should give a "provisional" DSM-IV diagnosis, as if this qualifier doesn't exist, or that we aren't doing a good job if we don't "know" the "truth." In CHT, we prefer discussing characteristics, strengths, and needs, not focusing on labels. No matter how hard we try, psychology is not going to be a "hard science" for some time (until *Star Trek* tricorders become readily available!), and we need to recognize the limitations of our methods. When you are making diagnoses, you need to consider the reliability and validity of the disorder criteria used to establish diagnosis, as well as the methods used for obtaining the information. Research has suggested that training in semistructured interview techniques results in fairly good reliability (Sonuga-Barke, 1998), but even if the data are reliable, you must consider whether the information is valid. Most agree that multimethod–multisource approaches lead to more accurate diagnoses and interventions (Hale et al., 1998). We see some parents who minimize a child's behavior problem, others who exaggerate it, and others who just don't see the problem, because they are unaware of it or do not see it in the different setting—all problems incurred during the use of informant ratings of behaviors (see Merrell, 1999). When one considers the low agreement rate between parent and teacher informants, and the high comorbidity rates between IDs and EDs, complex, multifaceted approaches to assessment and intervention are required (McConaughy & Skiba, 1993).

Given these issues, it is extremely difficult to determine whether children really fall into one diagnostic category or another (i.e., whether they have "pure" disorders). Indeed, comorbidity between disorders unfortunately appears to be the norm rather than the exception, with rates ranging from 19% to 75% (Sonuga-Barke, 1998). Even this broad range of comorbidity rates is telling: If we can't decide what a disorder is, and accurately determine whether it is comorbid with other disorders, what good is a categorical system at all? For one thing, children with comorbid disorders are twice as likely to receive psychiatric services (Costello et al., 1996), and comorbidity helps clinicians determine etiology, course, and treatment (Angold, Costello, & Erkanli, 1999). Meta-analyses results reveal that comorbidity is not due to referral bias, rater expectancy effects, or use of multiple informants; nor is it the result of multiple or nonspecific symptoms (Angold et al., 1999). Categories and their comorbidities appear to serve a useful purpose: They give us a template to explore each child's unique characteristics and to determine how he or she differs from the category exemplar (a fictitious child who serves as conceptual anchor). But be careful, and don't make children try to "fit" into a category if they don't. You're always safer describing cognitive and behavioral functioning than justifying categorical labels.

Although categorical diagnoses and comorbidity appear to be verifiable phenomena, it is critical to use a developmental perspective when determining diagnoses. The variability in comorbidity rates described above is probably related to the developmental manifestations of the overt symptoms displayed by children, which may change according to their age and gender. For instance, among young children with disruptive behavior problems, boys tend to show more externalizing symptoms and girls to show more internalizing ones in adolescence. As behaviors tend to be correlated moderately over time and to increase with age, but tend to decrease as the time between observations increases (Roberts & Del Vecchio, 2000), ongoing assessment and regular monitoring is critical for helping children with emotional or behavior disorders. Understanding the relationship between symptom development and expression requires a certain flexibility in thought and practice, as we have suggested in the CHT model. In CHT, we try to determine how much of a problem is related to the individual's characteristics, and how much of it is related to and shaped by environmental contingencies. Exploring this canalization of behavior helps us recognize the developmental continuum of psychopathology (Grossman et al., 2003), but the relationship between the etiology and behaviors displayed is seldom a linear one (Sonuga-Barke, 1998); it demands that we embrace variability and comorbidity in child psychopathology, not dismiss it. The question we often face in clinical practice is not an "either–or" one, but a "how much" one.

In the following sections, we examine some common childhood disorders that pose risks for both cognitive and psychosocial disturbance, and offer several intervention recommendations for each. However, as you review this material, it is critical to recognize that no particular pattern or sign on psychological or neuropsychological tests provides you with unequivocal evidence that a child has a particular psychopathological disorder (Tramontana & Hooper, 1997). It is up to you to conduct comprehensive CHT evaluations with multiple measures and data sources to ensure diagnostic accuracy. The cursory examination that follows should serve to further your interest in and exploration of the neuropsychology of childhood psychopathology, because this area is growing at a phenomenal rate. Although resources are limited at this time, we predict that entire books will be written about this important subject in the very near future.

SELECTED CHILDHOOD PSYCHOPATHOLOGIES

Mental Retardation/Pervasive Developmental Disorders

Characteristics and Comorbidities

Psychologists in the schools are often called upon to identify and treat comorbid emotional and behavior problems in children with mental retardation (MR) and PDDs. Despite the high prevalence of psychiatric comorbidity found for these children with MR/DD (Rojahn & Tasse, 1996), few clinicians receive extensive training in MR/PDDs and associated disorders (Silka & Hauser, 1997). They must rely on psychologists and other professionals to help formulate comprehensive treatment programs. For complex comorbid MR/PDD cases, neuropsychological evaluation of patterns of performance and aberrant behaviors can enhance diagnostic accuracy, which may be the single most important determinant of intervention success (Mulick & Hale, 1996). As children with MR/PDDs often have a broad array of problems and needs, careful examination and interdisciplinary coordination is required. Children with MR/PDDs seldom show uniform patterns of performance on measures—the so-called "flat profile" thought to be characteristic of the population with MR. Instead, children with these disorders are just as complex as those with the higher-incidence disorders discussed throughout this book. After a thorough diagnostic workup, you will collaborate with other team members to develop interventions that address medical, language, motor, adaptive, academic, and behavioral needs. The physician may suggest a trial of psychotropic medication. Careful neuropsychological and behavioral monitoring of medication response using multiple tools and informants is critical, especially if multiple medications are used for neurological and psychiatric symptoms (Lewis, Aman, Gadow, Schroeder, & Thompson, 1996).

Characteristics and Treatment of Autism

Children with PDDs such as autism (AU) and Asperger syndrome (AS) are difficult to assess and treat, largely because behavioral interference with performance on standardized tests may limit the utility of these measures, and necessitate the use of behavioral observation and interviews to formulate diagnostic impressions (Mulick & Hale, 1996). Knowing the characteristics and behavioral manifestations of these disorders is an important first step. Characterized by impaired communication skills, poor sociability, and a limited range of interests and activities, children with AU have many associated features, including inattention, sensory–motor deficits, concrete thought, perseveration, affective blunting, poor insight, and sleep disturbance (Rapin & Katzman, 1998).

Most children with PDDs display signs of neuropsychological deficits (Hooper, Boyd, Hynd, & Rubin, 1993), but there is considerable debate whether dysfunctional hemispheric (Sussman & Lewandowski, 1990), cerebellar and brainstem (Courchesne, 1995), or cortical–subcortical integration (Horwitz, Rumsey, Grady, & Rapoport, 1988) systems could account for their associated deficits. Neurological abnormalities are common in the AU spectrum disorders, including abnormal gyri patterns, increased brain size (especially in the posterior regions), increased ventricular size, smaller corpus callosum, and cerebellar abnormalities (Eliez & Reiss, 2000). Interestingly, while the corpus callosum is smaller than expected in AU, the enlarged occipital, temporal, and parietal areas are due to *excessive* white matter (Filipek, 1999). They tend to have microscopic abnormalities in both the cortex and subcortical structures, including the anterior cingulate, hippocampus, amygdala, and cerebellum (Filipek, 1999). The amygdala is of particular interest, given its relationship with "social intelligence" and the finding that children with AU do not use this region during mentalistic inferences (Baron-Cohen et al., 2000). The increased caudate volume observed in AU, similar to that in OCD and Tourette syndrome, could account for the compulsive and ritualistic behavior observed in this population (Cody, Pelphrey, & Piven, 2002). Although the prefrontal cortex appears to be hypermetabolic in AU, the left posterior temporal and parietal lobes are characteristically hypometabolic (Peterson, 1995), despite the excessive white matter in these regions. Given the large number of brain areas associated with AU, it is fairly reasonable to speculate that there are many subtypes of AU spectrum disorders or PDDs, each with its own unique pathophysiology and treatment course.

Unless they are "high-functioning," children with AU often have low overall intelligence. Also, their speech and language may be impaired or delayed—characterized by intonation problems, neologisms, pronoun reversal, meaningless echolalia, and pragmatic deficits affecting social reciprocity and conversation exchange (Bailey, Phillips, & Rutter, 1996). They have poor motor and language imitation skills, limited sequential processing, and difficulty shifting cognitive sets, but may have good rote recall, as suggested by common finding of immediate and delayed echolalia (Hooper & Tramontana, 1997). Unlike most children with developmental aphasia, individuals with AU show an aversion to social contact or exchange. They show facial processing deficits, such as looking at lips instead of eyes (Joseph & Tanaka, 2003) and using the inferior temporal lobe to process faces, as if they were objects (Schultz et al., 2000). They also have poor eye contact, limited interest or use of social cues, abnormal preoccupations and rituals, stereotypic or repetitive behavior patterns, and a need for environmental consistency (Hooper et al., 1993).

Given the neurological problems in AU, it is not surprising to find that these children have significant attention, memory, and executive function deficits (Hughes, Russell, & Robbins, 1994). Children with AU may be specifically deficient in verbal working memory (Pennington & Ozonoff, 1996), possibly related to the frontal functions of temporal ordering or sequential processing of information (Bennetto, Pennington, & Rogers, 1997). However, other deficits have been noted, including perseveration (Liss et al., 2001) and problems with cognitive flexibility or shifting cognitive sets (Rinehart, Bradshaw, Brereton, & Tonge, 2002). In an attempt to link executive and social functioning or "mindblindness" (Baron-Cohen, 1995) deficits in AU, researchers have used "theory-of-mind" tasks to assess their understanding of the beliefs, thoughts, desires, and intentions of others (Klin, 2000). Liss and colleagues (2001) suggest that poor use of verbal rules and mediation to solve executive and social problems leads to social impairments in AU. The consensus is that children with AU and AS show theory-of-mind deficits (Jolliffe & Baron-Cohen, 1999), with poorer performance for children with AU suggested (Ziatas, Durkin, & Pratt, 1998).

Certainly delays in most areas of academic functioning can be expected, and depending on the severity of these delays, a functional curriculum may be advised. Adaptive behavior is likely to be limited, especially in the areas of language and social activities, even in high-functioning individuals. Children with AU have difficulty with auditory perception, vocabulary, verbal memory, verbal fluency, and articulation (Klin, Volkmar, Sparrow, Cicchetti, & Rourke, 1995), so speech and language services, in addition to augmented communication techniques, will be necessary for most of these children. Because of the possible cerebellar involvement in some children with AU (Courchesne, 1995), they may have difficulty with motor coordination, balance, gait, and implicit learning. Careful monitoring of these behaviors, in conjunction with physical and/or occupational therapy, is good practice. For learning and behavior problems, strict operant conditioning procedures have been shown to be effective with children with AU (Lovaas, 1996), but systematic monitoring is required to ensure efficacy. Stereotypic behaviors and/or self-injurious behaviors may require intensive behavioral and possibly psychotropic medication interventions. It may be important to use functional analysis to determine whether the aberrant behaviors are driven by proximal (internal) or distal (external) reinforcement (Hale, Mulick, & Rojahn, 1995). For instance, Hale and colleagues (1995) used structural equation modeling to show that proximal reinforcement predicted stereotypic behaviors and some self-injurious behaviors. However, some self-injurious behaviors were also driven by distal or environmental contingencies, as were all aggressive behaviors. This suggests that distal behaviors may be more amenable to operant control, whereas proximal behaviors may require a combination of behavioral and psychotropic interventions (Hale et al., 1995). By identifying and operationalizing key problem behaviors, administering formal and informal cognitive measures, and systematically observing the behaviors during baseline and treatment conditions, psychologists in schools can help others monitor treatment response.

Assessment and Treatment of Asperger Syndrome

Although the differentiation of AU and AS is controversial (see In-Depth 8.2), there is evidence suggesting that children with these disorders have different etiologies and clinical courses (Klin & Volkmar, 1997), as well as unique patterns of neuropsychological strengths and deficits. Although intellectual measures can be used for this discrimination, as children with AU are generally lower-functioning than those with AS, variable subtest patterns often preclude interpretation of level of performance (e.g., IQ), especially if unique strengths (e.g., savant syndrome) or weaknesses are present (Pring, Hermelin, & Heavey, 1995). Distinguishing high-functioning AU from AS on the basis of verbal–performance or verbal–nonverbal reasoning score differences has been recom-

IN-DEPTH 8.2. Are AU and AS the Same Disorder?

It is important to note that not all mental health professionals concur with our presentation of the differences between AU and AS. Most claim that the distinction between AU and AS is primarily one of severity (Wing, 1998). Although this is certainly plausible, and several studies have supported this conclusion, let us try to explain some of the contradictory research. The major difference in the definitions of AU and of AS is that language is "preserved" in AS. What does "preserved language" in AS look like? Based on the arguments about right-hemisphere language functions we have presented in Chapter 2, we would suggest that language is not preserved in AU or AS, but that children with AS might do better than those with AU on standardized *left*-hemisphere language tasks. Their obvious verbosity and good grammatical skills could lead clinicians to think that their language is adequate, but impairments in pragmatics and socioemotional discourse are apparent in AS (Adams, Green, Gilchrist, & Cox, 2002). Remember when your professor taught you to be careful about scoring Wechsler Intelligence Scale for Children (WISC) Verbal responses, because verbose kids tend to get inflated scores? Well, this probably applies to children with AS as well. Another finding that has been used to claim that AU and AS are similar is related to early language development, which has been found to be delayed in both high-functioning AU and AS (Meyer & Minshew, 2002); again, this suggests to many observers that the difference is one of severity. However, we would expect delayed language development in children with right-hemisphere dysfunction, and then would expect them to develop rote, pedantic, and circumscribed language and interests with time. This would account for the equivalent language processes in early development, and for greater language skills later in children with AS than in those with AU on standardized tests.

As noted earlier, children with AU have a particular strength on Block Design, and visual-perceptual weaknesses are common for children with AS. However, Gilchrist and colleagues (2001) reported comparable Block Design scores for both groups, suggesting that this distinction was not reliable. However, this may have been because the two groups had comparable Performance IQs, or because the two groups performed the task differently (the group with AU making *local* errors, and the group with AS making *global* errors). Recall that Block Design error analysis is necessary for interpretation; problems with pattern are related to left-hemisphere functions, while problems with spatial configuration are related to right-hemisphere ones (Suchan et al., 2002). This renders the overall score meaningless in making the distinction between AU and AS. Finally, it is not uncommon for researchers to define high-functioning AU and AS on the basis of intelligence test scores, and then, controlling for global or verbal IQ, to find no difference between the two groups (e.g., Miller & Ozonoff, 2000). Yet this well-known problem with circularity severely limits the utility of these and similar findings, as we have discussed in previous chapters.

Obviously, among the major limitations for PDD research are the diagnostic techniques used for subject inclusion: The children with AU and AS are often diagnosed on the basis of overt behaviors displayed, diagnostic interviews, and rating scales. What if we used brain-based neuropsychological differences instead, and then determined how many children met AU and AS criteria? Consistent with this argument, Green et al. (2002) suggest that syndrome coherence should not be sought at the functional level; instead, researchers and clinicians should focus on biological factors in relation to genetic and environmental causes of these disorders. Throughout this book, we have seen that focusing solely on overt behaviors gets us in diagnostic and treatment hot water.

Most of the research reported earlier was on individuals with AU or groups of subjects defined as having AU and AS, and the variable criteria used to diagnose the disorders probably limit the generalizability of findings. We argue that a distinction between left-hemisphere dysfunction (AU) and right-hemisphere dysfunction (AS) may be useful, but there are certainly cortical–subcortical interactions influencing these disorders as well. One physiological distinction worth noting is the white matter differences between the groups. Could excessive white matter in AU and white

(continued)

IN-DEPTH 8.2. *(continued)*

matter deficits in AS lead to qualitative differences between the conditions? Recall that AU morphological findings suggest increased white matter (particularly in the left posterior regions) and a smaller corpus callosum (Filipek, 1999), and that AS symptoms indicate characteristic right-hemisphere white matter dysfunction (Volkmar et al., 2000). Our earlier description of white matter as being the streets and superhighways of the brain suggests that maybe children with AU have too much uncoordinated information being processed by various parts of the brain at once; hence they become overloaded by stimuli and have difficulty with perceptual integration. Their lower-level processes remain intact, but their higher-level concept formation processes are impaired (Frith, 1991). In AS, the white matter disruption may lead to poor connectedness of ideas, which would account for these children's pedantic and impoverished verbosity, poor adaptation to novelty, and peculiar interests. Both groups would display executive deficits, but different types of deficits and causes for their problems. Children with AU may display perseverative, fixated, and ritualistic behaviors (i.e., symptoms suggestive of OCD), while those with AS may exhibit inattention, impulsivity, and poor novel problem solving (i.e., symptoms suggestive of ADHD). This would be consistent with findings that children with AU have greater interests in sameness, whereas those with AS have more circumscribed interests (Meyer & Minshew, 2002).

In any case, the hypothesis we present is merely a possibility that must be explored empirically before definitive conclusions can be drawn about the differences between AU and AS. When we begin to focus on neurophysiological and neuropsychological symptoms to define PDDs, we may gain a greater understanding of the differences between AU and AS. However, once again, it is interesting to note that we find somewhat similar behavioral outcomes with possibly different etiologies—ones that might benefit from different intervention strategies.

---

mended. Children with AU show lower verbal than visual-perceptual/performance skills, whereas verbal skills are a strength for those with AS (Ehlers et al., 1997; Joseph, Tager-Flusberg, & Lord, 2002; Klin et al., 1995; Lincoln, Courchesne, Allen, Hanson, & Ene, 1998; Minshew, Goldstein, & Siegal, 1997). Nonverbal performance and Arithmetic deficits are typically found in AS, but children with AU show poor verbal skills and a strength in Block Design (Ehlers et al., 1997). This has led some to suggest that children with AU have left-hemisphere dysfunction (Fein, Humes, Kaplan, Lucci, & Waterhouse, 1984), while those with AS have right-hemisphere dysfunction (Ellis, Ellis, Fraser, & Web, 1994).

Children with AS also have more impaired visual–spatial perception, visual memory, nonverbal concept formation, fine and gross motor skills, and visual–motor integration (Klin et al., 1995). Although children with AS are said to have language strengths, they are likely to present with idiosyncratic, agrammatical, and pedantic speech; preferences for rote, automatized verbal information; prosopagnosia; and marked difficulties with visual-perceptual–motor skills, prosody, and novel problem solving (Ghaziuddin & Gerstein, 1996; Klin et al., 1995; Kracke, 1994). Consistent with case study findings showing right-hemisphere white matter damage in AS (Volkmar, Klin, Schultz, Rubin, & Bronen, 2000), you may want to consider AS to be a more severe form of the "nonverbal learning disorder" syndrome described by Rourke (1994) and colleagues.

The differential neurocognitive and psychological deficits experienced by children with AS may be revealed through a comprehensive neuropsychological evaluation (Tsai, 1992). Children with AS are likely to display discordant/divergent language deficits, in which they have difficulty with understanding inference, implicit messages, metaphor, humor, and prosody. Despite being highly verbal, children with AS are likely to miss the "gist" of social discourse, and to have significantly more academic and social problems in the middle childhood to adolescent years. In support of these "nontraditional" language deficits, Gilchrist and colleagues (2001) found that verbal rituals, stereotyped utterances, and inappropriate questions were similar among those with AU and AS, but that children with AS had less echolalia and pronominal reversal. In addition to language issues, neuropsychological testing should allow for examination of frontal, right frontal, and right posterior brain functions, including the dorsal and ventral visual streams. This would include an examination of executive functions, working memory, attention, novel problem-solving and fluid reasoning skills, implicit receptive and expressive language, receptive and expressive prosody, and visual–spatial as well as visual object memory. Signs of neglect and anosagnosia could be present, so careful observation and history should be acquired. Look for signs of poor hygiene, poor cleaning habits, and inattention, especially to the left side of stimuli. Children with AS and right-hemisphere ("nonverbal") learning disorders often show neglect in subtle ways. For instance, their writing may drift to the right side of the page. The history may also reveal difficulty with early language acquisition, but their parents will often report that they "caught up" quickly once they began to speak.

As you would expect from their symptoms of right parietal dysfunction, these children are also clumsy and uncoordinated (Ghaziuddin, Butler, Tsai, & Ghaziuddin, 1994). These children are likely to have right-hemisphere-based constructional apraxia and to display graphomotor deficits secondary to dorsal stream spatial problems, as evidenced by their difficulty with throwing and catching a ball (Green et al., 2002). Both physical (gross motor) and occupational (fine motor) therapy are often required. Other than graphomotor deficits affecting handwriting, these children are likely to display few academic difficulties early in school, but they begin to falter when rote learning is no longer emphasized (Rourke, 1994). However, their social skills are likely to be dramatically impaired, and socioemotional problems are likely to be significant. Children with AS have more social interests than those with AU (Happe & Frith, 1996), but they have comparable impairments. As a result, intensive cognitive-behavioral therapy, behavior management, and social skills instruction can be helpful. Although AS is not an executive dysfunction syndrome, children with AS may benefit from metacognitive instruction to improve self-monitoring and control.

Learning Disorders

Characteristics and Comorbidities

As described earlier in the book, there are many causes and interventions for children with learning disabilities (LDs), but the relationship between LD subtypes and psychosocial functioning is only in its infancy. Although extensive research on children with LDs has occurred over the last three decades, early studies examining psychosocial functioning in this population produced limited results, because subtypes were ignored and children with LDs were treated as a homogeneous group (Rourke, 1994). Even with this approach, numerous studies using undifferentiated samples with LDs have revealed that they are at greater risk for social, emotional, and behavioral disorders (for a review, see Bryan, 1991); however, other studies have been inconclusive. Inconsistent study results may be related to the use of heterogeneous group designs, as differences between the groups with LDs and the control groups were often ones of severity (Rourke, 2000). For instance, longitudinal research suggests that children with a single LD (e.g., reading) are more likely to experience internalizing behavior problems, whereas children with multiple LDs (e.g., reading, math, and writing) are more likely to display disruptive behavior disorders (Prior, Smart, Sanson, & Oberklaid, 1999). Poor socioemotional adjustment is common in children with LDs, and is greatest among those with multiple LDs (White, Moffitt, & Silva, 1992). These findings would fit nicely with the developmental lag model of LDs (Fakouri, 1991), in which the more disabling children's LDs are, the more likely it is that they will display problematic behavior.

Although the developmental lag model received widespread recognition in the early literature on LDs, and is still popular among some school psychologists, longitudinal and cross-sectional studies confirm that children with LDs experience specific neuropsychological *deficits* (Francis, Shaywitz, Stuebing, Shaywitz, & Fletcher, 1994) and certain patterns of psychosocial functioning (Fuerst & Rourke, 1995). With each year that passes, more evidence emerges supporting the model of developmental deficits as opposed to developmental lag. However, even these deficit-based LD subtype studies have been limited, because researchers have often used ability–achievement discrepancy to determine participant eligibility—a problem discussed repeatedly in this text. As neurophysiological and neuropathological evidence supports the heterogeneous nature of this population (Lyon & Rumsey, 1996), neuropsychological assessment is likely to enhance identification of and intervention for these disorders, because specific cognitive deficits and associated emotional and behavioral problems may not be addressed during typical LD evaluations. Moving from a discrepancy-based LD determination to a neuropsychological one allows us to see achievement deficits as an outcome of an underlying processing deficit. This "inside-to-outside" approach for diagnosing LDs (Denckla, 1996) could allow for more accurate identification of LD subtypes, and determine the variability in academic and behavioral outcomes displayed by children with similar patterns of performance.

Many children with LDs may experience persistent maladaptive behavior patterns, but a large proportion appear to experience no significant signs of psychopathology (see Rourke & Fuerst, 1991). Rourke (2000) and his colleagues have identified subtypes on the basis of Wechsler Intelligence Scale for Children (WISC) Verbal–Performance discrepancies or Wide Range Achievement Test (WRAT) Arithmetic–Reading/Spelling discrepancies. Several of these subtype studies have described a pattern of arithmetic deficits with nonverbal LDs, lower WISC Performance than Verbal scores, right-hemisphere deficits, and psychopathology. This subtype has problems with speech prosody; with affective, tactile, and visual-perceptual/organizational skills; with affect recognition and production; and with novel problem solving. As a result, these children may experience significant psychopathology (Fuerst & Rourke, 1991; Manoach, Sandson, & Weintraub, 1995; Rourke & Fuerst, 1996; Semrud-Clikeman & Hynd, 1990; White et al., 1992), similar to that seen in AS (described earlier). Their processing weaknesses are likely to lead to social skills deficits, because they may misinterpret the affect and motivation of others (Loveland, Fletcher, & Bailey, 1990). Although both internalizing and externalizing pathology has been noted in children with nonverbal LDs, they appear to be at particular risk for IDs (Rourke, 2000). Given this association among the right hemisphere, emotional functioning, and psychopathology (Borod et al., 1998), we should not be surprised to find that child behavior problems are more closely related to "nonverbal" than to "verbal" development (Plomin, Price, Eley, Dale, & Stevenson, 2002), and that more children with nonverbal LDs and arithmetic deficits are likely to receive individual counseling as part of their individualized education plans (Davis, Parr, & Lan, 1997). Interestingly, Rourke and his colleagues have taken a position similar to ours, in that "nonverbal" doesn't quite reflect the complexity of right-hemisphere dysfunction. They note that white matter dysfunction leads to concept formation and problem-solving deficits, regardless of modality, and that semantic and pragmatic linguistic deficits are also found in children with nonverbal LDs (Rourke, 2000).

Although the evidence supporting the relationship between nonverbal LDs and psychopathology fits well with our understanding of how the hemispheres work, as white matter dysfunction is likely to lead to problems with intermodal/interregional communication and integration (Rourke, 1987; Semrud-Clikeman & Hynd, 1990), several questions about this relationship need exploration. First, these studies seldom differentiate between anterior and posterior deficits in this population; nonverbal LDs are seen as "whole" right-hemisphere matter problems. This is undoubtedly the case for some children, but what about those with right *frontal* dysfunction? Do they differ from those with right *posterior* problems? Another issue has to do with the type of psychopathology displayed by children with nonverbal LDs. Why do some develop IDs while others display EDs? In addition, what about comorbid IDs and EDs? Could this be related to the frontal–posterior distinction alluded to above?

In our research, we have been using neuropsychological tests to examine the relationship between psychopathology and right frontal versus right posterior dysfunction. Preliminary results that suggest the group with right frontal dysfunction has more inattentive and disinhibited ADHD-type symptoms, whereas the group with right posterior dysfunction displays inattention and other symptoms much more like Rourke's nonverbal LD syndrome (Hale, Rosenberg, Hoeppner, & Gaither, 1997). This is somewhat consistent with other research, which has found that children with nonverbal LDs often display signs of attention deficit (Voeller, 1986), and that those with anterior dysfunction are more likely to experience hyperactivity and EDs, whereas those with posterior dysfunction experience AN (Nussbaum, Bigler, Koch, & Ingram, 1988). Inattention may be a symptom of right-hemisphere dysfunction, but separating the anterior from the posterior type could be critical, as only the former is likely to benefit from stimulant medication.

Another question has to do with the differences between children who develop psychosocial problems and those who don't experience significant psychopathology. Although we could suggest that environmental factors play a role (as they do with all children), this suggestion needs further examination. We must examine why some children with apparent neuropsychological deficits develop certain psychopathological disorders, others develop a few problems, and still others seem to adapt quite well. We also need to see whether some children with similar neuropsychological profiles develop different patterns of socioemotional adjustment. Another question about nonverbal LD research has to do with the developmental progression of the disorder. Our cross-sectional research suggests that there may be a developmental difference between those with verbal and nonverbal LDs, with the latter group becoming more pathological over time (Hale et al., 1997), but others have found that patterns of psychopathology are consistent across age groups (Fuerst & Rourke, 1995); thus the results are inconclusive (Rourke, 2000). Finally, the finding that mechanical arithmetic is deficient in nonverbal LDs provides us with only a hypothetical relationship between math deficits and psychopathology. We presume that the right posterior problems (i.e., dorsal stream) are what lead to symptoms of nonverbal LDs and math deficits—but there are at least three different causes for mathematics disorders as discussed in Chapter 6, and some children in these studies may have had procedural math deficits due to right frontal dysfunction and difficulty with problem solving.

Although there is clearly evidence that children with nonverbal LDs have psychosocial difficulties, some children with reading or language-based LDs, presumed to be the results of left-hemisphere dysfunction, may have difficulty with affect and social perception as well (Loveland et al., 1990). In fact, Rourke and Fuerst (1991) reported that a large portion of their Verbal < Performance group also displayed psychopathology, especially IDs (e.g., DE, AN, withdrawal, somatic complaints). This is consistent with the finding that children with left-hemisphere impairments experience internalizing symptoms such as dysphoria, anxiety, and withdrawal (Glossner & Koppell, 1987; Nussbaum, Bigler, & Koch, 1986). In particular, children with receptive language deficits—which we have associated with several types of LDs—are more likely to experience psychopathology than those with expressive deficits (Whitehurst & Fischel, 1994). Although such children are probably accurate at reading nonverbal cues in social discourse, they may experience limited verbal comprehension, resulting in a tendency to withdraw from social exchange (Baker & Cantwell, 1987b; Nussbaum & Bigler, 1986). Some researchers have suggested that language impairment alone leads to problematic behavior (Rice, 1993), but others have concluded that the associated LDs are what lead to psychopathology (Beitchman, Brownlie, & Wilson, 1996; Lynam, Moffitt, & Stouthamer-Loeber, 1993; Tomblin, Zhang, & Buckwalter, 2000), especially of the internalizing type. Children with language and reading disorders are more likely to be seen as withdrawn, anxious, fearful, and depressed (Boetsch, Green, & Pennington, 1996; Cohen, Menna, et al., 1998; Smart, Sanson, & Prior, 1996).

Given the earlier arguments that left-hemisphere dysfunction could lead to negative affect, it is not surprising that DE and other IDs could occur in children with reading and language disorders. However, reading disorders have been associated with both IDs and EDs, with girls more likely to display the former and boys the latter (Willcutt & Pennington, 2000). Numerous studies suggest that language and reading disorders often lead to EDs, especially CD, and that this tendency increases with age (Beitchman et al., 1996). In one child psychiatry sample, over 40% had undiagnosed language and learning impairment, and those with undetected receptive language problems were more likely to be diagnosed with ADHD and to have externalizing problems such as aggression and delinquent behavior (Cohen, Barwick, Horodezky, Vallance, & Im, 1998). Could the failure to accurately diagnose and treat the language and learning problems of these children lead to feelings of frustration, anger, and alienation, and eventually to antisocial behavior? It is possible that some children with LDs develop psychopathology because of the way their brains process social and emotional information, but other children may develop problems in response to repeated academic and social failure, which could be the case for those with left-hemisphere-based CD. Further research is needed to address these important questions of whether the psychopathological disorders precede, follow, or occur concurrently with the LDs (Spreen, 1989), because the former would require interventions that address socioemotional processing deficits (e.g., social skills instruction), while the latter would need better academic instruction, environmental adaptations, and counseling to foster coping with the disorders.

Assessment and Treatment of Learning Disorders

Previous LD subtype research has been limited, because studies have used only a particular disorder (i.e., learning impairment), have examined only a particular population (i.e., psychiatric sample), or have used Verbal–Performance discrepancies or arithmetic–verbal/spelling deficit patterns in constructing subtypes. Consistent with material presented in earlier chapters, these categorical approaches or dichotomies may not be accurate. Children with LDs who have right-hemisphere deficits are also likely to display reading/spelling deficits (Branch, Cohen, & Hynd, 1995) and language deficits (Bryan & Hale, 2001). In addition to facial and prosodic deficits, these children may have psychosocial difficulties because they rely on successive rather than semantic processing of verbal information (Fisher & DeLuca, 1997). In addition, arithmetic calculation (Batchelor, Gray, & Dean, 1990) and reading/spelling skills (Branch et al., 1995) appear to be bilaterally subserved in children with LDs, and different pathways for processing academic information may be used in populations with different LDs. As described in earlier chapters, different academic skill assets and deficits are associated with the posterior–anterior and left–right axes, and differential diagnosis is needed to understand the nature in which these children process both academic and socioemotional information.

Accurate identification of LD subtypes remains a critically important task for the psychologist applying neuropsychological principles in the schools. Using a neuropsychological CHT orientation to interpret these characteristics can serve as a foundation during collaborative problem solving with teachers and parents. As discussed earlier, lateralization research suggests that we need to rethink our understanding of how the hemispheres work together on complex tasks (Banich & Heller, 1998). We must consider alternative intellectual and neuropsychological assessment methods to ensure accurate evaluation of routinized versus novel and receptive versus executive skills. Assessment of intellectual patterns of performance from this new perspective (i.e., convergent/concordant/crystallized vs. divergent/discordant/fluid) may be necessary to understand hemispheric differences in the development of psychopathology in children with LDs. As discussed in Chapter 3, thorough neuropsychological assessment of such children's assets and deficits, academic skills, and psychosocial adjustment can provide meaningful insight for clinicians and educators working with this heterogeneous population.

Despite conflicting findings, it seems apparent that children with LDs are at risk for psychosocial problems that can lead to psychological disturbance (Voeller, 1994). There are a host of reasons why this may be so. Although some researchers have focused on the psychological effects of labeling and learned helplessness, even these apparently "environmental" causes may have physiological effects on subcortical structures such as the amygdala (Schneider et al., 1996). As noted earlier, research has shown left-hemisphere activation to be associated with positive affect, and right-hemisphere activation with negative affect; these results suggest that the former is the "approach" hemisphere, and the latter is the "avoidant" hemisphere (Davidson & Fox, 1988). Could it be possible that left-hemisphere dysfunction leads to internalizing symptoms such as withdrawal, and right-hemisphere dysfunction leads to disinhibition? Research findings on individuals with brain damage and individuals undergoing anesthetization of the hemispheres generally support the idea that when the left hemisphere is underactive, "catastrophic" or negative affect emerges, and when the right is underactive, "indifferent" or impulsive behavior emerges (Sackheim et al., 1982).

Although inconsistent findings are worth noting, this leads us to an important conclusion: Not all psychosocial outcomes for children with LDs are based solely on neuropsychological characteristics. Instead, it is more likely that these characteristics interact with environmental determinants of behavior to result in degrees of psychosocial adjustment or maladjustment. With this caveat in mind, let's look at some possible psychosocial outcomes associated with having a right-hemisphere versus a left-hemisphere LD ("frontal" LD—i.e., ADHD—will be a discussed in a subsequent section).

As described earlier, children with a right-hemisphere disorder are likely to rely on rote, automatic, well-learned skills in academic and social situations. Their early language may be delayed, but they will quickly acquire an expansive vocabulary that they may not use appropriately. They will thrive on the structure, drill, and repetition of early school experiences, and will probably get good grades in early elementary school. However, as structure decreases and the complexity of academic material increases, poor performance is more likely. Math computation can be impaired in problem solving and spatial domains, and word problems may be difficult because the children have difficulty distinguishing between relevant and irrelevant information. We have seen these children excel on written math computation worksheets, only to fail on word problems because they don't know how to "set up" the problems. Although their word attack and recognition skills may be quite good, and they may memorize sight words quite well, these children typically use a phonemic approach on all unknown words. Language and reading comprehension will show a distinct pattern of deficits associated with implicit/inferential communication. Ask a typical elementary school fact or detail question, and these children will know the answer, but higher-order questions asked in later grades will be difficult for them. Handwriting will often be awkward and messy, and difficulties with organization and coherence in written expression may be apparent.

Because these children are typically good students and highly verbal, teachers and parents may not initially see their social problems, but they typically have few friends and seem isolated or rejected by others. When discussing dinosaurs, for instance, children with right-hemisphere dysfunction may repeat the many types and their individual characteristics—maybe even provide details, such as head circumference and number of teeth! However, they are unlikely to exchange ideas and information in a reciprocal fashion, or to adjust their dialogue according to the conversation context. Because they have difficulty reading nonverbal cues and prosody, they are likely to misinterpret subtle nuances during social exchange (e.g., rolling eyes, raised eyebrows, sighs, excited vocal tone). They may also be disinhibited and inattentive, lacking awareness of their own state and the environment. As performance variability on nonverbal measures increases, the more likely children are to display signs of internalizing and/or externalizing psychopathology (Greenway & Milne, 1999). As depicted in Case Study 8.1, Buck displayed many of the learning and behavioral characteristics of a child with a "right-hemisphere" LD.

CASE STUDY 8.1. Buck's Baseball Blunder

Buck was an 11-year-old boy who displayed a classic right-hemisphere pattern of performance on intellectual, neuropsychological, and psychosocial measures. He had fairly good verbal skills, scoring above average on the WISC-III Information and Vocabulary subtests, but his performance on the Comprehension subtest was poor, and his "SCAD" (Symbol Search, Coding, Arithmetic, and Digit Span) profile was also low. Buck scored in the low average range on the Picture Completion and Picture Arrangement subtests, while his Block Design and Object Assembly skills were poor: Two configuration errors were noted on Block Design, and he failed to complete any of the abstract Object Assembly items. CHT results revealed poor fluid reasoning, spatial perception, and nonverbal memory, as well as inconsistent executive functions. Interestingly, Buck had adequate visual memory for meaningful stimuli and faces, suggesting that his ventral stream was adequate. His mathematics skills were poor (due to computation and spatial errors), but his word reading was in the superior range, and his reading comprehension was average.

Behavior ratings, observation, and interview revealed that Buck had social difficulties because he talked incessantly, often made off-task or irrelevant comments, had poor eye contact, and complained that others were whispering or yelling when talking with him. It did not help that he had very poor hygiene (due to self-neglect) and that his gross and fine motor skills were quite poor (because of poor visual-perceptual feedback to the motor system). Noting his social difficulties, his parents had encouraged him to join a Little League team. After all, baseball was Buck's favorite sport, and he studied the statistics of his favorite players, such as batting averages and earned run averages. He tried to play baseball, but was quickly relegated to the bench for most games. When Buck did play, he made several errors; his batting average was abysmal; and he often sat alone on the end of the bench. After a missed catch that resulted in a broken nose, Buck quit the game, and the parents decided to seek a school evaluation. The teacher reported that Buck was "fine—one of my best students," struggling only in math and writing class. She minimized any social problems, as he was "fine" during supplemental math instruction. However, the day before he was scheduled for a private evaluation, Buck was suspended from school for hitting a "bully," and he was severely depressed upon presentation. Needless to say, we recommended intensive behavioral, social skills, and counseling support following our evaluation.

For children with left-hemisphere dysfunction, poor crystallized and language skills are likely. However, the real difficulties for these children lie in their poor automaticity and routinization skills. Academic skills are likely to be impaired in some or all areas, but they may do relatively well in math calculation. Word problems may be more difficult only because of the linguistic requirements, and learning of math facts is likely to be impaired. They will often use finger counting or hash marks in an attempt to arrive at answers. They may seem somewhat scattered or withdrawn, seemingly in their "own world." They can have difficulty comprehending oral communication, and may frequently ask for repetition or not follow directions; this may lead some to suggest that they have an "attention deficit." Their limited fluency and word-finding problems make others say, "Come on, spit it out." As a result of limited language comprehension and expression, children with a left-hemisphere disorder are likely to seem like "nice kids" but quiet— the type of children that few consider as having any socioemotional problems. They may choose an apparently adaptive strategy of relying on nonverbal visual and prosodic cues during social situations to understand others. Because they are adept at reading these cues, they are likely to develop verbal skills that are likely to support or adopt the group position, and likely to comply with social group norms. But their limited or variable verbal skills, especially when combined with their academic deficits, could lead to a tendency to withdraw in social situations and show depressive symptoms. Over time, as they experience repeated academic failure and the resultant social difficulties associated with it (we have often heard children with performance skills in the superior range call themselves "dumb"), these children may develop signs of oppositional defiant disorder (ODD) or CD, especially as they grow older. As depicted in Case Study 8.2, Steve displayed many of the learning and behavioral characteristics of a child with a "left-hemisphere" LD.

Internalizing and Externalizing Disorders

We now look at research on children with IDs and EDs, and evaluate the neuropsychological patterns found for each. As you read the heading, you may be wondering why we put IDs and EDs in the same section. The fact is that for many children, it is not uncommon to find comorbidity among these apparently opposite conditions (Semrud-Clikeman & Hynd, 1990). Children with IDs (e.g., DE) and EDs (e.g., CD) represent a heterogeneous population that may have associated neuropsychological deficits, and both IDs and EDs are likely to coexist with LDs. Children with IDs or EDs can display differential patterns of performance solely on the basis of poor motivation or persistence on task. For instance, children with IDs may receive lower scores on tasks requiring sustained attention or psychomotor speed, and children with CD or other EDs may put forth little effort on tasks or show inconsistent patterns not reflective of their true level of functioning. To complicate matters further, IDs and EDs represent fairly distinct factors in research (Achenbach, 2001), but the prevalence of comorbid IDs and EDs is relatively high (Baron, Fennell, & Voeller, 1995). In a meta-analysis of the literature, Angold and colleagues (1999) found that CD/ODD and ADHD were more closely associated with DE than with AN symptoms, but that DE symptoms were more likely to be related to AN than to CD/ODD. This suggests that DE + AN and DE + CD/ODD may represent different subtypes warranting further investigation. Children with AN show more ADHD symptoms than controls (Baving, Laucht, & Schmidt, 2002), but it is unclear whether their ADHD is comorbid with or secondary to their AN.

For much of the 20th century, children were not thought to have "adult" disorders such as DE. With the understanding that IDs such as DE, AN, dysphoria, withdrawal, and somatic complaints occur in children, we have begun to explore the associated neuropsychological deficits in this population. These deficits can easily lead to misdiagnosis, with such children being seen as

CASE STUDY 8.2. Steve's Best Friend

Steve was an 8-year-old boy referred for a psychological evaluation because the teacher felt he had "dyslexia." Described as a pleasant, compliant, and "sweet" boy, Steve was said to have no psychosocial problems, but he was failing most of his academic subjects. Except for word problems, math was said to be a relative strength for Steve, and he was only in the below-average range in this area during formal testing. His word attack skills were quite poor, and he couldn't do pseudoword decoding, but his reading fluency was fairly good on easy passages, and his reading comprehension was pretty good unless he had many word recognition errors. Surprisingly, he did quite well with writing, largely because he wrote creative and interesting prose. However, the passage he wrote received limited credit for vocabulary, grammar, capitalization, and punctuation. Cognitive testing revealed that Steve had significant strengths on the fluid, visual, and short-term/working memory subtests, but he did poorly on the crystallized, auditory processing, long-term memory, and processing speed measures. CHT results revealed poor auditory processing skills and both receptive and expressive language problems. His expressive language was notable for circumlocutions, poor fluency, and semantic paraphasias. Steve had limited crystallized knowledge, but only minor retrieval problems. A comparison of motor, visual, and visual–motor processing revealed that his problem was related to motor (left-hemisphere) rather than spatial processes, suggesting possible dyspraxic symptoms. The interview revealed similar fine motor deficits, left–right confusion, and dressing dyspraxia. His Block Design performance, while in the average range, was notable for reversal, inversion, and rotation errors, but he performed all items quickly.

On the parent ratings, Steve was noted as having few problems, but clinical elevations were found on measures of anxiety, depression, withdrawal, and attention problems. The last of these appeared to be related to language or mood rather than to ADHD, given his strong working memory performance and executive functions. Additional personality testing suggested that Steve had poor self-esteem and a preference for solitary activities, such as watching television and playing with his "best friend"—his dog. He reported having many "friends," but he was not close to anyone outside his immediate family and spent little time with other children outside of school. Good relationships were noted with parents and the teacher. In addition, to academic interventions, we suggested that Steve receive individual counseling to address self-esteem and affect issues. The teacher was encouraged to help Steve work with a "study buddy" in the class, and to provide him with leadership opportunities in areas of his interest and success. We also recommended that Steve become involved in group activities, such as team sports and an environmental group he had expressed interest in.

"slow" or "inattentive." Children with DE have poorer selective attention and working memory (Landro, Stiles, & Sletvold, 2001), suggesting possible executive and frontal dysfunction. Because executive function problems in DE may be due to the same brain areas affected in ADHD (see the section on ADHD, below), differential diagnosis is particularly important, as the medications used to treat these disorders affect different neurotransmitter systems. Interestingly, although those with IDs such as DE and AN tend to have lower overall dorsolateral prefrontal activity and increased orbital activity (Baxter et al., 2001; Mayberg, 2001), these individuals tend to use the dorsolateral prefrontal and Broca's areas during problem solving instead of relying on automatic processing (Johnson et al., 1999; Mayberg, 2001); these findings suggest internally directed self-talk and possibly rumination, which interfere with efficient performance. This internal dialogue may in part account for their propensity to be self-focused and avoid social contact. Individuals with IDs tend to be *overstimulated*, as discussed earlier, so reducing external stimuli is adaptive for them.

Given the change in our understanding of DE in children, it is not surprising that researchers are discovering that pediatric mania is not as rare as once thought (Biederman et al., 2000).

Children with bipolar disorder (BP) show elated mood, grandiosity, racing thoughts, hypersexuality, and decreased need for sleep (Geller et al., 1998). Although individuals with BP have adequate intellectual skills, impaired performance skills can be seen during acute episodes, and attention, inhibition, verbal memory, verbal fluency, and executive function deficits are typical (Clark, Iversen, & Goodwin, 2002; Lebowitz, Shear, Steed, & Strakowski, 2001; Quraishi & Frangou, 2002), but they do not differ from children with ADHD in hyperactivity or distractibility (Geller et al., 1998). In addition, there is no consistent difference on these measures between individuals with BP and unipolar DE (Quraishi & Frangou, 2002). Although this is a fairly consistent finding, these mood disorders differ on emotional tests, with results suggesting that individuals with mania respond to positive stimuli, whereas those with DE respond to negative stimuli (Murphy & Sahakian, 2001). Comorbidity of child BP is common, especially with ADHD, CD, and AN (Papolos & Papolos, 2000). The most substantial overlap is between BP and ADHD (Biederman et al., 1996), and this comorbidity may represent a distinct subtype that is different from other types of ADHD (Faraone, Biederman, Mennin, Wozniak, & Spencer, 1997). In pediatric BP, rapid cycling of mood is commonplace (Geller et al., 1998), suggesting extreme emotional lability, which can lead to explosive, aggressive outbursts and additional diagnoses of CD (Biederman et al., 2000). Given the symptoms and high rates of comorbidity displayed in child BP, differentiating BP from ADHD and/or CD is a difficult task—but a critical one, given the differences in psychopharmacological treatment for these disorders (Biederman et al., 2000).

As would be expected, given the wide array of symptoms associated with IDs, understanding the neuropsychological characteristics of this heterogeneous population is further complicated by an examination of the neurological findings reported in In-Depth 8.3.

By definition, CD and ODD are likely to gain the attention of parents and teachers alike, but the neuropsychological characteristics of these EDs may go undetected because intervention efforts may focus on the overt disruptive behaviors. A majority of delinquents have neuropsychological deficits (Teichner & Golden, 2000), and approximately half have experienced traumatic brain injury (Hux, Bond, Skinner, Belau, & Sanger, 1998), but the brain areas affected and types of deficits displayed vary among studies. Deficits in executive function suggest behavioral dyscontrol (P. M. Cole, Usher, & Cargo, 1993), which is typical of children with both CD and ADHD (Pennington & Ozonoff, 1996). Several studies have found frontal deficits to be common in CD and antisocial disorders (Enns, 1998; Hurt & Naglieri, 1992; Kandel & Freed, 1989; Seguin, Pihl, Harden, Tremblay, & Boulerice, 1995). These executive deficits could account for the fearless, disinhibited, stimulus-seeking characteristics of children with CD, which lead to aggressive and antisocial behavior (Raine, 2002). Although some suggest that assessment of executive and other neuropsychological functions is important for identifying CD (Szatmari et al., 1990; Toupin, Dery, Pauze, Mercier, & Fortin, 2000), controlling for the effects of ADHD may limit the utility of frontal or executive function measures in differential diagnosis (Pennington & Ozonoff, 1996).

As with the other disorders explored in this chapter, there may be several subtypes of children with CD. For instance, whereas many children with CD show authority, school, and alcohol/drug abuse problems, some children may show signs of a comorbid mood disorder, while others show antisocial behavior associated with thought disorder symptoms (Pena, Megargee, & Brody, 1996). Could these differences be associated with right- and left-hemisphere processes? CD has been associated with nonverbal LDs, but delinquents have been found to have persistent verbal deficits (Moffitt, Lynam, & Silva, 1994) or lower overall intellectual functioning (Raine, 1993; White et al., 1994). Verbal deficits interfere with abilities to solve problems, mediate verbal situations, and learn in school (Teichner & Golden, 2000). Consistent with the arguments above that a hemispheric equilibrium is important in overall adjustment, children with large Verbal–

IN-DEPTH 8.3. Brain Functioning and IDs

IDs have been associated with neurological soft signs (Shaffer et al., 1985) and left-hemisphere dysfunction, especially in the left frontal region (Baker & Cantwell, 1987b; George, Ketter, & Post, 1994; Glossner & Koppell, 1987). As noted earlier, internalizing symptoms have also been associated with right-hemisphere dysfunction (Brumback & Weinberg, 1990; Kluger & Goldberg, 1990). Increased left-hemisphere functioning has been associated with manic states, whereas the reverse is true for right-hemisphere hyperactivation and DE episodes (Sackheim et al., 1982). Electrophysiological studies have suggested that right-hemisphere activation results in AN or negative affect (Heller, Nitschke, & Miller, 1998), whereas left-hemisphere activation has been associated with positive affect (Davidson, 1995). Decreased left-hemisphere functioning has been associated with DE, but mania/hostile behavior can result from right-hemisphere damage (Robinson, Kubos, Starr, Rao, & Price, 1984). These findings would be entirely consistent with Davidson's (1995) left/positive/approach–right/negative/withdrawal arguments about hemispheric functions. For instance, right-hemisphere dysfunction would lead to deficits in the withdrawal system (Davidson, 1998), which in turn would lead to uncontrollable, impulsive approach behaviors; this is entirely consistent with current thinking on ADHD, as we note later in this chapter. Could this suggest that there must be an *equilibrium* between hemispheres for typical affect and behavior? For instance, a child with very high right-hemisphere and very low left-hemisphere functions would show the greatest likelihood of DE. If this is indeed the case, then as the discrepancy between right- and left-hemisphere functions increases, so does the likelihood of psychopathology.

Although we can think of the left–right axis as being critical for the manifestation of IDs, the posterior–anterior dimension is likely to play a role as well. DE has also been associated with dorsolateral prefrontal and dorsal anterior cingulate hypofunctioning, which leads to executive dysfunction, response biases, working memory deficits, and poor stimulus monitoring (Liotti & Mayberg, 2001; Mayberg, 2001). This could account for the similarity between DE and inattentive ADHD (see later discussion). Prefrontal hypermetabolic activity has been associated with AN and AN with DE, especially in the orbital cortex (Drevets & Raichle, 1995; Mayberg, 2001), suggesting overly controlled and inhibited behavior. Similar to our two-axis model described in Chapter 2, Heller (1993) suggests that the left–right frontal quadrants represent the valence (pleasant–unpleasant) axis, whereas the arousal axis (high–low) has to do with right posterior functioning; increased right frontal activity and decreased right parietal activity are associated with DE. Shenal, Harrison, and Demaree (2003) also use a quadrant approach to suggest that left frontal dysfunction leads to anhedonia, euthymia, limited expressive language, emotional sequencing problems, behavioral slowing, and limited social initiation. Right frontal dysfunction is related to emotional lability and self-regulation. Right posterior dysfunction leads to indifference, poor affect perception, decreased arousal, and DE symptoms. Although empirical investigation is needed, this quadrant approach is what is needed to tease out the right frontal–right posterior issues in nonverbal LDs.

Performance splits, *in either direction*, have higher rates of delinquency than those whose Verbal and Performance skills are comparable (Walsh, Petee, & Beyer, 1987). Despite conflicting evidence regarding the relationship of brain dysfunction to CD, these children experience higher rates of LDs and suffer more brain injuries than other children (Tramontana & Hooper, 1997). Whether these conditions are the causes or the results of CD remains to be seen, but the brain–behavior correlates of CD/ODD are beginning to be recognized, as highlighted in In-Depth 8.4.

Future research will need to explore the complex interaction of hemispheric strengths and deficits to determine whether differences are more likely to result in IDs, EDs, or both. This exploration will be furthered by research attempts to explore posterior–anterior differences as well.

IN-DEPTH 8.4. Brain Functioning and EDs

Children with CD/ODD are a heterogeneous group who display a wide array of neuropsychological assets and deficits. Are there commonalities among these children that could explain their disruptive behavior? As we have suggested previously, the orbital prefrontal cortex, amygdala, and anterior cingulate play an important role in emotion regulation. Orbital frontal damage has been associated with impulsive aggression (Giancola, 1995), and individuals who display violent behavior show frontal hypometabolism (Pliszka, 1999). However, unlike ADHD, which is probably related to catecholamine dysfunction (see the section on ADHD), CD—like DE—has been associated with serotonergic dysfunction (Lahey, Hart, Pliszka, Applegate, & McBurnett, 1993); this could account for the comorbidity between IDs and EDs. In addition to the frontal lobes, medial temporal lobe and limbic structures have been associated with anger and aggression (Bear, 1991). Dysfunction in the right hemisphere, with primary control over autonomic functions (Raine, 2002), has been implicated in conduct problems. Studies of antisocial and violent populations using functional magnetic resonance imaging (Raine et al., 2001) and neuropsychological tests (Day & Wong, 1996) reveal decreased right-hemisphere functioning. However, as noted earlier, there has been a strong association among language problems, LDs, and EDs, with lower left-hemisphere activity found for children with ODD (Baving, Laucht, & Schmidt, 2002) and CD (Moffitt, 1993). Some have suggested that spatial and early learning problems lead to skills' crowding the left hemisphere, which could explain the verbal, spatial, and global IQ deficits seen in delinquents (Raine, Yaralian, Reynolds, Venables, & Mednick, 2002).

It is possible that the difference between the right-hemisphere dysfunction and left-hemisphere dysfunction in delinquents may be related to the type of delinquency they display. Because children with right-hemisphere dysfunction have limited social information-processing skills (Rourke, 2000), they may be more likely to show *undersocialized* conduct problems (Loney, Frick, Mesha, & McCoy, 1998). Children with right-hemisphere CD would lack insight into their own behavior or the behavior of others; these may be the type of children who fail to show remorse for their actions. However, those with left-hemisphere dysfunction may have *socialized* conduct problems. They understand the nature of their acts and abide by antisocial norms. The distinction between undersocialized and socialized delinquency could reflect child- and adolescent-onset subtype differences, as only the former subtype is likely to display neuropsychological deficits (Clarizio, 1997). Consistent with this argument, Hinshaw (1992) notes that the relationship between antisocial behavior and academic underachievement becomes evident only in adolescence.

But do these findings apply to children with right, left, and/or frontal dysfunction? As discussed later in connection with ADHD, frontal factors are likely to play a primary or an additive role, but additional investigation is needed. As for the right–left differences, it is possible that children with CD and right-hemisphere dysfunction show early social problems and then begin to fail their academic subjects because of the complexity of the curriculum and unstructured instruction, as discussed previously. It is also possible that school failure becomes associated with CD in the left-hemisphere dysfunction group in adolescence, because the CD follows the continued failure and alienation that results from their language-based LD. Could this be an explanation for undersocialized versus socialized CD? This certainly warrants further investigation, as the diagnostic and treatment implications would be profound. Differentiating between the direct and indirect effects of brain dysfunction remains a critical task for the practitioner, especially when one considers the transactional and dynamic interplay among the brain, behavior, and environment (Tramontana & Hooper, 1997).

Although the search for brain–behavior relationships in these populations will undoubtedly continue, it is important to recognize that behavioral outcome is always a result of the complex interaction of neuropsychological and environmental determinants, as it is with all of the disorders we have discussed. Neuropsychological assessment can play an important role in helping determine whether neuropsychological assets or deficits exist in children with IDs and/or EDs, and if so, whether the patterns of performance are affected by psychological or other treatments. For instance, even if counseling is warranted, could the neuropsychological characteristics affect a child's response to the therapist, the therapist–child relationship, or the therapeutic strategies implemented? The research presented above suggests that children will respond variably to the same therapeutic techniques, strategies, and behaviors during individual or group counseling. Because children with LDs are likely to display a wide variety of neuropsychological and socio-emotional issues, using the CHT model during counseling will allow you to adjust your behavior and treatment orientation/strategies to meet each child's unique therapeutic needs.

As we conclude our discussion of the psychosocial aspects of various disorders, you may have recognized that we have only alluded briefly to the posterior–anterior axis. The remainder of this chapter examines the consummate anterior disorder—where "learning disabilities" is given the different categorical name of ADHD, and which involves the frontal–subcortical systems discussed earlier.

Attention-Deficit/Hyperactivity Disorder

Characteristics and Comorbidities

A plethora of research on the heterogeneous, disabling disorder of ADHD has been conducted in the last 30 years, but there is still considerable debate about its causes and treatment. Viewpoints may be conflicting because most of the research has been descriptive, exploratory, and atheoretical (Taylor, 1996). As ADHD is variable in presentation and treatment course, we present a series of arguments in the following paragraphs supporting the assertion that there are a number of ADHD subtypes. Specifically, we suggest that there are a number of "primary" ADHD subtypes (the "true" ADHD types that respond to stimulant medication treatment), as well as "secondary" ADHD subtypes that do not respond to medication and have different underlying causes. Given this premise, let's explore the literature that supports and refutes our position.

In addition to the hallmark symptoms of inattention and/or hyperactivity–impulsivity, children with ADHD frequently have comorbid LDs and behavior disorders. Tannock (1998) notes that comorbidity rates range from 50% to 80% of children with ADHD, with 40%–90% displaying disruptive behavior disorders, and approximately 15%–25% displaying mood disorders, anxiety disorders, and/or LDs. Metanalyses results confirm that comorbid ADHD + CD is more common than ADHD + DE, and that there is little overlap between the two groups (Angold et al., 1999), suggesting the possibility of at least two comorbid subtypes. Inattentive ADHD often occurs concomitantly with LDs (Marshall, Hynd, Handwerk, & Hall, 1997) and IDs such as DE (Biederman, Newcorn, & Sprich, 1991). Children with the hyperactive–impulsive ADHD subtype are more likely to receive comorbid diagnosis of EDs such as ODD or CD (Jensen, Martin, & Cantwell, 1997), but LDs are common in this population as well (Decker, McIntosh, Kelly, Nicholls, & Dean, 2001). Of the LD subtypes discussed in earlier chapters, children with ADHD are more likely to have written language disorders than other types of LDs (Mayes, Calhoun, & Crowell, 2000), but comorbid reading and/or math problems are also likely. Although empirical evidence suggests ADHD subtypes are distinct from one another (Goodyear & Hynd, 1992), only subtle differences are found among them (Faraone, Biederman, Weber, & Russell, 1998), suggesting that the DSM-IV ADHD criteria may not be sufficient when questions of comorbidity obfuscate accurate diagnosis or confound treatment results.

Given that the right frontal lobe is involved in attention networks and working memory (Smith & Jonides, 1999), neuropsychological evaluation of attention, working memory, and executive functions may be helpful in differential diagnosis and management of ADHD (Barkley, 1997). Because they have difficulty planning, organizing, regulating, evaluating, and changing their behavior (Hale et al., 1998), these children do not allocate or regulate effort in accordance with task demands, leading to slow and variable responding (Douglas, 1999; Scheres, Oosterlaan, & Sergeant, 2001). Numerous reviews and studies have shown ADHD to be characterized by deficits in attention, inhibition, interference, temporal relationships, planning, mental flexibility, maintaining/shifting cognitive set, and reaction time/processing speed (Barkley, Edwards, Laneri, Fletcher, & Metevia, 2001; Grodzinsky & Barkley, 1999; Nigg, Blaskey, Huang-Pollock, & Rappley, 2002; Seidman, Biederman, Faraone, Weber, & Ouellette, 1997; Shallice et al., 2002). The hyperactive–impulsive type has generally been found to involve less neuropsychological impairment than the inattentive or combined types (e.g., Chhabildas, Pennington, & Willcutt, 2001), with the combined type showing the greatest impairment (e.g., Houghton et al., 1999; Klorman et al., 1999). Recent research has started to discriminate between subtypes, with measures of executive function, working memory, and processing efficiency associated with the inattentive and combined types, whereas inhibition measures help identify the hyperactive–impulsive type (Hale, Bertin, & Brown, 2004; Rucklidge & Tannock, 2002).

Given the association between frontal–subcortical structures and LDs, we are not surprised to find that comorbid ADHD and LDs result in greater executive function deficits (Lazar & Frank, 1998; Seidman, Biederman, Monuteaux, Doyle, & Faraone, 2001). As discussed in Chapter 5, reading fluency has been associated with many of the brain structures affected in ADHD. As a result, it is not surprising that studies have shown high rates of comorbidity between ADHD and reading disorders (Shaywitz, Fletcher, & Shaywitz, 1995), with results suggesting that phonological awareness, verbal working memory, verbal retrieval, and processing speed should be considered for differential diagnosis (Pennington, Groisser, & Welsh, 1993; Purvis & Tannock, 2000; Rucklidge & Tannock, 2002; Weiler, Bernstein, Bellinger, & Waber, 2000). Whereas some math deficits seen in ADHD appear to be of the frontal–procedural–working memory type discussed in Chapter 6 (see Zentall & Smith, 1993), math deficits associated with the inattentive type of ADHD could be caused by a more posterior, nonverbal LD syndrome (Marshall et al., 1997). This distinction would appear to fit nicely with the math disorder subtypes discussed in Chapter 6. However, before you think that executive deficits are the result of learning or behavior problems, it is important to note that studies have controlled for these problems and still found executive deficits in children with ADHD (Nigg, Hinshaw, Carte, & Treuting, 1998).

Some clinicians may prefer to use behavioral approaches for diagnosis of ADHD, but we suggest that attention, working memory, and executive function measures should be used to supplement behavioral approaches. Notice that we say "supplement" rather than "substitute," as measures of executive function do not consistently discriminate between children with ADHD and those with other psychiatric disorders (Pennington & Ozonoff, 1996; Sergeant, Geurts, & Oosterlaan, 2001). Although these measures have good positive predictive power, their negative predictive power is only modest, and they have limited specificity (Doyle, Biederman, Seidman, Weber, & Faraone, 2000; Grodzinsky & Barkley, 1999); these factors suggest that it is best to use a battery of related measures to diagnose ADHD (Perugini, Harvey, Lovejoy, Sandstrom, & Webb, 2000). Thus we believe that accurate diagnosis of ADHD is likely to require neuropsychological testing, behavioral observation and ratings, and diagnostic interviews. However, it is important to consider that the limitations of neuropsychological measures in detecting ADHD could be related to the behavioral/interview diagnostic approaches used in these studies to define groups, whereas ADHD (especially the inattentive type) could be due to other causes not detected through such approaches (e.g., DE, parietal dysfunction). Measures may become more specific and sensitive when we start to determine what "true" ADHD is, and start to link subtype behavior and neuropsychological performance to frontal–subcortical circuits, as suggested in In-Depth 8.5 and Table 8.1.

In attempts to further delineate attention, working memory, and executive function deficits in ADHD, several models have emerged, three of which we will discuss briefly. Barkley's (1997) ADHD model posits that disinhibition and poor task persistence, due to prefrontal–subcortical circuit dysfunction, result in executive impairments in self-regulation, working memory, internalization of speech, temporal relationships, planning, goal-directed behavior, and problem solving. Barkley suggests that the inattentive type of ADHD, with symptoms of daydreaming, lethargy, staring, confusion, and passivity, is due to problems with focused or selective attention, rather than to the frontal–subcortical circuit dysfunction seen in the other ADHD subtypes—a point

IN-DEPTH 8.5. ADHD as a Frontal–Subcortical Circuit Disorder

Although ADHD was once thought to be simply a behavior disorder, a growing body of evidence highlighted in Table 8.1 highlights that ADHD is clearly a frontal-subcortical disorder. Consistent with findings of executive function deficits in ADHD, frontal–subcortical abnormalities found in children with ADHD include asymmetric/dysmorphic conditions (Hynd, Semrud-Clikeman, Lorys, Novey, & Eliopulos, 1990), abnormal electrical activity (Novak, Solanto, & Abikoff, 1995), and lowered cerebral blood flow (Ernst et al., 1994; Lou, Henriksen, & Bruhn, 1984; Lou, Henriksen, Bruhn, Borner, & Nielsen, 1989; Zametkin et al., 1993). In particular, the right frontal lobe, dorsolateral and orbital prefrontal cortex, or frontal cortical–subcortical systems may be differentially impaired (Voeller, 2001). As noted earlier, the right frontal lobe has been related to attention, whereas the orbital frontal cortex and striatum have been related to inhibition (Semrud-Clikeman et al., 2000; Starkstein & Kremer, 2001; Vaidya et al., 1998). Dopaminergic deficiencies may lead to frontal/striatal hypometabolism in children with ADHD (Rubia et al., 1999), which would account for the salutary effects of the dopamine agonist methylphenidate (Lou et al., 1989; Vaidya et al., 1998).

A comparison of dorsolateral–dorsal cingulate–striatal and orbital–ventral cingulate–striatal frontal–subcortical circuits suggests that the former may be related to the inattentive type, whereas the disinhibited hyperactive–impulsive type could be related to the latter, with the combined type having both areas affected (Goldberg, 2001; Hale, Bertin, & Brown, 2004). However, as noted earlier, others suggest that the inattentive type is related to parietal dysfunction and nonverbal LDs, and indeed this may be the case for many children diagnosed with ADHD. However, we would argue that children with this type of attention problem will be unlikely to respond to medication, because their symptoms are actually secondary to parietal lobe dysfunction. This is consistent with research suggesting that children with the frontal type of ADHD respond to stimulant medication, but those with greater occipital–parietal involvement do not (Filipek et al., 1997). As stimulants have therapeutic effects because they are dopamine agonists (Swanson, Castellanos, Murias, LaHoste, & Kennedy, 1998), it is not surprising that children with ADHD and IDs are less likely to respond to stimulant medication (DuPaul, Barkley, & McMurray, 1994), possibly because their attention problems are associated with serotonin dysfunction and DE (e.g., Lahey et al., 1993).

TABLE 8.1. Frontal–Subcortical Structures Implicated in ADHD

Source	Finding
Frontal lobe	
Casey et al. (1997)	Frontal volume/right frontal involvement
Castellanos et al. (1996)	
Filipek et al. (1997)	
Hynd et al. (1990)	
Semrud-Clikeman et al. (2000)	
Basal ganglia	
Casey et al. (1997)	Left or right caudate
Castellanos et al. (1994)	
Castellanos et al. (1996)	
Filipek et al. (1997)	
Hynd et al. (1993)	
Aylward et al. 1996)	Left or total globus pallidus
Casey et al. (1997)	
Castellanos et al. (1996)	
Semrud-Clikeman et al. (2000)	
Singer et al. (1993)	
Max et al. (2002)	Ventral putamen
Anterior cingulate	
Rubia et al. (1999)	Anterior cingulate
Corpus callosum	
Baumgardner et al. (1996)	Anterior and/or posterior corpus callosum
Giedd et al. (1994)	
Hynd et al. (1991)	
Semrud-Clikeman et al. (1994)	
Cerebellum	
Castellanos et al. (1996)	Cerebellar reductions

echoed in a controversial review by Milich, Balentine, and Lyman (2001). In addition, Pennington and Ozonoff's (1996) executive function review seems to concur with Barkley's argument; these authors suggest that only measures of motor inhibition may be specific to ADHD. As discussed earlier, children with ADHD perform poorly on several components of Mirsky's (1996) model of attention. However, this model reveals that multiple brain areas are involved in the focus/execute (striatum/superior temporal/inferior parietal), encode (hippocampus/amygdala), shift (prefrontal/anterior cingulate), and sustain/stability (reticular formation/thalamus) attention elements, which are measured by many of the instruments discussed in Chapter 4. Mirsky's model certainly reveals the complexity of attention processes and their interactions with other constructs (e.g., memory and executive function), but this confounding of attention with other constructs possibly limits the utility of the model in clinical practice. We would argue that children with "real" ADHD have difficulty with what Posner and Raichle (1994) describe in their model as the anterior alerting/vigilance and executive/processing networks (i.e., frontal–subcortical circuits), but not the posterior orienting network (i.e., parietal function). Of course, differential diagnosis still needs to consider the attention and executive deficits found in DE, but distinguishing frontal (executive measures) from parietal (dorsal stream measures) ADHD is an important consideration in differential diagnosis. Differentiating between parietal and frontal ADHD symptoms is difficult, as the inferior parietal–ventral frontal connections and the superior parietal–dorsal frontal connections operate in a reciprocal manner (Starkstein & Kremer, 2001). This suggests that regardless of the area primarily affected, deficits can be expected in both. Is it the parietal dysfunction that is affecting frontal attention, working memory, and executive functions, or the opposite? Is the problem a "bottom-up" (i.e., parietal) or a "top-down" (i.e., frontal) one? This is the diagnostic question you must answer with your CHT evaluation; as we have noted, the intervention strategies and treatment course will be different, depending on the primary area affected.

In conclusion, there has been much research on ADHD, and while there is still debate on the etiology and treatment of the disorder, some emerging trends suggest that it is a frontal–subcortical circuit disorder. Several important questions remain, however—questions that we hope will be addressed in future neurophysiological, neuropharmacological, and neuropsychological research. We feel that these critical diagnostic and treatment questions include the following:

• Given our earlier discussion of AS, could the difference between ADHD and AS be one between right frontal and right posterior dysfunction, respectively? Or could the difference be related to frontal white matter hypoactivity (ADHD) versus right-hemisphere white matter dysfunction (AS)? Can measures of executive and dorsal stream function separate these distinct children with attention problems?

• Could the association between ADHD and IDs such as DE be related to the parietal attention network and nonverbal LDs, or is this association related to the frontal executive problems found in both DE and ADHD? Can you differentiate between the inattention due to ADHD and DE, so the proper medication treatment is attempted? Given that AN is likely to be caused by too much orbital prefrontal activity, and the hyperactive–impulsive type of ADHD by too little, how do you make sure that a child's fidgety behavior isn't just nervousness?

• As the highest comorbidity rate for ADHD is with EDs, could both ADHD and ED be related to underactive or hypoactive cortical functioning? Is the difference between them related to differences between cortical and subcortical causes of hypoactivity? How can you design instruction and interventions that maximize the cortical functioning level in these children, so they are available for learning?

• How do you differentiate among ADHD, OCD, and Tourette syndrome, as these disorders are also likely to show attention and executive deficits suggestive of frontal–subcortical circuit dysfunction? How do you discriminate between underactive (i.e., ADHD) and overactive (i.e., OCD) orbital frontal–subcortical circuits, especially when both these disorders occur comorbidly with Tourette syndrome? Could dysregulation (either an excess or an absence) of attention, impulse control, and motor activity be found in all of these disorders, suggesting a similar underlying pathophysiology?

• How do you discriminate between dorsolateral–subcortical and executive deficits in ADHD and childhood schizophrenia? Do the left frontal and temporal/hippocampal functions of long-term memory encoding, language processing, object recognition, and categorization help differentiate ADHD from childhood schizophrenia? Or does adequate response inhibition combined with executive deficits best predict childhood schizophrenia?

Obviously, until these questions are addressed by systematic research, we are left with the available clinical tools and our clinical acumen to guide our practice. However, these questions are presented in an attempt to guide your thinking about diagnostic and treatment issues. An advantage of the CHT approach is that you will quickly recognize it if you have gone down the wrong diagnostic path with a child. The CHT model suggests the use of neuropsychological and other measures to explore each of these possibilities in a child who presents with inattention, impulsivity, and/or hyperactivity. Through ongoing data collection and monitoring, you can assure treatment efficacy for the children you serve.

Assessment and Treatment of ADHD

As we have noted earlier, the multidimensional nature of attention disorders suggests that interview and behavior rating scales may have limited utility in differential diagnosis of ADHD subtypes and determining medication treatment effects. Because children with ADHD have different intentional and inhibitory capacities (Denckla, 1996), vary across cognitive dimensions (Fletcher et al., 1996), and may perform poorly on tasks because of comorbid deficits (Morris, 1996), a thorough evaluation of the neuropsychological, academic, and behavioral characteristics of children who have ADHD with or without comorbid diagnoses can ensure accurate diagnosis and successful management of all disorders (Teeter & Semrud-Clikeman, 1995). Obviously, the neuropsychological assessment of ADHD should focus on the integrity of the frontal–subcortical systems involved in attention, inhibition, and executive control. However, a complete evaluation may be necessary to rule out auditory processing, language, visual-perceptual (right parietal), and other psychiatric disorders, such as ODD/CD, DE, AN, and thought disorder. Given the poor agreement between parent and teacher ratings of ADHD behaviors, and the limited utility of standardized rating scales in differential diagnosis of ADHD subtypes (Hale, How, DeWitt, & Coury, 2001), we feel that a neuropsychological assessment of ADHD symptoms should be included in evaluations of all children with attention problems.

For treatment, most studies confirm that the dopamine agonist methylphenidate (Ritalin) and other stimulants are highly effective in treating the associated executive and behavior deficits. However, a meta-analysis of 74 studies revealed substantial medication effects on behavioral but not academic outcomes, with little evidence that behavioral effects translated into academic gains (Purdie, Hattie, & Carroll, 2002). Why would a medication that is highly effective in reducing the problem behaviors associated with ADHD have little impact on academic achievement? We believe that this is because most medication management strategies typically rely on behavior observations and ratings in the classroom and home to determine treatment effects, and little attention is paid to the effects of medication on cognition. Although medication response can be systematically monitored through direct child observation or administration of rating scales (Greenhill et al., 1996), cognitive and behavior domains are often affected differentially by medications, even at the same dose (Hale et al., 1998; Hoeppner et al., 1997). The best dose for behavior may have a limited or even a detrimental effect on cognitive functioning (Swanson, Cantwell, Lerner, McBurnett, & Hanna, 1991). Neuropsychological assessment and consultation may be necessary, because many children respond to psychotropic medication in an idiosyncratic manner, especially when comorbid LDs and behavior disorders are present (Hale et al., 1998).

Given that children with ADHD respond differentially to medication, and that some doses may have a detrimental effect on learning (e.g., the "zombie" effect), the psychologist must be ready to help monitor treatment response for physicians. We have developed a multimethod double-blind placebo medication trial protocol designed to monitor methylphenidate dose–response relationships for children with ADHD (see Hale et al., 1998; Hale, Fiorello, et al., 2001; Hoeppner et al., 1997). During the trials, neuropsychological, behavioral, and observational data are collected over a 4-week period of baseline, placebo, and low and high doses of methylpheni-date. Following all data collection, the "blind" is broken, data are summarized, and the variables are rank-ordered across conditions from 1 (best performance) to 4 (lowest performance) to ensure that each measure has equal weight in determining response. The data are subjected to separate nonparametric analyses to determine statistical response. A summary report, including a response graph and recommendations, is provided to help referring physicians determine clinical response.

Figure 8.1 depicts the medication trial results for Doug, with lower ranks indicating better performance and behavior. After several unsuccessful attempts to treat his learning and behavior problems with different stimulant medications, school interventions, and behavior therapy, Doug was referred for the medication trial service. As can be seen, Doug's neuropsychological perfor-mance was better on 5 mg of methylphenidate, whereas his behavioral response was optimal on the 10 mg dose. Subsequent to the trial, Doug was successfully treated with a low medication dose and adjunctive behavior therapy to help control his out-of-seat, off-task, and calling-out be-haviors. Your skills in research design and measurement can be used to help physicians design similar trials to optimize psychotropic medication titration or monitor untoward effects for chil-dren with ADHD. This is the intervention part of CHT, where you hypothesize that medication will work, set up a data collection strategy, analyze the medication effects on and off medicine, and then help determine whether the treatment is effective. Although you may choose to use behavioral observations and/or ratings to help make this judgment, we feel it is critical to include some measure of cognitive or academic functioning as well, given the findings presented above.

Even if stimulant treatment is effective, it is not the cure-all that some hope it is. Medication just makes a child more available to learn from the environment (Silver, 1990). In addition to med-ication management to ameliorate attention and executive deficits, academic and behavioral strat-egies will be necessary for all children with ADHD, especially if a lower dose is chosen to opti-mize cognition. Learning strategies and metacognitive interventions are unlikely to be highly effective when children are unmedicated, because of the executive deficits described earlier. However, as adjuncts to medication management, they can be highly effective in improving self-monitoring and awareness, mental flexibility, organizational strategies, inhibition, and persis-tence. Table 8.2 provides a number of interventions for children with ADHD and other executive function disorders.

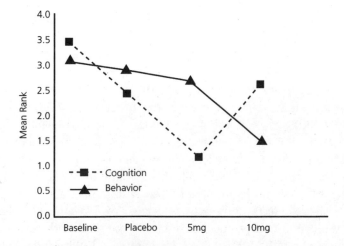

FIGURE 8.1. Medication trial results for Doug V.

TABLE 8.2. Interventions for Metacognitive Processing and Executive Functions

Presenting problem	Goal of intervention	Intervention	Reference
Poor use of metacognitive strategies	Teach metacognitive strategy use	Think-alouds	Davey, 1983 (p. 286)[a]
		Self-regulated strategy development	Graham & Harris, 1999 (p. 286)[a]
		Mnemonics	Alsopp, 1999 (p. 287)[a]
		Cognitive behavior modification	Meichenbaum, 1977, 1983 (p. 287)[a]
		Child-generated strategies	Naglieri & Gottling, 1995
	Stimulate metacognitive strategy use with priming/ prelearning activities	Anticipation guide	Adapted from Tierney & Readance, 1999 (p. 427)[b]
		Semantic feature analysis: Concepts, vocabulary	Adapted from Anders & Bos, 1986; and Bos, Anders, Filip, & Jaffe, 1989 (p. 484)[b]
		Semantic maps: Advance organizers	Bos & Vaughn, 2001 (p. 486)[b]
Poor use of academic strategies	Improve note taking	Cornell Method	Pauk, 1993 (p. 288)[a]
		Three-column method	Saski, Swicegood, & Carter, 1983 (p. 288)[a]
		"AWARE" method	Suritsky & Hughes, 1993 (p. 288)[a]
	Improve test preparation and test-taking strategies	"PIRATES" test-taking strategy	Adapted from Hughes & Schumaker, 1991 (p. 471)[b] and (p. 297)[a]
		"PORPE" strategy for test preparation and comprehension	Simpson & Stahl, 1987 (p. 315)[a]

[a]Described in Goldstein and Mather (2001).
[b]Described in Mather and Jaffe (2002).
AWARE, Arrange to take notes, Write quickly, Apply cues, Review notes as soon as possible, Edit notes; PIRATES, Prepare to succeed, Inspect the instructions, Read, remember, and reduce; Answer or abandon, Turn back; Estimate; Survey; PORPE, Predict, Organize, Rehearse, Practice, Evaluate.

Behavioral strategies, such as contingency management and behavioral contracting, are based largely on the operant conditioning techniques described in Chapter 4 (see In-Depth 4.1). They have been shown to be highly useful as adjunctive therapies to medication, but again to have limited effects without it (Greenhill et al., 1996). This is because medication may serve as an "establishing operation" necessary for a child with ADHD to respond to the discriminative stimulus. Without the beneficial effects of medication, the child is less likely to attend to a discriminative stimulus (e.g., teacher direction) or to inhibit a behavior (e.g., calling out an answer), possibly because the medication also strengthens response to reinforcement and extinction interventions (Johansen, Aase, Meyer, & Sagvolden, 2002). Case Study 8.3 describes this important interaction between medication and behavioral interventions.

CASE STUDY 8.3. Getting Terry's Behavior under Stimulus Control

Terry was an 8-year-old boy who was seen initially for a prereferral intervention consultation after re-peated physical altercations with his peers. When Terry was observed in the classroom, momentary time sampling made it clear that he was frequently inattentive to task materials or the teacher (off-task behav-ior 55%, vs. 15% for a control peer) and that his motor activity was high (60%, vs. 10% for the control peer). He had nine (impulsive) call-outs during a 20-minute block of instruction, whereas the control peer had none. However, functional analysis (done through observation and teacher data collection) re-vealed that Terry only engaged in inappropriate peer interactions when the other children were either standing around their desks or lining up to go to lunch, recess, or other out-of-class events. Typically, Terry would become very animated and excited at these times. He'd start showing increased body move-ment and gestures, and would begin talking in a loud voice. Then he would often bump into someone, or another child would bump into him. The subsequent verbal exchange would inevitably lead to a shov-ing match, and one time a fight broke out. In the subsequent interview and follow-up consultation with the teacher, we decided to use differential reinforcement of incompatible behavior (DRI) whenever the children had to line up in the classroom. The other incidents could (we hoped) be reduced by the use of teacher proximity and interference. For the DRI program, we taught Terry to put his hands in his pock-ets whenever he stood up to get in line. When the teacher gave the direction for the class to rise, she would tap on his desk, and he would put his hands in his pockets on his way to the line. Verbal praise was used as a reinforcer.

After 1 week, we met again. The event-recording data produced by the teacher suggested that Terry had learned the operant behavior, but was using it inconsistently in the classroom. The teacher said she thought he was not sufficiently motivated by the praise, so we added 5 minutes of computer time at the end of each day for each time Terry complied with the DRI behavior. Two weeks later, the teacher stopped me (Hale) in the hall, and we went to her room to look at the data. Some days Terry earned 15–20 minutes of computer time, yet other days he earned no time. The teacher was upset be-cause she felt that Terry's inconsistent performance was related to home problems or that he was being oppositional, but in reality his variable performance was what I had expected all along. The subsequent neuropsychological evaluation, including measures of attention, working memory, and executive func-tions, revealed the telltale signs of dorsolateral and orbital dysfunction associated with the combined type of ADHD. After the parents and teacher were helped to understand the condition, and various treatment options were offered, Terry underwent a double-blind placebo-controlled medication trial of methylphenidate. After the trial, the physician decided to choose the best dose to optimize cognition, and thereafter the DRI procedure worked without a problem. Apparently Terry's executive functions needed to be maximized for him to respond consistently to the behavioral treatment. Because the "brain boss" was now online, he could now easily recognize the discriminative stimuli (teacher direction and tap on desk), and the reinforcer (praise or computer time) was highly effective.

CASE STUDY PRESENTATION

In Appendix 8.1, you will find a sample case report that highlights how neuropsychological assess-ment can provide additional insights for management of a child with numerous concerns. Report-writing styles may vary, based on the school setting and administration. Some of you may choose to write reports that all can understand, while others may prefer to write reports at a professional level and provide a brief supplemental letter for parents. Regardless of the style you select, it is important to emphasize the functional characteristics of the individual, listing positive findings before deficits. Ensure that you integrate history, observation, intellectual/cognitive, achieve-ment, and psychosocial data, especially in the summary section. You should limit discussion of complex statistics in the report, and you may want to avoid any references to brain structures. Your knowledge of neuropsychology only helps you formulate diagnostic impressions and treatment options; it is not necessary to put a lot of references to brain areas in your report.

Recommendations should be based on findings and tailored to address referral questions and/or problems uncovered during your CHT evaluation. We don't see recommendations as diagnostic–prescriptive, so we tend to provide more recommendations and options than are needed. For some cases, the assessment is only the first step in developing a collaborative problem-solving relationship with the teacher, parent, and other professionals. After the report is presented, a follow-up consultation could be designed to address specific questions and concerns regarding the unique strengths and needs of the child, or to brainstorm ideas for intervention and monitoring of medication response as the next step in CHT. Although the teacher and parents may ultimately carry out many of the interventions, as consultant you should collect additional information during follow-up meetings or provide services directly to the child as needed.

As we have repeated throughout this book, for neuropsychological principles to be effectively applied in school settings, you must recognize that the assessment, interpretation, report writing, and feedback session are merely the beginnings of a successful intervention. It is up to you to work collaboratively with others to ensure that your understanding of neuropsychological principles is translated into effective interventions for the children you serve. CHT involves testing hypotheses not only about a child's neuropsychological strengths and weaknesses, but also about intervention. Even if your initial problem-solving intervention is less than optimal, you can recycle it as necessary until you achieve an intervention that successfully helps a child overcome his or her deficits. Despite all the promise of neuropsychological principles, it is up to you as a scientist-practitioner to reach the ultimate goal, making sure you meet the unique needs of the children you serve.

NEUROPSYCHOLOGICAL CONSULTATION

Identifying Information

Name: Nathan Smith
Chronological age: 10 years, 11 months
Referral source: Ms. Brooke
Referral diagnosis: ADHD, predominantly inattentive type (provisional)

Reason for Referral

Nathan was referred for an evaluation because of continued academic and interpersonal relationship difficulties and a poor response to methylphenidate treatment.

Relevant Background Information

Nathan's birth and developmental histories were unremarkable, other than Ms. Brooke's reporting low Apgar scores at 1 minute. Developmental milestones were reportedly achieved within normal limits, but he may have had slight language delays. The medical history is positive for chronic ear infections, overweight problems, and a right frontal injury at age 7. Nathan reported that he tripped and fell against a coffee table. Although he was "confused" and "upset" by the incident, there was no reported loss of consciousness, headache, nausea, or vomiting, and he was released from the emergency room after receiving six sutures.

Nathan lives with his mother, stepfather, and typically developing 9-year-old brother. The parents were divorced 5 years ago, and the boys have regular visitation with their biological father. Relationships are reportedly adequate, but family members spend little time with each other. Nathan did not discuss his family other than to mention occasional fights with his sibling. Nathan said that he had many friends, but could only name one, and admitted that he and this friend seldom spend time together outside of school. Ms. Brooke reported that Nathan has difficulty with peer relationships and "doesn't seem to get it" with his same-age peers, instead preferring to play with younger neighborhood children or spend time alone in his room.

School records and parental report indicated that Nathan did well in preschool, but had attention problems in the early elementary years. Nathan had more difficulty upon entering middle school, and he occasionally failed mathematics and science tests. Nathan reported that he has problems understanding material, and that when taking tests he cannot remember "what to do." Although reading had previously been a strength, Nathan's grades have dropped recently, because "the teacher asks too many hard questions." The teacher report indicated that Nathan wants to do well in school and tries to get along with others, but that he is somewhat aloof and withdrawn.

Instruments Administered

Wechsler Intelligence Scale for Children—Third Edition (WISC-III)
Differential Ability Scales (DAS), Matrices subtest
Wisconsin Card Sorting Test (WCST)
Stroop Color–Word Test
Conners Continuous Performance Test II (CPT-II)
Boston Naming Test (BNT)

(continued)

    Controlled Oral Word Association Test (COWAT)
    Wisconsin Verbal Selective Reminding Test (WSRT)
    Test of Memory and Learning (TOMAL), Nonverbal subtests
    Trail Making Test (TMT), Parts A and B
    Developmental Test of Visual–Motor Integration
    Wechsler Individual Achievement Test—Second Edition
    Achenbach Child Behavior Checklist (CBCL) and Youth Self-Report Form
    Clinical interview

Assessment Observations

Nathan presented for testing as a slightly overweight boy with blond hair and glasses. Although Nathan was polite and compliant during the evaluation, he responded only when directly questioned and did not engage in spontaneous conversation. His articulation was clear, but he rarely paused between phrases, and he repeated himself on occasion. When responding to verbal test items, Nathan's sentence structure was simple, and he often talked his way through nonverbal problems. Although his verbalizations were often indirect and circumlocutious, suggesting possible retrieval difficulties, his answers were not bizarre, tangential, or confabulatory. Visual–motor tasks appeared to be difficult for Nathan, as he rubbed his eyes several times. Nathan's attention and concentration skills varied by the stimulus materials presented, with verbal items receiving more interest than nonverbal ones. However, he was not impulsive, perseverative, or easily frustrated, and he appeared to put forth consistent effort throughout the evaluation. His motor activity was typical, but his affect was generally flat. These observations suggest that the results are reliable and valid indicators of Nathan's current level and pattern of functioning.

Assessment Results and Clinical Impressions

Cognitive/Neuropsychological Functioning

On the WISC-III (mean = 100, standard deviation = 15; higher scores = better performance), a measure of intellectual functioning, Nathan had significant scatter on several subtests and the global scores. When a youth displays this variable pattern of performance, it is best to interpret factor standard scores (SSs) and/or subtest scores. At this level of analysis, Nathan was within the average range for the Verbal Comprehension and Freedom from Distractibility/Working Memory factors (both SSs = 98), but his Processing Speed factor score was low average (SS = 88), and his Perceptual Organization factor score was in the borderline range (SS = 77).

An evaluation of Nathan's pattern of performance revealed fairly well-developed receptive and expressive language skills, but he often spoke at length before arriving at a correct answer. He appeared to have a good fund for factual information, missing only science-related items. His expressive vocabulary was age-appropriate, but he was somewhat concrete in his responses, which would account for his difficulty on verbal concept formation tasks assessing categorical relationships among word pairs and social knowledge or reasoning. His auditory attention and concentration skills were age-appropriate when he was asked to recall digits or solve simple oral arithmetic problems; he had more difficulty with mental manipulation of information when asked to recall digits backward or solve multistep problems. On tests of verbal learning, retrieval, and fluency, Nathan's performance was within normal limits suggesting adequate encoding and retrieval of words from long-term memory.

Unlike his adequate verbal skills, Nathan's visual-perceptual skills were relatively impaired across the WISC-III Performance subtests. Although he demonstrated adequate visual scanning speed of abstract stimuli on one subtest, Nathan had more difficulty reproducing simple abstract symbols quickly

(continued)

and efficiently, determining missing parts in pictures, sequencing pictures presented in disarray, replicating block design patterns from a model, and especially synthesizing puzzles without a template. Subsequent examination on a different measure of nonverbal and fluid reasoning was accordingly low. On tests of visual–motor integration and psychomotor speed, Nathan's performance was below average, but fairly consistent with his other nonverbal skills. His performance on tests tapping working memory for visual stimuli and encoding of visual–spatial information into long-term memory was below average, and he displayed variable performance on several visual measures. His recognition of faces from memory was significantly better than his memory for spatial locations.

For attention, memory, and executive functions, Nathan's performance was mostly within normal limits. He had difficulty sustaining attention, as indicated by omission errors, variable response times, and limited tendency toward risk taking on a continuous performance task. This suggests limited arousal, which could account for his slow but accurate performance on tests of psychomotor reproduction. His performance on memory tests suggests adequate verbal and visual working and long-term memory processes, and only mild difficulty with retrieval of visual–spatial information. Although retention, mental manipulation, or retrieval of auditory information may be somewhat difficult for Nathan, no consistent weakness was demonstrated. He had no difficulty on an executive function task that requires inhibiting automatic response of reading words to name the color of ink they are printed in. He quickly learned sorting principles, maintained response sets, and shifted categories easily with few perseverative errors on another executive function measure. On a measure that requires psychomotor speed to draw lines and mental flexibility to shift between numbers and letters, Nathan was slightly below average. However, these results would be expected, given his performance on the other graphomotor measures.

Academic Functioning

Although Nathan is reportedly functioning below grade level in his academic subjects, his overall standardized achievement performance was within normal limits for reading, mathematics, and written language domains. Given his cognitive/neuropsychological performance, Nathan would not appear to qualify for learning disability services at this time. Although he displayed good word attack and phonemic analysis skills, and responded well to comprehension items requiring recall of factual information, Nathan had the most difficulty with reading comprehension items requiring inference and implicit comprehension. Nathan had more difficulty on the written mathematics computation section than he did on orally presented math problems, and column/spatial errors were evident during computation. His spelling errors were mostly phonemic or homophone equivalents, and he did have more problems with irregular sight words. Nathan had no difficulty with written language, but his sample was similar to his spoken language—lengthy and poorly organized. However, Nathan had no difficulty with grammar and punctuation.

Psychosocial/Behavioral Screening

The screening of behavioral functioning revealed a discrepancy between Nathan's self-perception and Ms. Brooke's ratings. Whereas Nathan rated himself in the average range across domains, Ms. Brooke rated him in the clinical range on the CBCL Attention Problems and Social Problems subscales, borderline on the Withdrawn subscale, and clinically elevated on the Aggressive Behavior subscale. The Total and Internalizing scores were in the clinical range, whereas the Externalizing score was borderline clinical. Ms. Brooke endorsed items suggesting that Nathan is inattentive, labile, and withdrawn. As noted above, she indicated that he has difficulty with peer relationships and prefers playing with younger children. He can become oppositional, defiant, and aggressive at times, occasionally destroying his own or someone else's property. Although this suggests that Nathan may be minimizing his problems, he may have limited awareness of his difficulties. In addition, Ms. Brooke may see an increased need for intervention, and therefore her responses may be somewhat elevated. Despite this contrast, Nathan, Ms.

(continued)

Brooke, and the teacher all reported difficulty with peer and adult relationships warranting clinical attention. Further psychological and/or psychiatric evaluation appears to be warranted.

Summary and Recommendations

Nathan is a 10-year, 11-month-old male referred for neuropsychological consultation because of continued academic and relationship difficulties and a poor response to methylphenidate treatment. Nathan's pattern of performance suggests difficulty with perceptual analysis and synthesis, maintaining part–whole configurations, and holistic reasoning. Difficulty with global spatial relationships probably leads to graphomotor problems, with poor visual feedback to the motor system. Occupational therapy and graduated guidance during handwriting instruction may be helpful. Subsequent hypothesis-testing results confirm that higher-level nonverbal reasoning skills or fluid abilities are impaired. This suggests that Nathan will have the greatest difficulty learning novel or complex information, whether it is auditory–verbal or visual–motor in nature. In addition, flexibility in thought will be limited as the quantity or complexity of stimuli increases. This pattern will also interfere with Nathan's ability to sustain attention for extended periods, which may be already limited for some auditory and many visual stimuli. He may show limited attention to himself or his environment, but this inattention appears to be secondary to his processing issues. It does not appear to be a primary attention deficit amenable to stimulant medication treatment. Accordingly, Nathan would benefit from classroom tape-recording and note-taking services (the latter might be accomplished by a peer buddy system). Although Nathan's mathematics computation skills are somewhat below those of his same-age peers, he is likely to have the most difficulty when required to comprehend abstract concepts, draw inferences, or make predictions about academic material. The complexity of his oral and written expression is likely to be limited as well, especially when he is given little structure or guidance with which to proceed. As communication pragmatics and drawing inferential conclusions are likely to be difficult for Nathan, he may benefit from speech and language therapy in these areas. Task analysis (breaking tasks down) and hierarchical ordering of higher-level assignments will be critical for Nathan. As this pattern of performance rarely results in poor academic achievement until the later grades, it is not surprising that Nathan is having substantial difficulty at this time. In addition, this may be the reason why he does not currently meet criteria for a learning disability and should be re-evaluated on a regular basis to monitor academic progress. Individuals with this type of learning disorder often experience deficits in perception of facial affect and speech prosody, which could account for the Nathan's lack of friendships and periodic confrontations with peers and adults. He may benefit from structured therapeutic role-play techniques designed to help him identify affective behavior and communicate effectively with others. Social skills instruction and participation in group activities are highly recommended. Further psychological, psychiatric, occupational therapy, and/or speech and language evaluation may be helpful for comprehensive examination of his cognitive, language, and socioemotional needs. I will be available for further discussion of Nathan's current functioning and intervention options at your earliest convenience. Thank you for the consult.

References

Aaron, P. G. (1997). The impending demise of the discrepancy formula. *Review of Educational Research, 67*, 461–502.

Abbott, R. D., & Berninger, V. W. (1993). Structural equation modeling of relationships among developmental skills and writing skills in primary- and intermediate-grade writers. *Journal of Educational Psychology, 85*, 478–508.

Achenbach, T. M. (1991). *Manual for the Teacher Report Form and 1991 Profile*. Burlington, VT: University Associates in Psychiatry.

Achenbach, T. M. (2001). Challenges and benefits of assessment, diagnosis, and taxonomy for clinical practice and research. *Australian and New Zealand Journal of Psychiatry, 35*, 263–271.

Adams, C., Green, J., Gilchrist, A., & Cox, A. (2002). Conversational behavior of children with Asperger syndrome and conduct disorder. *Journal of Child Psychology and Psychiatry, 43*, 679–690.

Adams, M. J. (1990). *Beginning to read*. Cambridge, MA: MIT Press.

Adolphs, R., Tranel, D., Damasio, H., & Damasio, A. R. (1995). Fear and the human amygdala. *Journal of Neuroscience, 15*, 5879–5891.

Allen, S. J., & Graden, J. L. (2002). Best practices in collaborative problem solving for intervention design. In A. Thomas & J. Grimes (Eds.), *Best practices in school psychology IV* (Vol. 1, pp. 565–582). Bethesda, MD: National Association of School Psychologists.

American Educational Research Association, American Psychological Association, & National Council on Measurement in Education. (1999). *Standards for educational and psychological testing*. Washington, DC: Author.

American Psychiatric Association. (1994). *Diagnostic and statistical manual of mental disorders* (4th ed.). Washington, DC: Author.

American Psychiatric Association. (2000). *Diagnostic and statistical manual of mental disorders* (4th ed., text rev.). Washington, DC: Author.

Americans with Disabilities Act (ADA). 42 U.S.C. § 12101 et seq. (1990).

Anastasi, A., & Urbina, S. (1997). *Psychological testing* (7th ed.). Upper Saddle River, NJ: Prentice Hall.

Anderson, V. (1998). Assessing executive functions in children: Biological, psychological, and developmental considerations. *Neuropsychological Rehabilitation, 8*, 319–349.

Angold, A., Costello, E. J., & Erkanli, A. (1999). Comorbidity. *Journal of Child Psychology and Psychiatry, 40*, 57–87.

Ashlock, R. B. (1998). *Error patterns in computation* (7th ed.). Upper Saddle River, NJ: Merrill/Prentice Hall.

Avons, S. E., & Hanna, C. (1995). The memory-span deficit in children with specific reading disability: Is speech rate responsible? *British Journal of Developmental Psychology, 13*, 303–311.

Aylward, E. H., Reiss, A. L., Reader, M. J., Singer, H. S., Brown, J. E., & Denckla, M. B. (1996). Basal ganglia volumes in children with attention-deficit hyperactivity disorder. *Journal of Child Neurology, 11*, 112–115.

Ayres, R. R., & Cooley, E. J. (1986). Sequential versus simultaneous processing on the K-ABC: Validity in predicting learning success. *Journal of Psychoeducational Assessment, 4*, 211–220.

Badecker, W., Rapp, B., & Caramazza, A. (1996). Lexical morphology and the two orthographic routes. *Cognitive Neuropsychology, 13*, 161–175.

Badian, N. A. (1997). Dyslexia and the double deficit hypothesis. *Annals of Dyslexia, 47*, 69–87.

Bailey, A., Phillips, W., & Rutter, M. (1996). Autism: Towards an integration of clinical, genetic, neuropsychological, and neurobiological perspectives. *Journal of Child Psychology and Psychiatry, 37*, 89–126.

Baker, L., & Cantwell, D. P. (1987a). Comparison of well, emotionally-disordered, and behaviorally-disordered children with linguistic problems. *Journal of the American Academy of Child and Adolescent Psychiatry, 26*, 193–203.

Baker, L., & Cantwell, D. P. (1987b). A prospective psychiatric follow-up of children with speech/language disorders. *Journal of the American Academy of Child and Adolescent Psychiatry, 26*, 546–553.

Baldo, J. V., Shimamura, A. P., Delis, D. C., Kramer, J., & Kaplan, E. (2001). Verbal and design fluency in patients with frontal lobe lesions. *Journal of the International Neuropsychological Society, 7*, 586–596.

Bandura, A. (1978). The self system in reciprocal determinism. *American Psychologist, 33*, 344–358.

Banich, M. T., & Heller, W. (1998). Evolving perspectives on lateralization of function. *Current Directions in Psychological Science, 7*, 1–2.

Barker, T. A., Torgesen, J. K., & Wagner, R. K. (1992). The role of orthographic processing skills on five different reading tasks. *Reading Research Quarterly, 27*, 334–345.

Barkley, R. A. (1997). *ADHD and the nature of self-control.* New York: Guilford Press.

Barkley, R. A., Edwards, G., Laneri, M., Fletcher, K., & Metevia, L. (2001). Executive functioning, temporal discounting, and sense of time in adolescents with attention deficit hyperactivity disorder (ADHD) and oppositional defiant disorder (ODD). *Journal of Abnormal Child Psychology, 29*, 541–556.

Baron, I. S. (2000). Clinical implications and practical applications of child neuropsychological evaluations. In K. O. Yeates, H. D. Ris, & H. G. Taylor (Eds.), *Pediatric neuropsychology: Research, theory, and practice* (pp. 439–454). New York: Guilford Press.

Baron, I. S., Fennell, E. B., & Voeller, K. K. S. (1995). *Pediatric neuropsychology in the medical setting.* New York: Oxford University Press.

Baron-Cohen, S. (1995). *Mindblindness: An essay on autism and theory of mind.* Cambridge, MA: MIT Press.

Baron-Cohen, S., Ring, H. A., Bullmore, E. T., Wheelwright, S., Ashwin, C., & Williams, S. C. R. (2000). The amygdala theory of autism. *Neuroscience and Biobehavioral Reviews, 24*, 355–364.

Basso, A., Burgio, F., & Caporali, A. (2000). Acalculia, aphasia and spatial disorders in left and right brain-damaged patients. *Cortex, 36*, 265–280.

Batchelor, E. S., Gray, J. W., & Dean, R. S. (1990). Empirical testing of a cognitive model to account for neuropsychological functioning underlying arithmetic problem solving. *Journal of Learning Disabilities, 23*, 38–42.

Baumgardner, T. L., Singer, H. S., Denckla, M. B., Rubin, M. A., Abrams, M. T., Colli, M. J., et al. (1996). Corpus callosum morphology in children with Tourette syndrome and attention deficit hyperactivity disorder. *Neurology, 47*, 477–482.

Bavelier, D., Corina, D., Jezzard, P., Clark, V., Karni, A., Lalwani, A., et al. (1998). Hemispheric specialization for English and ASL: Left invariance–right variability. *NeuroReport, 9*, 1537–1542.

Baving, L., Laucht, M., & Schmidt, M. H. (2002). Frontal brain activation in anxious school children. *Journal of Child Psychology and Psychiatry, 43*, 265–274.

Baxter, D. M., & Warrington, E. K. (1994). Measuring sysgraphia: A graded-difficulty spelling test. *Behavioral Neurology, 7*, 107–116.

Baxter, L. R., Clark, E. C., Iqbal, M., & Ackermann, R. F. (2001). Cortical–subcortical systems in the medication of obsessive–compulsive disorder: Modeling the brain's mediation of a classic "neurosis." In D. G. Lichter & J. L. Cummings (Eds.), *Frontal–subcortical circuits in psychiatric and neurological disorders.* New York: Guilford Press.

Beach, R. (1993). *A teacher's introduction to reader-response theories.* Urbana, IL: National Council of Teachers of English.

Bear, D. (1991). Neurological perspectives on aggressive behavior. *Journal of Neuropsychiatry and Clinical Neurosciences, 3*, S3–S8.

Beauchaine, T. P. (2001). Vagal tone, development, and Gray's motivational theory: Toward an integrated model of autonomic nervous system functioning in psychopathology. *Development and Psychopathology, 13*, 183–214.

Beauregard, M., Chertkow, H., Bub, D., Murtha, S., Dixon, R., & Evans, A. (1997). The neural substrate for concrete, abstract, and emotional word lexica: A positron emission tomography study. *Journal of Cognitive Neuroscience, 9,* 441–461.

Beck, I. L., & McKeown, M. G. (1981). Developing questions that promote comprehension: The story map. *Language Arts, 58,* 913–918.

Beeman, M. (1993). Semantic processing in the right hemisphere may contribute to drawing inferences from discourse. *Brain and Language, 44,* 80–120.

Beeman, M., & Chiarello, C. (Eds.). (1998). *Right hemisphere language comprehension: Perspectives from cognitive neuroscience.* Mahwah, NJ: Erlbaum.

Beery, K. E. (1997). *Developmental Test of Visual–Motor Integration—Fourth Edition.* Cleveland, OH: Modern Curriculum.

Beitchman, J. H., Brownlie, E. B., & Wilson, B. (1996). Linguistic impairment and psychiatric disorder: Pathways to outcome. In J. H. Beitchman, N. J. Cohen, M. M. Konstantareas, & R. Tannock (Eds.), *Language, learning, and behavior disorders: Developmental, biological, and clinical perspectives* (pp. 493–514). New York: Cambridge University Press.

Belger, A., & Banich, M. T. (1998). Costs and benefits of integrating information between the two hemispheres: A computational perspective. *Neuropsychology, 12,* 380–398.

Benbow, C. P., & Lubinski, D. (1997). Psychological profiles of the mathematically talented: Some sex differences and evidence supporting their biological basis. In M. R. Walsh (Ed.), *Women, men, and gender* (pp. 271–287). New Haven, CT: Yale University Press.

Bennetto, L., Pennington, B. F., & Rogers, S. J. (1996). Intact and impaired memory functions in autism. *Child Development, 67,* 1816–1835.

Benton, A., & Tranel, D. (1993). Visuoperceptual, visuospatial, and visuoconstructive disorders. In K. M. Heilman & E. Valenstein (Eds.), *Clinical neuropsychology* (3rd ed., pp. 165–213). New York: Oxford University Press.

Berninger, V. W. (1994). Future directions for research on writing disabilities: Integrating endogenous and exogenous variables. In G. R. Lyon (Ed.), *Frames of reference for the assessment of learning disabilities* (pp. 419–440). Baltimore: Brookes.

Berninger, V. W. (1998). *Process Assessment of the Learner (PAL): Guides for intervention.* San Antonio, TX: Psychological Corporation.

Berninger, V. W. (2001). *Process Assessment of the Learner (PAL): Test battery for reading and writing.* San Antonio, TX: Psychological Corporation.

Berninger, V. W., & Abbott, R. D. (1992). The unit of analysis and the constructive processes of the learner: Key concepts for educational neuropsychology. *Educational Psychologist, 27,* 223–242.

Berninger, V. W., & Abbott, R. D. (1994). Redefining learning disabilities: Moving beyond ability–achievement discrepancies to failure to respond to validated treatment protocols. In G. R. Lyon (Ed.), *Frames of reference for the assessment of learning disabilities* (pp. 163–184). Baltimore: Brookes.

Berninger, V. W., Abbott, R. D., Abbott, S. P., Graham, S., & Richards, T. (2002). Writing and reading: Connections between language by hand and language by eye. *Journal of Learning Disabilities, 35,* 39–56.

Berninger, V. W., Abbott, R. D., Billingsley, & Nagy, F. W. (2001). Processes underlying timing and fluency of reading: Efficiency, automaticity, coordination, and morphological awareness. In M. Wolf (Ed.), *Dyslexia, fluency, and the brain* (pp. 383–414). Timonium, MD: York Press.

Berninger, V. W., Mizokawa, D. T., & Bragg, D. T. (1991). Theory-based diagnosis and remediation of writing disabilities. *Journal of School Psychology, 29,* 57–79.

Bernstein, J. H. (2000). Developmental neuropsychological assessment. In K. O. Yeates, M. D. Ris, & H. G. Taylor (Eds.), *Pediatric neuropsychology: Research, theory, and practice* (pp. 405–438). New York: Guilford Press.

Bever, T. G., & Chiarello, R. J. (1974). Cerebral dominance in musicians and nonmusicians. *Science, 185,* 537–539.

Biederman, J., Faraone, S., Mick, E., Wozniak, J., Chen, L., Ouellette, C., et al. (1996). Attention-deficit hyperactivity disorder and juvenile mania: An overlooked comorbidity? *Journal of the American Academy of Child and Adolescent Psychiatry, 35,* 997–1008.

Biederman, J., Mick, E., Faraone, S. V., Spencer, T., Wilens, T. E., & Wozniak, J. (2000). Pediatric mania: A developmental subtype of bipolar disorder? *Biological Psychiatry, 48,* 458–466.

Biederman, J., Newcorn, J., & Sprich, S. (1991). Comorbidity of attention deficit hyperactivity disorder with conduct, depression, anxiety, and other disorders. *American Journal of Psychiatry, 148,* 564–577.

Binder, J. R., Frost, J. A., Hammeke, T. A., Cox, R. W., Rao, S. M., & Prieto, T. (1997). Human brain language areas identified by functional magnetic resonance imaging. *Journal of Neuroscience, 17,* 353–362.

Binet, A., & Simon, T. (1905). Methodes nouvelles pour le diagnostic du niveau intellectuel anormaux. *L'Année Psychologique, 11*, 191–244.

Bjorklund, D. F., & Green, B. L. (1992). The adaptive nature of cognitive immaturity. *American Psychologist, 47*, 46–54.

Blanca, M. J., Zalabardo, C., Garcia-Criado, F., & Siles, R. (1994). Hemispheric differences in global and local processing dependent on exposure duration. *Neuropsychologia, 32*, 1343–1351.

Bley, N. S., & Thornton, C. A. (1995). *Teaching mathematics to students with learning disabilities* (3rd ed.). Austin, TX: PRO-ED.

Boetsch, E. A., Green, P. A., & Pennington, B. F. (1996). Psychosocial correlates of dyslexia across the life span. *Development and Psychopathology, 8*, 539–562.

Boll, T. J. (1993). *Children's Category Test.* San Antonio, TX: Psychological Corporation.

Bookheimer, S. Y., Zeffiro, T. A., Blaxton, T., Gaillard, W., & Theodore, W. (1995). Regional cerebral blood flow during object naming and word reading. *Human Brain Mapping, 3*, 93–106.

Bornstein, R. A. (1990). Neuropsychological test batteries in neuropsychological assessment. In A. A. Boulton & G. B. Baker (Eds.), *Neuropsychology* (pp. 281–310). Totowa, NJ: Humana Press.

Bornstein, R. A., Miller, H. B., & van Schoor, J. T. (1989). Neuropsychological deficit and emotional disturbance in brain-injured patients. *Journal of Neurosurgery, 70*, 509–513.

Borod, J. C., Cicero, B. A., Obler, L. K., Welkowitz, J., Erhan, H. M., Santschi, C., et al. (1998). Right hemisphere emotional perception: Evidence across multiple channels. *Neuropsychology, 12*, 446–458.

Bos, C. S., & Van Reusen, A. K. (1991). Academic interventions with learning-disabled students: A cognitive/metacognitive approach. In J. E. Obrzut & G. W. Hynd (Eds.), *Neuropsychological foundations of learning disabilities: A handbook of issues, methods, and practice* (pp. 659–683). Orlando, FL: Academic Press.

Bos, C. S., & Vaughn, S. (1998). *Strategies for teaching students with learning and behavior problems* (4th ed.). Needham Heights, MA: Allyn & Bacon.

Bottini, G., Corcoran, R., Sterzi, R., Paulesu, E., Schenone, P., Scarpa, P., et al. (1994). The role of the right hemisphere in the interpretation of figurative aspects of language: A positron emission tomography activation study. *Brain, 117*, 1241–1253.

Bowden, E. M., & Beeman, M. J. (1998). Getting the right idea: Semantic activation in the right hemisphere may help solve insight problems. Psychological *Science, 9*, 435–440.

Bowers, P. G. (1993). Text reading and rereading: Predictors of fluency beyond word recognition. *Journal of Reading Behavior, 25*, 133–153.

Bowers, P. G. (2001). Exploration of the basis for rapid naming's relationship to reading. In M. Wolf (Ed.), *Dyslexia, fluency, and the brain* (pp. 41–64). Timonium, MD: York Press.

Bowman, D. B., Markham, P. M., & Roberts, R. D. (2001). Expanding the frontier of human cognitive abilities: So much more than (plain) g! *Learning and Individual Differences, 13*, 127–158.

Boyce, W. T., Quas, J., Alkon, A., Smider, N. A., Essek, M. J., & Kupfer, D. J. (2001). Autonomic reactivity and psychopathology in middle childhood. *British Journal of Psychiatry, 179*, 144–150

Bracken, B. A. (1988). Ten psychometric reasons why similar tests produce dissimilar results. *Journal of School Psychology, 26*, 155–166.

Braden, J. P., & Kratochwill, T. R. (1997). Treatment utility of assessment: Myths and realities. *School Psychology Review, 26*, 475–485.

Bramlett, R. K., Murphy, J. J., Johnson, J., Wallingsford, L., & Hall, J. D. (2002). Contemporary practices in school psychology: A national survey of roles and referral problems. *Psychology in the Schools, 39*(3), 327–335.

Branch, W. B., Cohen, M. J., & Hynd, G. W. (1995). Academic achievement and attention-deficit/hyperactivity disorder in children with left- or right-hemisphere dysfunction. *Journal of Learning Disabilities, 28*, 35–43.

Breznitz, Z. (1997). Effects of accelerated reading rate on memory for text among dyslexic readers. *Journal of Educational Psychology, 89*, 289–297.

Breznitz, Z. (2001). The determinants of reading fluency: A comparison of syslexic and average readers. In M. Wolf (Ed.), *Dyslexia, fluency, and the brain* (pp. 245–276). Timonium, MD: York Press.

Brodmann, K. (1909). *Vergleichende lokalisationslehre der grosshirnrinde in ihren prinzipien dargestellt auf Grund des zellenbaues.* Leipzig: J. A. Barth.

Brody, N. (1997). Intelligence, schooling, and society. *American Psychologist, 52*, 1046–1050.

Browder, D. M., & Lalli, J. S. (1991). Review of research on sight word instruction. *Research in Developmental Disabilities, 12*, 203–228.

Bruck, M. (1987). The adult outcomes of children with learning disabilities. *Annals of Dyslexia, 37*, 252–263.

Brumback, R. A., & Weinberg, W. A. (1990). Pediatric behavioral neurology: An update on the neurologic aspects of depression, hyperactivity, and learning disabilities. *Pediatric Neurology, 8,* 677–703.

Bryan, K. L., & Hale, J. B. (2001). Differential effects of left and right hemisphere accidents on language competency. *Journal of the International Neuropsychological Society, 7,* 655–664.

Bryan, T. (1991). Social problems and learning disabilities. In B. Wong (Ed.), *Learning about learning disabilities* (pp. 190–231). San Diego, CA: Academic Press.

Bryden, M. P. (1988). Does laterality make any difference?: Thoughts on the relation between cerebral asymmetry and reading. In D. L. Molfese & S. J. Segalowitz (Eds.), *Brain lateralization in children: Developmental implications* (pp. 509–525). New York: Guilford Press.

Buckholdt, J. A. (2001). A short history of g: Psychometrics' most enduring and controversial construct. *Learning and Individual Differences, 13,* 101–114.

Bullock, J., & Walentas, N. (1989). *Touch Math instruction manual.* Colorado Springs, CO: Innovative Learning Concepts.

Burbaud, P., Degreze, P., Lafon, P., Franconi, J. M., Bouligand, B., Bioulac, et al. (1995). Lateralization of prefrontal activation during internal mental calculation: A functional magnetic resonance imaging study. *Journal of Neurophysiology, 74,* 2194–2200.

Butterworth, B. (1999). *The mathematical brain.* London: Macmillan.

Byrnes, J. P. (2001). *Minds, brains, and learning: Understanding the psychological and educational relevance of neuroscientific research.* New York: Guilford Press.

Cameron, A., Cubelli, R., & Della Sala, S. (2002). Letter assembling and handwriting share a common allographic code. *Journal of Neurolinguistics, 15,* 91–97.

Canli, T., Zhao, Z., Desmond, J. E., Kang, E., Gross, J., & Gabrieli, J. D. E. (2001). An fMRI study of personality influences on brain reactivity to emotional stimuli. *Behavioral Neuroscience, 115,* 33–42.

Caplan, D., Hildebrandt, N., & Makris, N. (1996). Location of lesions in stroke patients with deficits in syntactic processing in sentence comprehension. *Brain, 119,* 933–949.

Capote, H. A., Flaherty, L., & Lichter, D. G. (2001). Addictions and frontal-subcortical circuits. In D. G. Lichter, & J. L. Cummings (Eds.), *Frontal–subcortical circuits in psychiatric and neurological disorders* (pp. 231–259). New York: Guilford Press.

Caramazza, A., Miceli, G., Villa, G., & Romani, C. (1987). The role of the graphemic buffer in spelling: Evidence from acquired dysgraphia. *Cognition, 26,* 59–85.

Cardebat, D., Demonet, J. F., Viallard, G., Faure, S., Puel, M., & Celsis, P. (1996). Brain functional profiles in formal and semantic fluency tasks: A SPECT study in normals. *Brain and Language, 52,* 305–313.

Carlisle, J. F. (1987). The use of morphological knowledge in spelling derived forms by learning-disabled and normal students. *Annals of Dyslexia, 37,* 90–108.

Carnine, D., & Kinder, D. (1985). Teaching low-performing students to apply generative and schema strategies to narrative and expository material. *Remedial and Special Education, 6,* 20–29.

Carnine, D., Silbert, J., & Kame'enui, E. J. (1997). *Direct instruction reading.* Upper Saddle River, NJ: Prentice-Hall.

Carroll, J. B. (1993). *Human cognitive abilities: A survey of factor-analytic studies.* New York: Cambridge University Press.

Carroll, J. B. (1995). On methodology in the study of cognitive abilities. *Multivariate Behavioral Research, 30*(3), 429–452.

Carrow-Woolfolk, E. (1996). *Oral and Written Language Scales.* Circle Pines, MN: American Guidance Service.

Carrow-Woolfolk, E. (1999). *Comprehensive Assessment of Spoken Language.* Circle Pines, MN: American Guidance Service.

Casey, B. J., Trainor, R., Giedd, J., Vauss, J., Vaituzis, C. K., Hamburger, S., et al. (1997). The role of the anterior cingulate gyrus in automatic and controlled processes: A developmental neuroanatomical study. *Developmental Psychobiology, 30,* 61–69.

Castellanos, F. X., Giedd, J. N., Eckberg, P., Marsh, W. L., Vaituzis, A. C., Kaysen, D., et al. (1994). Quantitative morphology of the caudate nucleus in attention deficit hyperactivity disorder. *American Journal of Psychiatry, 151,* 1791–1796.

Castellanos, F. X., Giedd, J. N., Marsh, W. L., Hamburger, S. D., Vaituzis, A. C., Dickstein, D. P., et al. (1996). Quantitative brain magnetic resonance imaging in attention-deficit hyperactivity disorder. *Archives of General Psychiatry, 53,* 607–616.

Castles, A., & Coltheart, M. (1993). Varieties of developmental dyslexia. *Cognition, 47,* 149–180.

Cawley, J. F., Goodstein, H. A. Fitzmaurice, A. M., Lepore A., Sedlak, R., & Althaus, V. (1976). *Project MATH*. Tulsa, OK: Educational Development.

Cawley, J. F., & Miller, J. H. (1989). Cross-sectional comparisons of the mathematical performance of children with learning disabilities: Are we on the right track toward comprehensive programming? *Journal of Learning Disabilities, 22,* 250–254.

Cestnick, L. (2001). Cross-modality temporal processing deficits in developmental phonological dyslexics. *Brain and Cognition, 46,* 319–325.

Chafouleas, S. M., Riley-Tillman, T. C., & McGrath, M. C. (2002). *Making successful intervention decisions through testing intervention packages: A manual for conducting brief experimental analysis (BEA)*. Unpublished technical manual, University of Connecticut.

Chan, L. K. S., & Cole, P. G. (1986). The effects of comprehension monitoring training on the reading competence of learning disabled and regular class students. *Remedial and Special Education, 7,* 33–40.

Chan, L. K. S., Cole, P. G., & Barfett, S. (1987). Comprehension monitoring: Detection and identification of text inconsistencies by LD and normal students. *Learning Disability Quarterly, 10,* 114–124.

Chapman, S. G., Culhane, K. A., Levin, H. S., Harwood, H., Mendelsohn, F., Ewing-Cobbs, L., et al. (1992). Narrative discourse after closed head injury in children and adolescents. *Brain and Language, 43,* 42–65.

Chase, C. (1996). A visual deficit model of developmental dyslexia. In C. Chase, G. Rosen, & G. Sherman (Eds.), *Developmental dyslexia: Neural, cognitive, and genetic mechanisms*. Baltimore: York Press.

Cherney, L. R., & Canter, G. J. (1993). Informational content in the discourse of patients with probable Alzheimer's disease and patients with right brain damage. In M. L. Lemme (Ed.), *Clinical aphasiology* (pp. 123–134). Austin, TX: PRO-ED.

Chhabildas, N., Pennington, B. F., & Willcutt, E. G. (2001). A comparison of the neuropsychological profiles of the DSM-IV subtypes of ADHD. *Journal of Abnormal Child Psychology, 29,* 529–540.

Chiarello, C. (1998). On codes of meaning and the meaning of codes: Semantic assess and retrieval within and between hemispheres. In M. Beeman & C. Chiarello (Eds.), *Right hemisphere language comprehension: Perspectives from cognitive neuroscience* (pp. 141–160). Mahwah, NJ: Erlbaum.

Chiron, C., Jambaque, I., Nabbout, R., Lounes, R., Syrota, A., & Dulac, O. (1997). The right brain hemisphere is dominant in human infants. *Brain, 120,* 1057–1065.

Chochon, F., Cohen, L., van de Moortele, P. F., & Dehaene, S. (1999). Differential contributions of the left and right inferior parietal lobules to number processing. *Journal of Cognitive Neuroscience, 11,* 617–630.

Cipolotti, L., & Warrington, E. K. (1996). Does recognizing orally spelled words depend on reading?: An investigation into a case of better written than oral spelling. *Neuropsychologia, 34,* 427–440.

Clarizio, H. F. (1997). Conduct disorder: Developmental considerations. *Psychology in the Schools, 34,* 253–265.

Clark, F. L., Deshler, D. D., Schumaker, J. B., Alley, G. R., & Wagner, M. M. (1984). Visual imagery and self-questioning: Strategies to improve comprehension of written material. *Journal of Learning Disabilities, 17,* 145–149.

Clark, L., Iversen, S. D., & Goodwin, G. M. (2002). Sustained attention deficit in bipolar disorder. *British Journal of Psychiatry, 180,* 313–319.

Cleaver, R. L., & Whitman, R. D. (1998). Right hemisphere, white-matter learning disabilities associated with depression in an adolescent and young adult psychiatric population. *Journal of Nervous and Mental Disease, 186,* 561–565.

Clements, S. (1966). *Minimal brain dysfunction in children: Terminology and identification*. Washington, DC: U.S. Department of Health, Education and Welfare.

Cody, H., Pelphrey, K., & Piven, J. (2002). Structural and functional magnetic resonance imaging of autism. *International Journal of Developmental Neuroscience, 20,* 421–438.

Cohen, J. D., Botvinick, M., & Carter, C. S. (2000). Anterior cingulate and prefrontal cortex: Who's in control? *Nature Neuroscience, 3,* 421–424.

Cohen, L., Dehaene, S., Chochon, F., Lehericy, S., & Naccache, L. (2000). Language and calculation within the parietal lobe: A combined congnitive, anatomical and fMRI study. *Neuropsychologia, 38,* 1426–1440.

Cohen, M. (1997). *Children's Memory Scale*. San Antonio, TX: Psychological Corporation.

Cohen, N. J., Barwick, M. A., Horodezky, N. B., Vallance, D. D., & Im, N. (1998). Language, achievement, and cognitive processing in psychiatrically disturbed children with previously identified and unsuspected language impairments. *Journal of Child Psychology and Psychiatry, 39,* 865–877.

Cohen, N. J., Menna, R., Vallance, D. D., Barwick, M. A., Im, N., & Horodezky, N. B. (1998). Language, social cognitive processing, and behavioral characteristics of psychiatrically disturbed children with previously identified and unsuspected langauge impairments. *Journal of Child Psychology and Psychiatry, 39,* 853–864.

Cole, K. N., Dale, P. S., Mills, P. E., & Jenkins, J. R. (1993). Interaction between early intervention curricula and student characteristics. *Exceptional Children, 60,* 17–28.

Cole, P. M., Usher, B. A., & Cargo, A. P. (1993). Cognitive risk and its association with risk for disruptive behavior disorder in preschoolers. *Journal of Clinical Child Psychology, 22,* 154–164.

Collette, F., Salmon, E., Van der Linden, M., Chicherio, C., Belleville, S., Degueldre, C., et al. (1999). Regional brain activity during tasks devoted to the central executive of working memory. *Cognitive Brain Research, 7,* 411–417.

Coltheart, M. (2000). Deep dyslexia is right-hemisphere reading. *Brain and Language, 71,* 299–309.

Compton, D. L., Davis, C. J., DeFries, J. C., Gaycn, J., & Olson, R. K. (2001). Genetic and environmental influences on reading and RAN: An overview of results from the colorado twin study. In M. Wolf (Ed.), *Dyslexia, fluency, and the brain* (pp. 277–306). Timonium, MD: York Press.

Coney, J. (1998). Hemispheric priming in a reading task. *Brain and Language, 62,* 34–50.

Conners, C. K., & MHS Staff. (2000). *Conners Continuous Performance Test II.* Niagara Falls, NY: Multi-Health Systems.

Conway, A. R. A., & Engle, R. W. (1994). Working memory and retrieval: A resource-dependent inhibition model. *Journal of Experimental Psychology: General, 123,* 354–373.

Cooke, A., Zurif, E. B., Devita, C., Alsop, D., Koenig, P., Detre, J., et al. (2001). Neural basis for sentence comprehension: Grammatical and short-term memory components. *Human Brain Mapping, 15,* 80–94.

Corballis, M. C. (1996). Hemispheric interactions in temporal judgments about spatially separated stimuli. *Neuropsychology, 10,* 42–50.

Cornelissen, P. L., Hansen, P. C., Hutton, J. L., Evangelinou, V., & Stein, J. F. (1997). Magnocellular visual function and children's single word reading. *Vision Research, 38,* 471–482.

Costello, E. J., Angold, A., Burns, B. J., Stangl, D. K., Tweed, D. L., Erkanli, A., et al. (1996). The Great Smoky Mountains Study of Youth: Goals, design, methods, and the prevalence of DSM-III-R disorders. *Archives of General Psychiatry, 53,* 1129–1136.

Courchesne, E. (1995). New evidence of cerebellar and brainstem hypoplasia in autistic infants, children, and adolescents: The MRI imaging study by Hashimoto and colleagues. *Journal of Autism and Developmental Disorders, 25,* 19–22.

Cowell, S. F., Egan, G. F., Code, C., Harasty, J., & Watson, J. D. (2000). The functional neuroanatomy of simple calculation and number repetition: A parametric PET activation study. *Neuroimage, 12,* 565–573.

Crary, M. A., & Heilman, K. M. (1988). Letter imagery deficits in a case of pure apraxic agraphia. *Brain and Language, 34,* 147–156.

Crossman, D. L., & Polich, J. (1988). Hemispheric differences for orthographic and phonological processing. *Brain and Language, 35,* 301–312.

Cunningham, A. E., & Stanovich, K. E. (1998). Assessing print exposure and orthographic processing skill in children: A quick measure of reading experience. *Journal of Educational Psychology, 82,* 733–740.

Cunningham, J. W. (1979). An automatic pilot for decoding. *Reading Teacher, 32,* 420–424.

Czarnecki, E., Rosko, D., & Pine, E. (1998). How to call up notetaking skills. *Teaching Exceptional Children, 30,* 14–19.

Dalla Barba, G., Pariato, V., Jobert, A., Samson, Y., & Pappata, S. (1998). Cortical networks implicated in semantic and episodic memory: Common or unique? *Cortex, 34,* 547–561.

Damasio, H., Grabowski, T. J., Tranel, D., Hichwa, R. D., & Damasio, A. R. (1996). The neural basis of lexical retrieval. *Nature, 380,* 499–505.

D'Amato, R. C., Rothlisberg, B. A., & Rhodes, R. L. (1997). Utilizing a neuropsychological paradigm for understanding common educational and psychological tests. In C. R. Reynolds & E. Fletcher-Janzen (Eds.), *Handbook of clinical child neuropsychology* (pp. 270–295). New York: Plenum Press.

Daniele, A., Giustolisi, L., Silveri, M. C., Colosimo, C., & Gainotti, G. (1994). Evidence for a possible neuroanatomical basis for lexical processing of nouns and verbs. *Neuropsychologia, 32,* 1325–1341.

Das, J. P., Carlson, J., Davidson, M. B., & Longe, K. (1997). *PREP: PASS remedial program.* Seattle, WA: Hogrefe.

Das, J. P., Naglieri, J. A., & Kirby, J. R. (1994). *Assessment of cognitive processes: The PASS theory of intelligence.* Needham Heights, MA: Allyn & Bacon.

Das, J. P., & Varnhagen, C. K. (1986). Neuropsychological functioning and cognitive processing. In J. E. Obrzut & G. W. Hynd (Eds.), *Child neuropsychology: Vol. 1. Theory and research* (pp. 117–140). Orlando, FL: Academic Press.

Daselaar, S. M., Veltman, D. J., Rombouts, S. A.., Raaijmakers, R. B., & Jeroen, G. W. (2002). Medial temporal lobe activity during semantic classification using a flexible fMRI design. *Behavioral Brain Research, 136,* 399–404.

Davidson, R. J. (1995). Cerebral asymmetry, emotion, and affective style. In R. J. Davidson & K. Hugdahl (Eds.), *Brain asymmetry* (pp. 361–387). Cambridge, MA: MIT Press.

Davidson, R. J. (1998). Affective style and affective disorders: Perspectives from affective neuroscience. *Cognition and Emotion, 12,* 307–330.

Davidson, R. J. (2000). Affective style, psychopathology, and resilience: Brain mechanisms and plasticity. *American Psychologist, 55,* 1196–1214.

Davidson, R. J., & Fox, N. A. (1988). Frontal brain asymmetry predicts infants' response to maternal separation. *Journal of Abnormal Psychology, 98,* 127–131.

Davies, P. L., & Rose, J. D. (1999). Assessment of cognitive development in adolescents by means of neuropsychological tasks. *Developmental Neuropsychology, 15,* 227–248.

Davis, J. T., Parr, G., & Lan, W. (1997). Differences between learning disability subtypes classified using the revised Woodcock–Johnson Psychoeducational Battery. *Journal of Learning Disabilities, 30,* 346–352.

Day, R., & Wong, S. (1996). Anomalous perceptual asymmetries for negative emotional stimuli in the psychopath. *Journal of Abnormal Psychology, 105,* 648–652.

Dean, R. S. (1986). Neuropsychological aspects of psychiatric disorders. In J. E. Obrzut & G. W. Hynd (Eds.), *Child neuropsychology: Vol. 2. Clinical practice* (pp. 83–112). Orlando, FL: Academic Press.

Decker, S. L., McIntosh, D. E., Kelly, A. M., Nicholls, S. K., & Dean, R. S. (2001). Comorbidity among individuals classified with attention disorders. *International Journal of Neuroscience, 110,* 43–54.

Dehaene, S., & Cohen, L. (1995). Towards an anatomical and functional model of numerical processing. *Mathematical Cognition, 1,* 83–120.

Dehaene, S., & Cohen, L. (1997). Cerebral pathways for calculation: Double dissociation between rote verbal and quatitative knowledge of arithmetic. *Cortex, 33,* 219–250.

Dehaene, S., Naccache, L., Cohen, L., Bihan, D. L., Mangin, J. F., Poline, J. B., et al. (2001). Cerebral mechanisms of word masking and unconscious repetition priming. *Nature Neuroscience, 4,* 678–680.

Dehaene, S., Spelke, E., Pinel, P., Stanescu, R., & Tsivkin, S. (1999). Sources of mathematical thinking: Behavioral and brain-imaging evidence. *Science, 284,* 970–974.

Dehaene, S., Tzourio, N., Frak, V., Raynaud, L., Cohen, L., Mehler, J., et al. (1996). Cerebral activations during number multiplication and comparison: A PET study. *Neuropsychologica, 34,* 1097–1106.

Deiber, M. P., Honda, M., Ibanez, V., Sadato, N., & Hallett, M. (1999). Mesial motor areas in self-initiated versus externally triggered movements examined with fMRI: Effect of movement type and rate. *Journal of Neurophysiology, 81,* 3065–3077.

de la Paz, S. (1997). Strategy instruction in planning: Teaching students with learning and writing disabilities to compose persuasive and expository essays. *Learning Disability Quarterly, 20,* 227–248.

Delazer, M., Girelli, L., Semenza, C., & Denes, G. (1999). Numerical skills and aphasia. *Journal of the International Neuropsychological Society, 5,* 213–221.

Delis, D. C., Kaplan, E., & Kramer, J. H. (2001). *Delis–Kaplan Executive Function System.* San Antonio, TX: Psychological Corporation.

Delis, D. C., Kramer, J. H., Kaplan, E., & Ober, B. A. (1994). *CVLT-C: California Verbal Learning Test—Children's Version.* San Antonio, TX: Psychological Corporation.

Delis, D. C., Robertson, L., & Efron, R. (1986). Hemispheric specialization of memory for visual hierarchical stimuli. *Neuropsychologia, 24,* 205–214.

Demb, J. B., Boynton, G. M., & Heeger, D. J. (1998). Functional magnetic resonance imaging of early visual pathways in dyslexia. *Journal of Neuroscience, 18,* 6939–3951.

Demb, J. B., Desmond, J. E., Wagner, A. D., Vaidya, C. J., Glover, G. H., & Gabrielli, J. D. E. (1995). Semantic encoding and retrieval in the left inferior prefrontal cortex: A functional MRI study of task difficulty and process specificity. *Journal of Neuroscience, 15,* 5870–5878.

Demb, J. B., Poldrack, R. A., & Gabrieli, J. D. E. (1999). Functional neuroimaging of word processing in normal and dyslexic readers. In R. M. Klein & P. A. McMullen (Eds.), *Converging methods for understanding reading and dyslexia: Language, speech, and communication* (pp. 245–304). Cambridge, MA: MIT Press.

Denckla, M. B. (1996). Biological correlates of learning and attention: What is relevant to learning disability and attention-deficit hyperactivity disorder? *Journal of Developmental and Behavioral Pediatrics, 17,* 114–119.

Denckla, M. B., & Cutting, L. E. (1999). History and significance of rapid automatized naming. *Annals of Dyslexia, 49,* 29–42.

Dennis, M. (2000). Childhood medical disorders and cognitive impairment: Biological risk, time, development, and reserve. In K. O. Yeates, M. D. Ris, & H. G. Taylor (Eds.), *Pediatric neuropsychology: Research, theory, and practice* (pp. 3–24). New York: Guilford Press.

Deno, S. L. (1990). Individual differences and individual difference: The essential difference of special education. *Journal of Special Education, 24,* 160–173.

D'Esposito, M., Aquirre, G. K., Zarahn, E., Ballard, D., Shin, R. K., & Lease, J. (1998). Functional MRI studies of spatial and nonspatial working memory. *Cognitive Brain Research, 7,* 1–13.

Dewey, D., & Kaplan, B. J. (1994). Subtyping of developmental motor deficits. *Developmental Neuropsychology, 10,* 265–284.

DiSimoni, F. (1978). *Token Test for Children.* Hingham, MA: Teaching Resources Corporation.

Dixon, R. C. (1991). The application of sameness analysis to spelling. *Journal of Learning Disabilities, 24,* 285–291, 310.

Douglas, V. I. (1999). Cognitive control processes in attention-deficit/hyperactivity disorder. In H. C. Quay (Ed.), *Handbook of disruptive behavior disorders* (pp. 105–138). New York: Plenum Press.

Doyle, A. E., Biederman, J., Seidman, L. J., Weber, W., & Faraone, S. V. (2000). Diagnostic efficiency of neuropsychological test scores for discriminating boys with and without attention deficit-hyperactivity disorder. *Journal of Consulting and Clinical Psychology, 68,* 477–488.

Drevets, W. C., & Raichle, M. E. (1995). Positron emission tomographic imaging studies of human emotional disorders. In M. S. Gazzaniga (Ed.), *The cognitive neurosciences* (pp. 1153–1164). Cambridge, MA: MIT Press.

DuPaul, G. J., Barkley, R. A., & McMurray, M. B. (1994). Response of children with ADHD to methylphenidate: Interaction with internalizing symptoms. *Journal of the American Academy of Child and Adolescent Psychiatry, 33,* 894–903.

DuPaul, G. J., & Stoner, G. (1994). *ADHD in the schools: Assessment and intervention strategies.* New York: Guilford Press.

Dumont, R., Willis, J., & McBride, G. (2001). Yes, Virginia, there is a severe discrepancy clause, but is it too much ado about something? *The School Psychologist, 55*(1), 1, 4–13, 15.

Dumont, R., Willis, J., & Sattler, J. M. (2001). Differential ability scales. In J. M. Sattler (Ed.), *Assessment of children: Cognitive applications* (4th ed., pp. 506–545). San Diego, CA: Jerome M. Sattler.

Dunlap, W. P., & Brennan, A. H. (1979). Developing mental images of mathematical processes. *Learning Disability Quarterly, 2,* 89–96.

Dunn, L. M., & Dunn, L. M. (1997). *Peabody Picture Vocabulary Test—III.* Circle Pines, MN: American Guidance Service.

Eden, G. F., VanMeter, J. W., Rumsey, J. W., Maison, J., & Zeffiro, T. A. (1996). Functional MRI reveals differences in visual motion processing in individuals with dyslexia. *Nature, 382,* 66–69.

Eeds, M., & Cockrum, W. A. (1985). Teaching word meanings by expanding schemata vs. dictionary work vs. reading in context. *Journal of Reading, 28,* 492–97.

Ehlers, S., Nyden, A., Gillberg, C., Sandberg, A. D., Dahlgren, S. O., Hjelmquist, E., et al. (1997). Asperger syndrome, autism, and attention disorders: A comparative study of the cognitive profiles of 120 children. *Journal of Child Psychology and Psychiatry, 38,* 207–217.

Ehri, L. C., & Saltmarsh, J. (1995). Beginning readers outperform older disabled readers in learning to read words by sight. *Reading and Writing: An Interdisciplinary Journal, 7,* 295–326.

Eisele, J. A., Lust, B., & Aram, D. M. (1998). Presupposition and implication of truth: Linguistic deficits following early brain lesions. *Brain and Language, 61,* 376–394.

Elbert, J. C. (1993). Occurrence and pattern of impaired reading and written language in children with attention deficit disorders. *Annals of Dyslexia, 43,* 26–43.

Eliez, S., & Reiss, A. L. (2000). Annotation: MRI neuroimaging of childhood psychiatric disorders: A selective review. *Journal of Child Psychology and Psychiatry, 41,* 679–694.

Eliez, S., Rumsey, J. M., Giedd, J. N., Schmitt, J. E., Patwardhan, A. J., & Reiss, A. L. (2000). Morphological alteration of temporal lobe gray matter in dyslexia: An MRI study. *Journal of Child Psychology and Psychiatry, 41,* 637–644.

Elliott, C. D. (1990). *Differential Ability Scales: Administration and scoring manual.* San Antonio, TX: Psychological Corporation.

Elliott, R., Rees, G., & Dolan, R. J. (1999). Ventromedial prefrontal cortex mediates guessing. *Neuropsychologia, 37,* 403–411.

Ellis, H. D., Ellis, D. M., Fraser, W., & Deb, S. (1994). A preliminary study of right hemisphere cognitive deficits and impaired social judgments among young people with Asperger's syndrome. *European Child and Adolescent Psychiatry, 3,* 255–266.

Engelmann, S., & Carnine, D. (1981). *Corrective mathematics.* Chicago: Science Research Associates.

Engelmann, S., Carnine, D., & Steely, D. G. (1991). Making connections in mathematics. *Journal of Learning Disabilities, 24,* 292–303.

Engelmann, S., Hanner, S., & Johnson, G. (1999). Corrective reading. DeSoto, TX: Science Research Associates.

Englert, C. S. (1990). Unraveling the mysteries of writing through strategy instruction. In T. E. Scruggs & B. Y. L. Wong (Eds.), *Intervention research in learning disabilities* (pp. 186–223). New York: Springer-Verlag.

Englert, C. S. (1992). Writing instruction from a sociocultural perspective: The holistic, dialogic, and social enterprise. *Journal of Learning Disabilities, 25,* 153–172.

Englert, C. S., & Mariage, T. V. (1991). Shared understandings: Structuring the writing experience through dialogue. *Journal of Learning Disabilities, 24,* 330–342.

Englert, C. S., Raphael, T. E., Fear, K. L., & Anderson, L. M. (1988). Students' metacognitive knowledge about how to write informational texts. *Learning Disability Quarterly, 11,* 18–46.

Enns, R. A. (1998). Performance of incarcerated adolescents on the cognitive assessment system. *Developmental Disabilities Bulletin, 26,* 1–18.

Epstein, H. T. (2001). An outline of the role of brain in human cognitive development. *Brain and Cognition, 45,* 44–51.

Erchul, W. P., & Chewning, T. (1990). Behavioral consultation from a request-centered relational communication perspective. *School Psychology Quarterly, 5*(1), 1–20.

Erchul, W. P., & Martens, B. K. (2002). *School consultation: Conceptual and empirical bases of practice* (2nd ed.). New York: Kluwer Academic/Plenum Press.

Erchul, W. P., Raven, B. H., & Whichard, S. M. (2001). School psychologist and teacher perceptions of social power in consultation. *Journal of School Psychology, 39*(6), 483–497.

Ernst, M., Liebenauer, L. L., King, A. C., Fitzgerald, G. A., Cohen, R. M., & Zametkin, A. J. (1994). Reduced brain metabolism in hyperactive girls. *Journal of the American Academy of Child and Adolescent Psychiatry, 33,* 858–868.

Evans, M. A., Shedden, J. M., Hevenor, S. J., & Hahn, M. C. (2000). The effect of variability of unattended information on global and local processing: Evidence for lateralization at early stages of processing. *Neuropsychologia, 38,* 225–239.

Eysenck, H. J. (1983). The social application of Pavlovian theories. *Pavlovian Journal of Biological Science, 18,* 117–125.

Fakouri, M. E. (1991). Learning disabilities: A Piagetian perspective. *Psychology in the Schools, 28,* 70–76.

Farah, M. J. (1990). *Visual agnosia: Disorders of object recognition and what they tell us about normal vision.* Cambridge, MA: MIT Press.

Farah, M. J. (1995). Current issues in the neuropsychology of image generation. *Neuropsychologia, 33,* 1455–1471.

Faraone, S. V., Biederman, J., Mennin, D., Wozniak, J., & Spencer, T. (1997). Attention-deficit hyperactivity disorder with bipolar disorder: A familial subtype? *Journal of the American Academy of Child and Adolescent Psychiatry, 36,* 1378–1387.

Faraone, S. V., Biederman, J., Weber, W., & Russell, R. L. (1998). Psychiatric, neuropsychological, and psychosocial features of DSM-IV subtypes of attention-deficit/hyperactivity disorder: Results from a clinically referred sample. *Journal of the American Academy of Child and Adolescent Psychiatry, 37,* 185–193.

Faust, M. (1998). Obtaining evidence of language comprehension from sentence priming. In M. Beeman & C. Chiarello (Eds.), *Right hemisphere language comprehension: Perspectives from cognitive neuroscience* (pp. 161–186). Mahwah, NJ: Erlbaum.

Fawcett, A. J., & Nicholson, R. I. (1995). Persistent deficits in motor skill of children with dyslexia. *Journal of Motor Behavior, 27,* 235–240.

Fawcett, A. J., & Nicholson, R. I. (2001). Speed and temporal processing in dyslexia. In M. Wolf (Ed.), *Dyslexia, fluency, and the brain* (pp. 277–306). Timonium, MD: York Press.

Fein, D., Humes, M., Kaplan, E., Lucci, D., & Waterhouse, L. (1984). The question of left hemisphere dysfunction in infantile autism. *Psychological Bulletin, 95,* 258–281.

Felton, R. (1993). Effects of instruction on the decoding skills of children with phonological-processing problems. *Journal of Learning Disabilities, 26,* 583–589.

Felton, R., & Brown, I. S. (1990). Phonological processes as predictors or specific reading skills in children at risk for reading failure. *Reading and Writing: An Interdisciplinary Journal, 2,* 39–59.

Fennell, E. B., & Bauer, R. M. (1997). Models of inference in evaluating brain–behavior relationships in children. In C. R. Reynolds & E. Fletcher-Janzen (Eds.), *Handbook of clinical child neuropsychology* (2nd ed., pp. 204–218). New York: Plenum Press.

Fernald, G. M. (1988). *Remedial techniques in basic school subjects.* Austin, TX: PRO-ED.

Fiez, J. A. (1997). Phonology, semantics, and the role of the left inferior prefrontal cortex. *Human Brain Mapping, 5,* 79–83.

Fiez, J. A., & Petersen, S. E. (1998). Neuroimaging studies of word reading. *Proceedings of the National Academy of Sciences USA, 95,* 914–921.

Fiez, J. A., & Raichle, M. E. (1997). Linguistic processing. *International Review of Neurobiology, 41,* 233–254.

Filipek, P. A. (1999). Neuroimaging in the developmental disorders: The state of the science. *Journal of Child Psychology and Psychiatry, 40,* 113–128.

Filipek, P. A., Semrud-Clikeman, M., Steingard, R. J., Renshaw, P. F., Kennedy, D. N., & Biederman, J. (1997). Volumetric MRI analysis comparing attention-deficit/hyperactivity disorder and normal controls. *Neurology, 48,* 589–601.

Fink, G. R., Marshall, J. C., Halligan, P. W., & Dolan, R. J. (1999). Hemispheric asymmetries in global/local processing are modulated by perceptual salience. *Neuropsychologia, 37,* 31–40.

Fiorello, C. A., Hale, J. B., McGrath, M., Ryan, K., & Quinn, S. (2001). IQ interpretation for children with flat and variable test profiles. *Learning and Individual Differences, 13.*

Fiorello, C. A., Liebman, R. B., & Levine-Dawson, S. (1999, April). *Inclusion: What works? What doesn't?* Paper presented at the annual meeting of the National Association of School Psychologists, Las Vegas, NV.

Fisher, G. L., Jenkins, S. J., Bancroft, M. J., & Kraft, L. M. (1988). The effects of K-ABC-based remedial teaching strategies on word recognition skills. *Journal of Learning Disabilities, 21,* 307–312.

Fisher, N. J., & DeLuca, J. W. (1997). Verbal learning strategies of adolescents and adults with the syndrome of nonverbal learning disabilities. *Child Neuropsychology, 3,* 192–198.

Fitzmaurice-Hayes, A. (1984). Curriculum and instructional activities: Grades 2 through 4. In J. F. Cawley (Ed.), *Developmental teaching of mathematics for the learning disabled.* Rockville, MD: Aspen.

Flanagan, D. P., & Ortiz, S. O. (2001). *Essentials of cross-battery assessment.* New York: Wiley.

Flanagan, D. P., Ortiz, S. O., Alfonso, V. C., & Mascolo, J. T. (2002). *The achievement test desk reference (ATDR): Comprehensive assessment and learning disabilities.* Boston: Allyn & Bacon.

Fleischner, J. E. (1994). Diagnosis and assessment of mathematics learning disabilities. In G. R. Lyon (Ed.), *Frames of references for the assessment of learning disabilities* (pp. 441–458). Baltimore: Brookes.

Fleischner, J. E., Nuzum, M. B., & Marzola, E. S. (1987). Devising an instructional program to teach arithmetic problem-solving skills to students with learning disabilities. *Journal of Learning Disabilities, 20,* 214–217.

Fletcher, J. M., Francis, D. J., Stuebing, K. K., Shaywitz, B. A., Shaywitz, S. E., Shankweiler, D. P., et al. (1996). Conceptual and methodological issues in construct definition. In G. R. Lyon & N. A. Krasnegor (Eds.), *Attention, memory, and executive function* (pp. 17–42). Baltimore: Brookes.

Fletcher, J. M., Levin, H. S., & Landry. S. H. (1984). Behavioral consequences of cerebral insult in infancy. In C. R. Almli & S. Finger (Eds.), *Early brain damage* (pp. 189–213). Orlando, FL: Academic Press.

Fletcher, J. M., & Taylor, H. G. (1984). Neurological assessment of children: A developmental approach. *Texas Psychologist, 36,* 14–20.

Fletcher, P. C., Happe, F., Frith, U., Baker, S. C., Dolan, R. J., Frackowiak, R. S. J., et al. (1995). Other minds in the brain: A functional imaging study of "theory of mind" in story comprehension. *Cognition, 57,* 109–128.

Fletcher, P. C., Shallice, T., & Dolan, R. J. (1998). The functional roles of prefrontal cortex in episodic memory: I. Encoding. *Brain, 121,* 1239–1248.

Fletcher, P. C., Shallice, T., Frith, C. D., Frackowiak, R. S. J., & Dolan, R. J. (1998). The functional roles of prefrontal cortex in episodic memory: II. Retrieval. *Brain, 121,* 1249–1256.

Fletcher, J. M., Shaywitz, S. E., Shankweiler, D. P., Katz, L., Liberman, I. Y., Stuebing, K. K., Fowler, A. E., & Shaywitz, B. A. (1994). Cognitive profiles of reading disability: Comparisons of discrepancy and low achievement definitions. *Journal of Educational Psychology, 86,* 6–23.

Flor-Henry, P. (1990). Neuropsychology and psychopathology: A progress report. *Neuropsychology Review, 1,* 103–123.

Flynn, J., Deering, W., Goldstein, M., & Rahbar, M. (1992). Electrophysiological correlates of dyslexic subtypes. *Journal of Learning Disabilities, 25,* 133–141.

Folk, M. C., & Campbell, J. (1978). Teaching functional reading to the TMR. *Education and Training of the Mentally Retarded, 13,* 322–326.

Foorman, B. R., Francis, D. J., Shaywitz, S. E., Shaywitz, B. A., & Fletcher, J. M. (1997). The case for early reading intervention. In B. A. Blachman (Ed.), *Foundations of reading acquisition and dyslexia: Implications for early intervention* (pp. 243–264). Mahwah, NJ: Erlbaum.

Francis, D. J., Fletcher, J. M., & Rourke, B. P. (1988). Discriminant validity of lateral sensorimotor measures in children. *Journal of Clinical and Experimental Neuropsychology, 10,* 779–799.

Francis, D. J., Shaywitz, S. E., Stuebing, K. K., Shaywitz, B. A., & Fletcher, J. M. (1994). The easurement of change: Assessing behavior over time and within a developmental context. In G. R. Lyon (Ed.), *Frames of reference for the assessment of learning disabilities* (pp. 29–58). Baltimore: Brookes.

Francis, D. J., Shaywitz, S. E., Stuebing, K. K., Shaywitz, B. A., & Fletcher, J. M. (1996). Developmental lag versus deficit models of reading disability: A longitudinal, individual growth curves analysis. *Journal of Educational Psychology, 88,* 3–17.

Friebel, A. C., & Gingrich, C. K. (1972). *Math Applications Kit.* Chicago: Science Research Associates.

Frith, U. (Ed.). (1991). *Autism and Asperger syndrome.* New York: Cambridge University Press.

Fry, E., Polk, J., & Fountoukidis, D. (1984). *The reading teacher's book of lists.* Englewood Cliffs, NJ: Prentice-Hall.

Fuchs, D., Fuchs, L. S., Mathes, P. G., & Simmons, D. C. (1997). Peer-assisted learning strategies: Making classrooms more responsive to diversity. *American Educational Research Journal, 34,* 174–206.

Fuchs, L. S., & Fuchs, D. (1986). Effects of systematic formative evaluation: A meta-analysis. *Exceptional Children, 53*(3), 199–208.

Fuerst, D. R., & Rourke, B. P. (1991). Validation of psychosocial subtypes of children with learning disabilities. In B. P. Rourke (Ed.), *Neuropsychological validation of learning disability subtypes* (pp. 160–179). New York: Guilford Press.

Fuerst, D. R., & Rourke, B. P. (1995). Psychosocial functioning of children with learning disabilities at three age levels. *Child Neuropsychology, 1,* 38–55.

Fulbright, R. K., Jenner, A. R., Mencl, W. E., Pugh, K. R., Shaywitz, B. A., Shaywitz, S. E., et al. (1999). The cerebellum's role in reading: a functional MR imaging study. *American Journal of Neuroradiology, 20,* 1925–1930.

Galaburda, A. M. (1985). Developmental dyslexia: A review of biological interactions. *Annals of Dyslexia, 35,* 21–33.

Galaburda, A. M., LeMay, M., Kemper, T. L., & Geschwind, N. (1978). Right–left asymmetries in the brain. *Science, 199,* 852–856.

Galaburda, A. M., & Livingstone, M. (1993). Evidence for a magnocellular defect in developmental dyslexia. *Annals of the New York Academy of Sciences, 682,* 70–82.

Galliard, W. D., Pugliese, M., Brandin, C. B., Braniecki, S. H., Kondapaneni, P., Hunter, K., et al. (2001). Cortical localization of reading in normal children. *Neurology, 57,* 47–54.

Gardner, H. (1983). *Frames of mind: The theory of multiple intelligences.* New York: Basic Books.

Gazzaniga, M. S., Ivry, R. B., & Mangun, G. R. (1998). *Cognitive neuroscience: The biology of the mind.* New York: Norton.

Geary, D. C. (1993). Mathematical disabilities: Cognitive, neuropsychological, and gentic components. *Psychological Bulletin, 114,* 345–352.

Geary, D. C., Hamson, C. O., & Hoard, M. K. (2000). Numerical and arithmetical cognition: A longitudinal study of process and concept deficits in children with learning disability. *Journal of Experimental Child Psychology, 77,* 236–263.

Geary, D. C., Hoard, M. K., & Hamson, C. O. (1999). Numerical and arithmetical cognition: Patterns of functions and deficits in children at risk for a mathematical disability. *Journal of Experimental Child Psychology, 74,* 213–239.

Gehring, W. J., & Knight, R. T. (2000). Prefrontal–cingulate interactions in action monitoring. *Nature Neuroscience, 3,* 516–520.

Geller, B., Williams, M., Zimerman, B., Frazier, J., Beringer, L., & Warner, K. L. (1998). Prepubertal and early adolescent bipolarity differentiate from ADHD by manic symptoms, grandiose delusions, ultra-rapid or ultradian cycling. *Journal of Affective Disorders, 51,* 81–91.

Gentry, J. R. (1982). An analysis of developmental spellings: Gnys at wrk. *The Reading Teacher, 36,* 192–200.

George, M. S., Ketter, T. T., & Post, R. M. (1994). Prefrontal cortex dysfunction in clinical depression. *Depression, 2,* 59–72.

Gershberg, F. B., & Shimamura, A. P. (1995). Impaired use of organizational strategies in free recall following frontal lobe damage. *Neuropsychologia, 13,* 1305–1333.

Geschwind, N. (1983). Biological associations of left-handedness. *Annals of Dyslexia, 33,* 29–40.

Geschwind, N., & Galaburda, A. M. (1987). *Cerebral lateralization: Biological mechanisms, associations, and pathology*. Cambridge, MA: MIT Press.

Ghaziuddin, M., Butler, E., Tsai, L., & Ghaziuddin, N. (1994). Is clumsiness a marker for Asperger syndrome? *Journal of Intellectual Disability Research, 38*, 519–527.

Ghaziuddin, M., & Gerstein, L. (1996). Pedantic speaking style differentiates Asperger syndrome from high-functioning autism. *Journal of Autism and Developmental Disorders, 26*, 585–595.

Giancola, P. R. (1995). Evidence for dorsolateral and orbital prefrontal cortical involvement in the expression of aggressive behavior. *Aggressive Behavior, 21*, 431–450.

Giedd, J. N., Castellanos, F. X., Casey, B. J., Kozuch, P., King, A. C., Hamburger, S. D., et al. (1994). Quantitative morphology of the corpus callosum in attention deficit hyperactivity disorder. *American Journal of Psychiatry, 151*, 665–669.

Gilchrist, A., Green, J., Cox, A., Burton, D., Rutter, M., & LeCouteur, A. (2001). Development and current functioning in adolescents with Asperger syndrome: A comparative study. *Journal of Child Psychology and Psychiatry, 42*, 227–240.

Ginsburg, H. P. (1987). How to assess number facts, calculation, and understanding. In D. D. Hammill (Ed.), *Assessing the abilities and instructional needs of students* (pp. 483–503). Austin, TX: PRO-ED.

Gioia, G. A., Isquith, P. K., Guy, S. C., & Kenworthy, L. (2000). *Behavior Rating Inventory of Executive Function*. Odessa, FL: Psychological Assessment Resources.

Glass, E. W., & Glass, G. G. (1978). *Glass analysis for decoding only*. New York: Easier to Learn.

Glosser, G. (1993). Discourse production patterns in neurologically impaired and aged populations. In H. H. Brownell & Y. Joanette (Eds.), *Narrative discourse in neurologically impaired and normal aging populations* (pp. 191–212). San Diego, CA: Singular.

Glossner, G., & Koppell, S. (1987). Emotional–behavioral patterns in children with learning disabilities: Lateralized hemispheric differences. *Journal of Learning Disabilities, 20*, 365–368.

Glutting, J. J., Youngstrom, E. A., Ward, T., Ward, S., & Hale, R. L. (1997). Incremental efficacy of WISC-III factor scores in predicting achievement: What do they tell us? *Psychological Assessment, 9*, 295–301.

Gold, J. M., Berman, K. F., Randolph, T. E., Goldberg, T. E., & Weinberger, D. (1996). PET validation of a novel prefrontal task: Delayed response alternation. *Neuropsychology, 10*, 3–10.

Goldberg, A., Wolf, M., Cirino, P., Morris, R., & Lovett, M. (1998, July). *A test of the double-deficit hypothesis*. Paper presented at the annual meeting of the Society for the Scientific Study of Reading, San Diego, CA.

Goldberg, E. (2001). *The executive brain: Frontal lobes and the civilized mind*. New York: Oxford University Press.

Goldberg, E., & Costa, L. D. (1981). Hemispheric differences in the acquisition and use of descriptive systems. *Brain and Language, 14*, 144–173.

Goldberg, E., Harner, R., Lovell, M., Podell, K., & Riggio, S. (1994). Cognitive bias, functional cortical geometry, and the frontal lobes: Laterality, sex, and handedness. *Journal of Cognitive Neuroscience, 6*, 276–296.

Golden, C. J. (1997). The Nebraska Neuropsychological Children's Battery. In C. R. Reynolds & E. Fletcher-Janzen (Eds.), *Handbook of clinical child neuropsychology* (2nd ed., pp. 237–251). New York: Plenum Press.

Golden, C. J. (2002). *Stroop Color and Word Test*. Chicago: Stoelting.

Golden, C. J., Espe-Pfeifer, P., & Wachsler-Felder, J. (2000). *Neuropsychological interpretation of objective psychological tests*. New York: Kluwer Academic.

Golden, C. J., Freshwater, S. M., & Vayalakkara, J. (2000). The Luria Nebraska Neuropsychological Battery. In G. Groth-Marnat (Ed.), *Neuropsychological assessment in clinical practice: A guide to test interpretation and integration* (pp. 263–289). New York: Wiley.

Golden, C. J., Purisch, A., & Hammeke, T. (1985). *Manual for the Luria–Nebraska Neuropsychological Battery*. Los Angeles: Western Psychological Services.

Goldstein, S., & Mather, N. (2001). *Learning disabilities and challenging behaviors: A guide to intervention and classroom management*. Baltimore: Brookes.

Goldstein, S., & Reynolds, C. R. (Eds.). (1999). *Handbook of neurodevelopmental and genetic disorders in children*. New York: Guilford Press.

Good, R. H., III, Vollmer, M., Creek, R. J., Katz, L., & Chowdhri, S. (1993). Treatment utility of the Kaufman Assessment Battery for Children: Effects of matching instruction and student processing strength. *School Psychology Review, 22*, 8–26.

Goodglass, H., & Kaplan, E. (1987). *The assessment of aphasia and related disorders* (2nd ed.). Philadelphia: Lea & Febiger.

Goodyear, P., & Hynd, G. W. (1992). Attention-deficit disorder with (ADD/H) and without (ADD/WO) hyperactivity: Behavioral and neuropsychological differentiation. *Journal of Clinical Child Psychology, 21*, 273–305.

Gordon, C., & Braun, C. (1983). Using story schema as an aid to reading and writing. *Reading Teacher, 37,* 116–121.

Gordon, H. W., & Bogen, J. E. (1974). Hemispheric lateralization of singing after intracarotid sodium amylobarbitone. *Journal of Neurology, Neurosurgery and Psychiatry, 37,* 727–738.

Gordon, M. (1991). *The Gordon Diagnostic System.* Boulder, CO: Clinical Diagnostic Systems.

Gottfredson, L. S. (1997). Why g matters: The complexity of everyday life. *Intelligence, 24,* 79–132.

Gourovitch, M. L., Kirkby, B. S., Goldberg, T. E., Weinberger, D. R., Gold, J. M., Esposito, G., et al. (2000). A comparison of rCBF patterns during letter and semantic fluency. *Neuropsychology, 14,* 353–360.

Grabowski, A., & Nowicka, A. (1996). Visual–spatial–frequency model of cerebral asymmetry: A critical survey of behavioral and electrophysiological studies. *Psychological Bulletin, 120,* 434–449.

Graden, J. L., Zins, J. E., & Curtis, M. J. (Eds.). (1988). *Alternative educational delivery systems: Enhancing instructional options for all students.* Washington, DC: National Association of School Psychologists.

Grafman, J., Passafiume, D., Faglioni, P., & Boller, F. (1982). Calculation disturbances in adults with focal brain damage. *Cortex, 18,* 37–49.

Graham, S. (1992). Helping students with LD progress as writers. *Intervention in School and Clinic, 27,* 134–144.

Graham, S., & Freeman, S. (1986). Strategy training and teacher- vs. student-controlled study conditions: Effects on LD students' spelling performance. *Learning Disability Quarterly, 9,* 15–22.

Graham, S., & Harris, K. R. (1994). Implications of constructivism for teaching writing to students with special needs. *Journal of Special Education, 28,* 275–289.

Graham, S., Harris, K. R., & Loynachan. C. (1994). The spelling for writing list. *Journal of Learning Disabilities, 27,* 210–214.

Graham, S., Harris, K., MacArthur, C. A., & Schwartz, S. (1991). Writing and writing instruction for students with learning disabilities: Review of a research program. *Learning Disability Quarterly, 14,* 89–114.

Graham, S., & Voth, V. P. (1990). Spelling instruction: Making modifications for students with learning disabilities. *Academic Therapy, 25,* 447–457.

Grant, R. (1993). Strategic training for using text headings to improve students' processing of content. *Journal of Reading, 36,* 482–488.

Graves, A., & Hauge, R. (1993). Using cues and prompts to improve story writing. *Teaching Exceptional Children, 25,* 38–40.

Graves, D. H. (1994). *A fresh new look at writing.* Portsmouth, NH: Heinemann.

Gray, J. A. (1987). Perspectives on anxiety and impulsivity: A commentary. *Journal of Research in Personality, 21,* 493–509.

Green, D., Baird, G., Barnett, A. L., Henderson, L., Huber, J., & Henderson, S. E. (2002). The severity and nature of motor impairment in Asperger's syndrome: A comparison with specific developmental disorder of motor function. *Journal of Child Psychology and Psychiatry, 43,* 655–668.

Greene, G. (1994). The magic of mnemonics. *LD Forum, 19,* 34–37.

Greenhill, L. L., Abikoff, H. B., Arnold, L. E., Cantwell, D. P., Conners, C. K., Elliott, G., et al. (1996). Medication treatment strategies in the MTA study: Relevance to clinicians and researchers. *Journal of the American Academy of Child and Adolescent Psychiatry, 35,* 1304–1313.

Greenland, R., & Polloway, E. (1994). *Handwriting and students with disabilities: Overcoming first impressions.* (ERIC Document Reproduction Service No. ED378757)

Greenway, P., & Milne, L. (1999). Relationship between psychopathology, learning disabilities, or both and WISC-III subtest scatter in adolescents. *Psychology in the Schools, 36,* 103–108.

Greenwood, C. R., Carta, J. J., Kamps, D., Terry, B., & Delquadri, J. (1994). Development and validation of standard classroom observation systems for school practitioners: Ecobehavioral assessment systems software (EBASS). *Exceptional Children, 61*(2), 197–210.

Gregg, N. (1992). Expressive writing disorders. In S. R. Hooper, G. W. Hynd, & R. E. Mattison (Eds.), *Developmental disorders: Diagnostic criteria and clinical assessment* (pp. 127–172). Hillsdale, NJ: Erlbaum.

Grodzinsky, G. M., & Barkley, R. A. (1999). Predictive power of frontal lobe tests in the diagnosis of attention deficit hyperactivity disorder. *The Clinical Neuropsychologist, 13,* 12–21.

Gross-Tsur, V., Shalev, R. S., Manor, O., & Amir, N. (1995). Developmental right-hemisphere syndrome: Clinical spectrum of the nonverbal learning disability. *Journal of Learning Disabilities, 28,* 80–86.

Grossman, A. W., Churchill, J. D., McKinney, B. C., Kodish, I. M., Otte, S. L., & Greenough, W. T. (2003). Experience effects on brain development: Possible contributions to psychopathology. *Journal of Child Psychology and Psychiatry, 44,* 33–63.

Groth-Marnat, G. (2000a). Introduction to neuropsychological assessment. In G. Groth-Marnat (Ed.), *Neuropsy-*

chological assessment in clinical practice: A guide to test interpretation and integration (pp. 3–20). New York: Wiley.

Groth-Marnat, G. (Ed.). (2000b). *Neuropsychological assessment in clinical practice: A guide to test interpretation and integration*. New York: Wiley.

Groth-Marnat, G., Gallagher, R. E., Hale, J. B., & Kaplan, E. (2000). The Wechsler intelligence scales. In G. Groth-Marnat (Ed.), *Neuropsychological assessment in clinical practice: A guide to test interpretation and integration* (pp. 129–194). New York: Wiley.

Gruber, O., Indefrey, P., Steinmetz, H., & Kleinschmidt, A. (2001). Dissociating neural correlates of cognitive components in mental calculation. *Cerebral Cortex, 11*, 350–359.

Guilford, J. P. (1967). *The nature of human intelligence*. New York: McGraw-Hill.

Gurney, D., Gerstein, R., Dimino, J., & Carnine, D. (1990). Story grammar: Effective literature instruction for high school students with learning disabilities. *Journal of Learning Disabilities, 23*, 335–342.

Gutkin, T. B. (1999). Collaborative versus directive/prescriptive/expert school-based consultation: Reviewing and resolving a false dichotomy. *Journal of School Psychology, 37*(2), 161–190.

Hagborg, W. J., & Aiello-Coulter, M. (1994). The Developmental Test of Visual–Motor Integration—3R and teachers' ratings of written language. *Perceptual and Motor Skills, 79*, 371–374.

Hagin, R. A. (1997). Psychological problems that present as academic difficulties. *Child and Adolescent Psychiatric Clinics of North America, 6*, 473–488.

Hale, J. B., Bertin, M., & Brown, L. (2004). *Modeling frontal–subcortical circuits for ADHD subtype identification.* Unpublished manuscript.

Hale, J. B., & Fiorello, C. A. (2001). Beyond the academic rhetoric of *g*: Intelligence testing guidelines for practitioners. *The School Psychologist*, 113–139.

Hale, J. B., & Fiorello, C. A. (2002). Cross-battery cognitive assessment approaches to test interpretation: Are you a clumper or a splitter? *Communiqué, 31*(1), 37–40.

Hale, J. B., Fiorello, C. A., Bertin, M., & Sherman, R. (2003). Predicting math achievement through neuropsychological interpretation of WISC-III variance components. *Journal of Psychoeducational Assessment, 21*, 358–380.

Hale, J. B., Fiorello, C. A., Kavanagh, J. A., Hoeppner, J. B., & Gaither, R. A. (2001). WISC-III predictors of academic achievement for children with learning disabilities: Are global and factor scores comparable? *School Psychology Quarterly, 16*, 31–55.

Hale, J. B., Hoeppner, J. B., DeWitt, M. B., Coury, D. L., Ritacco, D. G., & Trommer, B. (1998). Evaluating medication response in ADHD: Cognitive, behavioral, and single-subject methodology. *Journal of Learning Disabilities, 31*, 595–607.

Hale, J. B., Hoeppner, J. B., & Fiorello, C. A. (2002). Analyzing Digit Span components for assessment of attention processes. *Journal of Psychoeducational Assessment, 20*, 128–143.

Hale, J. B., How, S. K., DeWitt, M. B., & Coury, D. L. (2001). Discriminant validity of the Conners scales for ADHD subtypes. *Current Psychology, 20*, 231–249.

Hale, J. B., & Kavanagh, J. A. (1991). Interagency cooperation in the schools: Multidisciplinary team member perceptions of participant input importance and level of cooperation. *Illinois School Research and Development, 27*, 132–142.

Hale, J. B., Mulick, J. A., & Rojahn, J. (1995, August). *The developmental progression of aberrant behavior in profound mental retardation.* Poster presented at the 103rd annual convention of the American Psychological Association, New York.

Hale, J. B., Naglieri, J., Kaufman, A. S., & Kavale, K. A. (2004). Specific learning disability classification in the new Individuals with Disabilities Education Act: The danger of good ideas. *The School Psychologist, 58*(1), 6–14.

Hale, J. B., Rosenberg, D., Hoeppner, J. B., & Gaither, R. (1997, April). *Cognitive predictors of behavior disorders in children with learning disabilities.* Paper presented at the annual convention of the National Association of School Psychologists, Anaheim, CA.

Hale, J. B., Willis, J., Dumont, R., Fiorello, C. A., & Rackley, C. (2004). *DAS subtest predictors of intellectual functioning.* Unpublished manuscript.

Hamann, S. B., Ely, T. D., Hoffman, J. M., & Kilts, C. D. (2002). Ecstasy and agony: Activation of human amygdala in positive and negative emotion. *Psychological Science, 13*, 135–141.

Happe, F. G. E., & Frith, U. (1996). Theory of mind and social impairment in children with conduct disorder. *British Journal of Developmental Psychology, 14*, 385–398.

Hari, R., Renvall, H., & Tanskanen, T. (2001). Left minineglect in dyslexic adults. *Brain, 124*, 1373–1380.

Harp, B. (1988). When the principal asks: "Why are your kids giving each other spelling tests?" *Reading Teacher,* *41,* 702–704.

Harris, K. R., & Graham, S. (1992). *Helping young writers master the craft: Strategy instruction and self-regulation in the writing process.* Cambridge, MA: Brookline Books.

Harris, K. R., & Graham, S. (1997). *Making the writing process work: Strategies for composition and self-regulation.* Cambridge, MA: Brookline.

Harris, M. J. (1991). Controversy and cumulation: Meta-analysis and research on interpersonal expectancy effects. *Personality and Social Psychology Bulletin, 17,* 316–322.

Harrison, P. L. (Ed.). (1996). 25th anniversary issue: Organizational change and school reform [Special issue]. *School Psychology Review, 25*(4).

Haslinger, B., Erhard, P., Weilke, F., Ceballos-Baumann, A. O., Bartenstein, P., Grafin von Einsiedel, H., et al. (2002). The role of lateral premoto–cerebellar–parietal circuits in moter sequence control: A parametric fMRI study. *Cognitive Brain Research, 13,* 159–168.

Hayes, A. M. F. (1985). Classroom implications. In J. F. Cawley (Ed.), *Cognitive strategies and mathematics for the learning disabled* (pp. 209–236). Rockville, MD: Aspen.

Heaton, R. K., Chellune, G. J., Talley, J. L., Kay, G. G., & Curtis, G. (1993). *Wisconsin Card Sorting Test (WCST) manual revised and expanded.* Odessa, FL: Psychological Assessment Resources.

Hecaen, H. (1976). Acquired aphasia in children and the ontogenesis of hemispheric functional specialization. *Brain and Language, 3,* 114–134.

Heckelman, R. G. (1986). N.I.M. revisited. *Academic Therapy, 21,* 411–420.

Heilman, K. M., Bowers, D., & Valenstein, E. (1993). Emotional disorders associated with neurological diseases. In K. M. Heilman & E. Valenstein (Eds.), *Clinical neuropsychology* (3rd ed., pp. 461–497). New York: Oxford University Press.

Heller, W. (1993). Neuropsychological mechanisms of individual differences in emotion, personality, and arousal. *Neuropsychology, 7,* 476–489.

Heller, W., Nitschke, J. B., & Miller, G. A. (1998). Lateralization in emotion and emotional disorders. *Current Directions in Psychological Science, 7,* 26–32.

Hellgren, L., Gillberg, C., & Gillberg, I. C. (1994). Children with deficits in attention, motor control and perception (DAMP) almost grown up: The contribution of various background factors to outcome at age 16 years. *European Child and Adolescent Psychiatry, 3,* 1–15.

Henson, R., Shallice, T., & Dolan, R. (2000). Neuroimaging evidence for dissociable forms of repetition priming. *Science, 287,* 1269–1272.

Herbster, A. N., Mintun, M. A, Nebes, R. D., & Becker, J. T. (1997). Regional cerebral blood flow during word and nonword reading. *Human Brain Mapping, 5,* 84–92.

Herrnstein, R. J., & Murray, C. (1994). *The bell curve: Intelligence and class structure in American life.* New York: Free Press.

Hertzig, M. E., & Shapiro, T. (1987). The assessment of nonfocal neurological signs in school-aged children. In D. E. Tupper (Ed.), *Soft neurological signs* (pp. 71–92). Orlando, FL: Grune & Stratton.

Heumann, J. E., & Hehir, I. (1994). *Intent/scope of LRE requirement.* 21 IDELR § 1152 (Office of Special Education Programs Memorandum No. 95-9).

Hickok, G., Bellugi, U., & Klima, E. S. (1996). The neurobiology of sign language and its implications for the neural basis of language. *Nature, 381,* 699–702.

Hiebert, J., & LeFevre, P. (1987). Conceptual and procedural knowledge in mathematics: An introductory analysis. In J. Hiebert (Ed.), *Conceptual and procedural knowledge in mathematics* (pp. 1–27). Hillsdale, NJ: Erlbaum.

Hillis, A. E., Kane, A., Tuffiash, E., Beauchamp, N. J., Barker, P. B., Jacobs, M. A., et al. (2002). Neural substrates of the cognitive processes underlying spelling: Evidence from MR diffusion and perfusion imaging. *Aphasiology, 16,* 425–438.

Hinojosa, J. A., Martin-Loeches, M., Munoz, F., Casado, P., Fernandez-Frias, C., & Pozo, M. A. (2001). Electrophysiolocial evidence of a semantic system commonly accessed by animals and tools categories. *Cognitive Brain Research, 12,* 321–328.

Hinshaw, S. P. (1992). Externalizing behavior problems and academic underachievement in childhood and adolescence: Causal relationships and underlying mechanisms. *Psychological Bulletin, 111,* 127–155.

Hitch, G. J., & McAuley, E. (1991). Working memory in children with specific mathematical learning disabilities. *British Journal of Psychology, 82,* 375–386.

Hittair-Delazer, M., Semenza, C., & Denes, G. (1994). Concepts and facts in calculation. *Brain, 117,* 715–728.

Hodges, J. R., & Marshall, J. C. (1992). Discrpant oral and written spelling after left hemisphere tumour. *Cortex, 28,* 643–656.

Hoeppner, J. B., Hale, J. B., Bradley, A., Byrns, M., Coury, D. L., & Trommer, B. L. (1997). A clinical protocol for determining methylphenidate dosage levels in ADHD. *Journal of Attention Disorders, 2,* 19–30.

Hooper, S. R., & Boyd, T. A. (1986). Neurodevelopmental learning disorders. In J. E. Obrzut & G. W. Hynd (Eds.), *Child neuropsychology: Vol. 2. Clinical practice* (pp. 15–58). Orlando, FL: Academic Press.

Hooper, S. R., Boyd, T. A., Hynd, G. W., & Rubin, J. (1993). Definitional issues and neurobiological foundations of selected severe neurodevelopmental disorders. *Archives of Clinical Neuropsychology, 8,* 279–307.

Hooper, S. R., Montgomery, J., Swartz, C., Reed, M. S., Sandler, A. D., Levine, M. D., et al. (1994). Measurement of written language expression. In G. R. Lyon (Ed.), *Frames of reference for the assessment of learning disabilities* (pp. 375–415). Baltimore: Brookes.

Hooper, S. R., & Tramontana, M. G. (1997). Advances in the neuropsychological bases of child and adolescent psychopathology: Proposed models, findings, and ongoing issues. In T. H. Ollendick & R. J. Prinz (Eds.), *Advances in clinical child psychology* (Vol. 19, pp. 133–175). New York: Plenum Press.

Horn, E. (1954). *Teaching spelling.* Washington, DC: American Educational Research Association.

Horn, J. L., & Cattell, R. B. (1967). Age differences in fluid and crystallized intelligence. *Acta Psychologica, 26,* 107–129.

Horwitz, B., Rumsey, J. M., & Donohue, B. C. (1998). Functional connectivity of the angular gyrus in normal reading and dyslexia. *Proceedings of the National Academy of Sciences USA, 95,* 8939–8944.

Horwitz, B., Rumsey, J. M., Grady, C. L., & Rapoport, S. I. (1988). The cerebral metabolic landscape in autism: Intercorrelations of regional glucose utilization. *Archives of Neurology, 45,* 749–755.

Hosp, J. L., & Reschly, D. J. (2002). Regional differences in school psychology practice. *School Psychology Review, 31,* 11–29.

Houck, C. K., & Billingsley, B. S. (1989). Written expression of students with and without learning disabilities: Differences across the grades. *Journal of Learning Disabilities, 22,* 561–572.

Hough, M. (1990). Narrative comprehension in adults with right and left hemisphere brain damage. *Brain and Language, 38,* 253–277.

Houghton, S., Douglas, G., West, J., Whiting, K., Wall, M., Langsford, S., et al. (1999). Differential patterns of executive function in children with attention-deficit/hyperactivity disorder according to gender and subtype. *Journal of Child Neurology, 14,* 801–805.

Howard, D., Patterson, K., Wise, R., Brown, W. D., Friston, K., Weiller, C., et al. (1992). The cortical localization of the lexicons. Positron emission tomography evidence. *Brain, 115,* 1769–1782.

Hughes, C., Russell, J., & Robbins, T. W. (1994). Evidence for executive dysfunction in autism. *Neuropsychologia, 32,* 477–492.

Hurt, J., & Naglieri, J. A. (1992). Performance of delinquent and nondelinquent males on planning, attention, simultaneous, and successive cognitive processing tasks. *Journal of Clinical Child Psychology, 48,* 120–128.

Hutchings, B. (1975). Low-stress subtraction. *The Arithmetic Teacher, 22,* 226–232.

Hutchings, B. (1976). *Low-stress algorithms.* Reston, VA: National Council of Teachers of Mathematics.

Hutchinson, N. L. (1993). Effects of cognitive strategy instruction on algebra problem solving of adolescents with learning disabilities. *Learning Disability Quarterly, 16,* 34–63.

Hux, K., Bond, V., Skinner, S., Belau, D., & Sanger, D. (1998). Parental report of occurrences and consequences of traumatic brain injury among delinquent and non-delinquent youth. *Brain Injury, 12,* 667–681.

Hynd, G. W., Hall, J., Novey, E. S., Eliopulos, D., Black, K., Gonzalez, J. J., et al. (1995). Dyslexia and corpus callosum morphology. *Archives of Neurology, 52,* 32–38.

Hynd, G. W., Hern, K. L., Novey, E. S., Eliopulos, D., Marshall, R., Gonzalez, J. J., et al. (1993). Attention-deficit hyperactivity disorder and asymmetry of the caudate nucleus. *Journal of Child Neurology, 8,* 339–347.

Hynd, G. W., Marshall, R. M., & Semrud-Clikeman, M. (1991). Developmental dyslexia, neurolinguistic theory, and deviations in brain morphology. *Reading and Writing: An Interdisciplinary Journal, 3,* 345–362.

Hynd, G. W., Semrud-Clikeman, M., Lorys, A., Novey, E. S., & Eliopulos, D. (1990). Brain morphology in developmental dyslexia and attention deficit disorder/hyperactivity. *Archives of Neurology, 47,* 919–926.

Idol, L., & Croll, V. J. (1987). Story-mapping training as a means of improving reading comprehension. *Learning Disability Quarterly, 10,* 214–229.

Idol-Maestas, L. (1985). Getting ready to read: Guided probing for poor comprehenders. *Learning Disability Quarterly, 8,* 243–254.

Individuals with Disabilities Education Act (IDEA). 20 U.S.C. § 1400 et seq. (1997).

Isaacs, E. B., Edmonds, C. J., Lucas, A., & Gadian, D. G. (2001). Calculation difficulties in children with very low birthweight. *Brain, 124,* 1701–1707.

Isaacson, S. (1988). Assessing the writing product: Qualitative and quantitative measures. *Exceptional Children, 54*(6), 528–534.

Isaacson, S. (1995). Written language. In P. J. Schloss, M. A. Smith, & C. N. Schloss, *Instructional methods for adolescents with learning and behavioral problems* (2nd ed., pp.200–224). Boston: Allyn & Bacon.

Iversen, S., & Tunmer, W. (1993). Phonological processing skills and the Reading Recovery program. *Journal of Educational Psychology, 85*, 112–126.

Ivry, R. B. (1993). Cerebellar involvement in the explicit representation of temporal information. *Annals of the New York Academy of Sciences, 682*, 214–230.

Ivry, R. B., Justus, T. C., & Middleton, C. (2001). The cerebellum, timing, and language: Implications for the study of dyslexia. In M. Wolf (Ed.), *Dyslexia, fluency, and the brain* (pp. 189–212). Timonium, MD: York Press.

Jackson, J. H. (1958). *Selected writings of John Hughlings Jackson*. New York: Basic Books.

Jenkins, I. H., Brooks, D. J., Nixon, P. D., Frackowiak, R. S. J., & Passingham, R. E. (1994). Motor sequence learning: A study with positron emission tomography. *Journal of Neuroscience, 14*, 3775–3790.

Jenkins, J. R., Heliotis, J. D., Stein, M. L., & Haynes, M. C. (1987). Improving reading comprehension by using paragraph restatements. *Exceptional Children, 54*, 54–59.

Jensen, A. R. (1998). *The g factor: The science of mental ability*. Westport, CT: Praeger.

Jensen, P. S., Martin, D., & Cantwell, D. P. (1997). Comorbidity in ADHD: Implications for research, practice, and DSM-V. *Journal of the American Academy of Child and Adolescent Psychiatry, 36*, 1065–1079.

Johansen, E. B., Aase, H., Meyer, A., & Sagvolden, T. (2002). Attention-deficit/hyperactivity disorder (ADHD) behaviour explained by dysfunctioning reinforcement and extinction processes. *Behavioral Brain Research, 130*, 37–45.

Johnson, D. D., & Pearson, P. D. (1984). *Teaching reading vocabulary*. New York: Holt, Rinehart & Winston.

Johnson, D. J. (1987). Disorders of written language. In D. J. Johnson & J. Blalock (Eds.), *Adults with learning disabilities: Clinical studies*. New York: Grune & Stratton.

Johnson, D. J., & Carlisle, J. F. (1996). A study of handwriting in written stories of normal and learning disabled children. *Reading and Writing, 8*, 45–59.

Johnson, D. J., & Myklebust, H. R. (1967). *Learning disabilities*. New York: Grune & Stratton.

Johnson, D. L., Wiebe, J. S., Gold, S. M., Andreasen, N. C., Hichwa, R. D., Watkins, L., et al. (1999). Cerebral blood flow and personality: A positron emission tomography study. *American Journal of Psychiatry, 156*, 252–257.

Johnson, M. H. (1999). Cortical plasticity: Implications for normal and abnormal cognitive development. *Development and Psychopathology, 11*, 419–437.

Jolliffe, T., & Baron-Cohen, S. (1999). The Strange Stories Test: A replication with high-functioning adults with autism or Asperger syndrome. *Journal of Autism and Developmental Disorders, 29*, 395–406.

Joseph, J., Noble, K., & Eden, G. (2001). The neurobiological basis of reading. *Journal of Learning Disabilities, 34*, 566–579.

Joseph, R. M., Tager-Flusberg, H., & Lord, C. (2002). Cognitive profiles and social-communicative functioning in children with autism spectrum disorder. *Journal of Child Psychology and Psychiatry, 43*, 807–821.

Joseph, R. M., & Tanaka, J. (2003). Holistic and part-based face recognition in children with autism. *Journal of Child Psychology and Psychiatry, 44*, 529–542.

Just, M. A., Carpenter, P. A., Keller, T. A., Eddy, W. F., & Thulborn, K. R. (1996). Brain activation modulated by sentence comprehension. *Science, 274*, 114–116.

Kahn, H. J., & Whitaker, H. A. (1991). Acalculia: An historical review of localization. *Brain and Cognition, 17*, 102–115.

Kail, R., & Hall, L. K. (1994). Processing speed, naming speed, and reading. *Developmental Psychology, 30*, 949–954.

Kamphaus, R. W. (1993). *Clinical assessment of children's intelligence: A handbook for professional practice*. Needham Heights, MA: Allyn & Bacon.

Kamphaus, R. W. (1998). Intelligence test interpretation: Acting in the absence of evidence. In A. Prifitera & D. H. Saklofske (Eds.), *WISC-III clinical use and interpretation: Scientist-practitioner perspectives* (pp. 39–57). San Diego, CA: Academic Press.

Kamphaus, R. W. (2001). *Clinical assessment of child and adolescent intelligence* (2nd ed.). Needham Heights, MA: Allyn & Bacon.

Kandel, E., & Freed, D. (1989). Frontal lobe dysfunction and antisocial behavior: A review. *Journal of Clinical Child Psychology, 45*, 404–413.

Kaplan, B. J., Dewey, D. M., Crawford, S. G., & Wilson, B. N. (2001). The term comorbidity is of questionable value in reference to developmental disorders: Data and theory. *Journal of Learning Disabilities, 34*, 555–565.

Kaplan, E. (1998). A process approach to neuropsychological assessment. In T. Boll & B. K. Bryant (Eds.), *Clinical neuropsychology and brain function: Research, measurement, and practice* (pp. 125–167). Washington, DC: American Psychological Association.

Kaplan, E., Fein, D., Kramer, J., Delis, D., & Morris, R. (1999). *WISC-III PI manual.* San Antonio, TX: Psychological Corporation.

Kapur, S., Rose, R. Liddle, P. F., Zipursky, R. B., Brown, G. M., Stuss, D., et al. (1994). The role of the left prefrontal cortex in verbal processing: Semantic processing or willed action. *NeuroReport, 5,* 2193–2196.

Katanoda, K., Yoshikawa, K., & Sugishita, M. (2001). A functional MRI study on the neural substrates for writing. *Human Brain Mapping, 13,* 34–42.

Kauffman, J. M., Hallahan, D. P., Haas, K., Brame T., & Boren, R. (1978). Imitating children's errors to improve their spelling performance. *Journal of Learning Disabilities, 11,* 217–222.

Kaufman, A. S. (1994). *Intelligent testing with the WISC-III.* New York: Wiley.

Kaufman, A. S., & Kaufman, N. L. (1983). *Kaufman Assessment Battery for Children: Interpretive manual.* Circle Pines, MN: American Guidance Service.

Kaufman, A. S., & Kaufman, N. L. (1993). *Kaufman Adolescent and Adult Intelligence Test.* Circle Pines, MN: American Guidance Service.

Kaufman, A. S., & Kaufman, N. L. (Eds.). (2001). *Specific learning disabilities and difficulties in children and adolescents: Psychological assessment and evaluation.* New York: Cambridge University Press.

Kavale, K. A., & Forness, S. R. (1995). *The nature of learning disabilities: Critical elements of diagnosis and classification.* Mahwah, NJ: Erlbaum.

Kavale, K. A., & Forness, S. R. (1996). Social skill deficits and learning disabilities: A meta-analysis. *Journal of Learning Disabilities, 29,* 226–237.

Kavale, K. A., & Forness, S. R. (1999). Effectiveness of special education. In C. R. Reynolds & T. B. Gutkin (Eds.), *The handbook of school psychology* (3rd ed., pp. 984–1024). New York: Wiley.

Kavale, K. A., & Reece, J. H. (1992). The character of learning disabilities. *Learning Disability Quarterly, 15,* 74–94.

Kearney, C. A., & Drabman, R. S. (1993). The write–say method for improving spelling accuracy in children with learning disabilities. *Journal of Learning Disabilities, 26,* 52–56.

Keefe, R. S. E. (1995). The contribution of neuropsychology to psychiatry. *American Journal of Psychiatry, 152,* 6–15.

Keeler, M. L., & Swanson, H. L. (2001). Does strategy knowledge influence working memory in children with mathematical disabilities? *Journal of Learning Disabilities, 34,* 418–434.

Keith, T. Z., Kranzler, J. H., & Flanagan, D. P. (2001). What does the Cognitive Assessment System (CAS) measure?: Joint confirmatory factor analysis of the CAS and the Woodcock–Johnson Tests of Cognitive Ability (3rd edition). *School Psychology Review, 30,* 89–119.

Keller, T. A., Carpenter, P. A., & Just, M. A. (2001). The neural bases of sentence comprehension: A fMRI examination of syntactic and lexical processing. *Cerebral Cortex, 11,* 223–237.

Kelly, M. S., Best, C. T., & Kirk, U. (1989). Cognitive processing deficits in reading disabilities: A prefrontal cortical hypothesis. *Brain and Cognition, 11,* 275–293.

Kennard, M. A. (1938). Reorganization of motor function in the cerebral cortex of monkeys deprived of motor and premotor areas in infancy. *Journal of Neurophysiology, 1,* 477.

Keogh, B. K. (1994). A matrix of decision points in the measurement of learning disabilities. In G. R. Lyon (Ed.), *Frames of references for the assessment of learning disabilities* (pp. 15–26). Baltimore: Brookes.

Khateb, A., Michel, C. M., Pegna, A. J., Thut, G., Landis, T., & Annoni, J. (2001). The time course of semantic category processing in the cerebral hemispheres: An electrophysical study. *Cognitive Brain Research, 10,* 251–264.

Kinsbourne, M. (1997). Mechanisms and development of cerebral lateralization in children. In C. R. Reynolds & E. Fletcher-Janzen (Eds.), *Handbook of clinical child neuropsychology* (2nd ed., pp. 102–119). New York: Plenum Press.

Kirk, S. A., & Bateman, B. (1962). Diagnosis and remediation of learning disabilities. *Exceptional Children, 29*(2), 73–78.

Kirk, S. A., Kirk, W. D., & Minskoff, E. H. (1985). *Phonic remedial reading lessons.* Novato, CA: Academic Therapy.

Kirk, S. A., McCarthy, J. J., & Kirk, W. D. (1968). *Illinois Test of Psycholinguistic Abilities (ITPA).* Urbana: University of Illinois Press.

Klin, A. (2000). Attributing social meaning to ambiguous visual stimuli in higher-functioning autism and Asperger syndrome: The social attribution task. *Journal of Child Psychology and Psychiatry, 41,* 831–846.

Klin, A., & Volkmar, F. R. (1997). The pervasive developmental disorders: Nosology and profiles of development.

In S. S. Luthar, J. A. Burack, D. Cicchetti, & J. R. Weisz (Eds.), *Developmental psychopathology: Perspectives on adjustment, risk, and disorder* (pp. 208–226). New York: Cambridge University Press.

Klin, A., Volkmar, F. R., Sparrow, S. S., Cicchetti, D. V., & Rourke, B. P. (1995). Validity and neuropsychological characterization of Asperger syndrome: Convergence with nonverbal learning disabilities syndrome. *Journal of Child Psychology and Psychiatry, 36,* 1127–1140.

Klingberg, T., Hedehus, M., Temple, E., Salz, T., Gabrieli, J. D., Moseley, M. E., et al. (2000). Microstructure of temporo-parietal white matter as a basis for reading ability: evidence from diffusion tensor magnetic resonance imaging. *Neuron, 25,* 493–500.

Klorman, R., Hazel-Fernandez, L. A., Shaywitz, S. E., Fletcher, J. M., Marchionne, K. E., Holahan, J. M., et al. (1999). Executive functioning deficits in attention-deficit/hyperactivity disorder are independent of oppositional or reading disorder. *Journal of the American Academy of Child and Adolescent Psychiatry, 38,* 1148–1155.

Kløve, H. (1963). *Grooved Pegboard.* Lafayette, IN: Lafayette Instrument.

Kluger, A., & Goldberg, E. (1990). IQ patterns in affective disorder, lateralized and diffuse brain damage. *Journal of Clinical and Experimental Neuropsychology, 12,* 182–194.

Kolb, B., & Fantie, B. (1997). Development of the child's brain and behavior. In C. R. Reynolds & E. Fletcher-Janzen (Eds.), *Handbook of clinical child neuropsychology* (2nd ed., pp. 17–41). New York: Plenum Press.

Kolb, B., & Whishaw, I. Q. (1990). *Fundamentals of human neuropsychology* (4th ed.). New York: Freeman.

Kopelman, M. D., Stevens, T. G., Foli, S., & Grasby, P. (1998). PET activation of the medial temporal lobe in learning. *Brain, 121,* 875–887.

Korkman, M., Kirk, U., & Kemp, S. (1998). *NEPSY: A developmental neuropsychological assessment manual.* San Antonio, TX: Psychological Corporation.

Kosslyn, S. M., Daly, P. F., McPeek, R. M., Alpert, N. M., Kennedy, D. N., & Caviness, V. S. (1993). Using locations to store shape: An indirect effect of a lesion. *Cerebral Cortex, 3,* 567–582.

Kracke, I. (1994). Developmental prosopagnosia in Asperger syndrome: Presentation and discussion of an individual case. *Developmental Medicine and Child Neurology, 36,* 873–886.

Kranzler, J. H. (2001). Commentary on "Is *g* a viable construct for school psychology?" *Learning and Individual Differences, 13,* 189–195.

Kranzler, J. H., & Keith, T. Z. (1999). Independent confirmatory factor analysis of the Cognitive Assessment System (CAS): What does the CAS measure? *School Psychology Review, 28,* 117–144.

Kratochwill, T. R., Elliott, S. N., & Callan-Stoiber, K. (2002). Best practices in school-based problem-solving consultation. In A. Thomas & J. Grimes (Eds.), *Best practices in school psychology IV* (Vol. 1, pp. 583–608). Bethesda, MD: National Association of School Psychologists.

Krishnan, H. R. (1999). Brain imaging correlates. *Journal of Clinical Psychiatry, 60,* 50–54.

Lahey, B. B., Hart, E. L., Pliszka, S., Applegate, B., & McBurnett, K. (1993). Neurophysiological correlates of conduct disorder: A rationale and review of research. *Journal of Clinical Child Psychology, 22,* 141–153.

Lahey, M. (1988). *Language disorders and language development.* New York: Macmillan.

Lahey, M., & Bloom, L. (1994). Variability and langauge learning disabilities. In G. P. Wallach & K. G. Butler (Eds.), *Language learning disabilities in school-age children and adolescents* (pp. 354–372). Needham Heights, MA: Allyn & Bacon.

Landro, N. I., Stiles, T. C., & Sletvold, H. (2001). Neurological function in nonpsychotic unipolar major depression. *Neuropsychiatry, Neuropsychology, and Behavioral Neurology, 14,* 233–240.

Langdon, D. W., & Warrington, E. K. (1997). The abstraction of numerical relations: A role for the right hemisphere in arithmetic? *Journal of the International Neuropsychological Society, 3,* 260–268.

Lazar, J. W., & Frank, Y. (1998). Frontal systems dysfunction in children with attention-deficit/hyperactivity disorder and learning disabilities. *Journal of Neuropsychiatry and Clinical Neurosciences, 10,* 160–167.

LeDoux, J. E. (1995). In search of an emotional system in the brain: Leaping from fear to emotion and consciousness. In M. S. Gazzaniga (Ed.), *The cognitive neurosciences* (pp. 1049–1061). Cambridge, MA: MIT Press.

Leavell, A., & Ioannides, A. (1993). Using character development to improve story writing. *Teaching Exceptional Children, 25,* 41–45.

Lebowitz, B. K., Shear, P. K., Steed, M. A., & Strakowski, S. M. (2001). Verbal fluency in mania. *Neuropsychology, Neuropsychiatry, and Behavioral Neurology, 14,* 177–182.

Leiner, H. C., Leiner, A. L., & Dow, R. S. (1993). Cognitive and language functions of the human cerebellum. *Trends in Neuroscience, 16,* 444–447.

Lenneberg, E. (1967). *Biological foundations of language.* New York: Wiley.

Lenz, B. K., & Hughes, C. A. (1990). A word identification strategy for adolescents with learning disabilities. *Journal of Learning Disabilities, 33,* 149–158.

Lerner, J. (2000). *Learning disabilities: Theories, diagnosis, and teaching strategies* (8th ed.). Boston: Houghton Mifflin.

Levine, M., Oberklaid, F., & Meltzer, L. (1981). Developmental output faillure: A study of low productivity in school-aged children. *Pediatrics, 67,* 18–25.

Levy, B. A. (2001). Moving the bottom: Improving reading fluency. In M. Wolf (Ed.), *Dyslexia, fluency, and the brain* (pp. 357–382). Timonium, MD: York Press.

Levy, B. A., Abello, B., & Lysynchuk, L. (1997). Transfer from word training to reading in context: Gains in reading fluency and comprehension. *Learning Disability Quarterly, 20,* 173–188.

Levy, L. (1974). Cerebral asymmetries as manifested in split-brain man. In M. Kinsbourne & W. L. Smith (Eds.), *Hemispheric disconnection and cerebral function.* Springfield, IL: Thomas.

Lewis, M. H., Aman, M. G., Gadow, K. D., Schroeder, S. R., & Thompson, T. (1996). Psychopharmacology. In J. W. Jacobson & J. A. Mulick (Eds.), *Manual of diagnosis and professional practice in mental retardation* (pp. 323–340). Washington, DC: American Psychological Association.

Lezak, M. D. (1988). IQ: RIP. *Journal of Experimental and Clinical Neuropsychology, 10,* 351–361.

Lezak, M. D. (1995). *Neuropsychological assessment* (3rd ed.). New York: Oxford University Press.

Lichter, D. G., & Cummings, J. L. (Eds.). (2001). *Frontal–subcortical circuits in psychiatric and neurological disorders.* New York: Guilford Press.

Liepmann, H. (1908). *Die linke hemisphare und das handeln: Drei aufsatze aus dem apraxiegebiet.* Berlin: Springer-Verlag.

Light, G. J., & DeFries, J. C. (1995). Comorbidity of reading and mathematics disabilities: Genetic and environmental etiologies. *Journal of Learning Disabilities, 28,* 96–106.

Lilienfeld, S. O., Waldman, I. D., & Israel, A. C. (1994). A critical examination of the use of the term and concept of comorbidity in psychopathology research. *Clinical Psychology: Science and Practice, 1,* 71–83.

Lincoln, A., Courchesne, E., Allen, M., Hanson, E., & Ene, M. (1998). Neurobiology of Asperger syndrome: Seven case studies and quantitative magnetic resonance imaging findings. In E. Schopler, G. B. Mesibov, & L. J. Kunce (Eds,), *Asperger syndrome or high-functioning autism?: Current issues in autism* (pp. 145–163). New York: Plenum Press.

Lindamood, P. C. (1994). Issues in researching the link between phonological awareness, learning disabilities, and spelling. In G. R. Lyon (Ed.), *Frames of reference for the assessment of learning disabilities* (pp. 351–374). Baltimore: Brookes.

Lindsley, O. R. (1991). Precision teaching's unique legacy from B. F. Skinner. *Journal of Behavioral Education, 1*(2), 253–266.

Liotti, M., & Mayberg, H. S. (2001). The role of functional neuroimaging in the neuropsychology of depression. *Journal of Clinical and Experimental Neuropsychology, 23,* 121–136.

Lipsky, D. K., & Gartner, A. (1995). *The evaluation of inclusive education programs.* (ERIC Document Reproduction Service No. ED385042)

Liss, M., Fein, D., Allen, D., Dunn, M., Feinstein, C., Morris, R., et al. (2001). Executive functioning in high-functioning children with autism. *Journal of Child Psychology and Psychiatry, 42,* 261–270.

Logan, G. (1997). Automaticity and reading: Perspectives from the instance theory of automatization. *Reading and Writing Quarterly, 13,* 123–146.

Lombardo, T. W., & Drabman, R. S. (1985). Teaching LD children multiplication tables. *Academic Therapy, 20,* 437–442.

Loney, B. R., Frick, P. J., Ellis, M., & McCoy, M. G. (1998). Intelligence, callous–unemotional traits, and antisocial behavior. *Journal of Psychopathology and Behavioral Assessment, 20,* 231–247.

Lou, H. C., Henriksen, L., & Bruhn, P. (1984). Focal cerebral hypoperfusion in children with dysphasia and/or attention deficit disorder. *Archives of Neurology, 41,* 825–829.

Lou, H. C., Henriksen, L., Bruhn, P., Borner, H., & Nielsen, J. (1989). Striatal dysfunction in attention deficit and hyperkinetic disorder. *Archives of Neurology, 46,* 48–52.

Lovaas, O. A. (1996). The UCLA young autism model of service delivery. In C. Maurice & G. Green (Eds.), *Behavioral intervention for young children with autism: A manual for parents and professionals* (pp. 241–248). Austin, TX: PRO-ED.

Lovegrove, W. (1993). *Visual transient system deficits in specific reading disability.* Paper presented at the biennial meeting of the Society for Research in Child Development, New Orleans, LA.

Loveland, K. A., Fletcher, J. M., & Bailey, V. (1990). Verbal and nonverbal communication of events in learning disability subtypes. *Journal of Clinical and Experimental Neuropsychology, 12,* 433–447.

Lovett, M. W., Borden, S. L., Deluca, T., Lacerenza, L., Benson, N. J., & Brackstone, D. (1994). Treating the core deficits of developmental dyslexia: Evidence of transfer-of learning following phonologically- and strategy-based reading training programs. *Developmental Psychology, 30,* 805–822.

Lovett, M. W., Steinbach, K. A., & Frijters, J. C. (2000). Remediating the core deficits of developmental reading disability: A double-deficit perspective. *Journal of Learning Disabilities, 33,* 334–358.

Lucchelli, F., & DeRenzi, E. (1993). Primary discalculia after a medial frontal lesion in the left hemisphere. *Journal of Neurology, 56,* 304–307.

Luria, A. R. (1973). *The working brain.* New York: Basic Books.

Luria, A. R. (1980a). *Higher cortical functions in man* (2nd ed.). New York: Basic Books.

Luria, A. R. (1980b). Neuropsychology in the local diagnosis of brain damage. *International Journal of Clinical Neuropsychology, 2,* 1–7.

Lynam, D., Moffitt, T. E., & Stouthamer-Loeber, M. (1993). Explaining the relation between IQ and delinquency: Class, race, test motivation, school failure, or self-control? *Journal of Abnormal Psychology, 102,* 187–196.

Lyon, G. R. (1995). Research initiatives in learning disabilities: Contributions from scientists supported by the National Institute of Child Health and Human Development. *Journal of Child Neurology, 10,* 120–126.

Lyon, G. R., Fletcher, J. M., Shaywitz, S. E., Shaywitz, B. A., Torgeson, J. K., Wood, F. B., et al. (2001). Rethinking learning disabilities. In C. E. Finn, A. J. Rotherham, & C. R. Hokanson (Eds.), *Rethinking special education for a new century* (pp. 259–287). Washington, DC: Progressive Policy Institute and The Thomas B. Fordham Foundation.

Lyon, G. R., & Moats, L. C. (1997). Critical conceptual and methodological considerations in reading intervention research. *Journal of Learning Disabilities, 30,* 578–588.

Lyon, G. R., & Rumsey, J. M. (Eds.). (1996). *Neuroimaging: A window to the neurological foundations of learning and behavior in children.* Baltimore: Brookes.

MacArthur, C., Schwartz, S., & Graham, S. (1991). Effects of reciprocal peer revision strategy in special education classrooms. *Learning Disabilities Research and Practice, 6,* 201–210.

MacMillan, D. L., Gresham, F. M., & Bocian, K. M. (1998). Discrepancy between definitions of learning disabilities and school practices: An empirical investigation. *Journal of Learning Disabilities, 31,* 314–326.

Macmann, G. M., & Barnett, D. W. (1997). Myth of the master detective: Reliability of interpretations for Kaufman's "intelligent testing" approach to the WISC-III. *School Psychology Quarterly, 12,* 197–234.

Majovski, L. V. (1997). Development of higher brain functions in children: Neural, cognitive, and behavioral perspectives. In C. R. Reynolds & E. Fletcher-Janzen (Eds.), *Handbook of clinical child neuropsychology* (2nd ed., pp. 17–41). New York: Plenum Press.

Makris, N., Meyer, J. W., Bates, J. F., Yeterian, E. H., Kennedy, D. N., & Caviness, V. S. (1999). MRI-based topographic parcellation of human cerebral white matter and nuclei: II. Rationale and applications with systematics of cerebral connectivity. *Neuroimaging, 9,* 18–45.

Manis, F. R., Doi, L. M., & Bhadha, B. (2000). Naming speed, phonological awareness, and orthographic knowledge in second graders. *Journal of Learning Disabilities, 33,* 325–333.

Manis, F. R., & Freedman, L. (2001). The relationship of naming speed to multiple reading measures in disabled and normal readers. In M. Wolf (Ed.), *Dyslexia, fluency, and the brain* (pp. 65–92). Timonium, MD: York Press.

Manis, F. R., Seidenburg, M. S., & Doi, L. M. (1999). See Dick RAN: Rapid naming and the longitudinal prediction of reading subskills in first and second graders. *Scientific Study of Reading, 3,* 129–157.

Manoach, D. S., Sandson, T. A., & Weintraub, S. (1995). The developmental social-emotional processing disorder is associated with right hemisphere abnormalities. *Neuropsychiatry, Neuropsychology, and Behavioral Neurology, 8,* 99–105.

Margolin, D. I., & Goodman-Shulman, R. (1992). Oral and written spelling impairments. In D. I. Margolin (Ed.), *Cognitive neuropsychology in clinical practice* (pp. 263–297). New York: Oxford University Press.

Markell, M. A., & Deno, S. L. (1997). Effects of increasing oral reading: Generalization across reading tasks. *Journal of Special Education, 31,* 233–250.

Marshall, R. M., Hynd, G. W., Handwerk, M. J., & Hall, J. (1997). Academic underachievement in ADHD subtypes. *Journal of Learning Disabilities, 30,* 635–642.

Marshall, R. M., Schafer, V. A., O'Donnell, L., Elliott, J., & Handwerk, M. L. (1999). Arithmetic disabilities and ADD subtypes: Implications for DSM-IV. *Journal of Learning Disabilities, 32,* 239–247.

Martin, A., Wiggs, C. L., & Weisberg, J. (1997). Modulation of human medial temporal lobe activity by form, meaning, and experience. *Hippocampus, 7,* 587–593.

Matarazzo, J. D. (1990). Psychological assessment versus psychological testing: Validation from Binet to school, clinic, and courtroom. *American Psychologist, 45,* 999–1017.

Mather, N., & Jaffe, L. E. (2002). *Woodcock–Johnson III: Reports, recommendations, and strategies.* New York: Wiley.

Max, J. E., Fox, P. T., Lancaster, J. L., Kochunov, P., Mathews, K., Manes, F. F., et al. (2002). Putamen lesions and the development of attention-deficit/hyperactivity symptoms. *Journal of the American Academy of Child and Adolescent Psychiatry, 41,* 563–571.

Mayberg, H. (2001). Depression and frontal–subcortical circuits: Focus on prefrontal–limbic interactions. In D. G. Lichter & J. L. Cummings (Eds.), *Frontal–subcortical circuits in psychiatric and neurological disorders* (pp. 177–206). New York: Guilford Press.

Mayer, E., Martory, M. D., Pegna, A. J., Landis, T., Delavelle, J., & Annoni, J. M. (1999). A pure case of Gerstmann syndrome with a subangular lesion. *Brain, 122,* 1107–1120.

Mayes, S. D., Calhoun, S. L., & Crowell, E. W. (2000). Learning disabilities and ADHD: Overlapping spectrum disorders. *Journal of Learning Disabilities, 33,* 417–424.

Mazzocco, M. M. M. (2001). Math learning disability and math LD subtypes: Evidence from studies of Turner syndrome, fragile X syndrome, and neurofibromatosis type 1. *Journal of Learning Disabilities, 34,* 520–533.

McBride, M.C. (1988). An individual double-blind crossover trial for assessing methylphenidate response in children with attention deficit disorder. *Journal of Pediatrics, 113,* 137–145.

McCloskey, M., Aliminosa, D., & Sokol, S. M. (1991). Facts, rules, and procedures in normal calculation: Evidence from multiple single-patient studies of impaired arithmetic fact retrieval. *Brain and Cognition, 17,* 154–203.

McConaughy, S. H., & Skiba, R. J. (1993). Comorbidity of externalizing and internalizing problems. *School Psychology Review, 22,* 421–436.

McDermott, P. A., Fantuzzo, J. W., & Glutting, J. J. (1990). Just say no to subtest analysis: A critique on Wechsler theory and practice. *Journal of Psychoeducational Assessment, 8,* 290–302.

McGhee, R. L. (2001). The McGhee prophecies: Commentary on "Is g a variable construct for school psychology?" *Learning and Individual Differences, 13,* 197–203.

McGregor, G., & Vogelsberg, R. T. (1998). *Inclusive schooling practices: A synthesis of the literature that informs best practices about inclusive schooling.* Pittsburgh, PA: Allegheny University of the Health Sciences.

McGrew, K. S., & Flanagan, D. P. (1998). *The intelligence test desk reference (ITDR): Gf-Gc cross-battery assessment.* Boston: Allyn & Bacon.

McGuigan, C. A. (1975). *The effects of a flowing words list vs. fixed words lists and the implementation of procedures in the Add-a-Word Spelling Program* (Working Paper No. 52). Seattle: University of Washington, Experimental Education Unit.

McLean, M. F., & Hitch, G. J. (1999). Working memory impairments in children with specific arithmetic learning difficulties. *Journal of Experimental Child Psychology, 74,* 240–260.

McNaughton, D., Hughes, C. A., & Clark, K. (1994). Spelling instruction for students with learning disabilities: Implications for research and practice. *Learning Disability Quarterly, 17,* 169–185.

McTighe, J., & Lyman, F. G., Jr. (1988). Cueing thinking in the classroom: The promise of theory-embedded tools. *Educational Leadership, 47,* 18–24.

Melroy, L. (1999, December). Manifest determination. *Communiqué, 28*(4), 8–9.

Menon, V., Boyette-Anderson, J. M., Schatzberg, A. F., & Reiss, A. L. (2002). Relating semantic and episodic memory systems. *Cognitive Brain Research, 13,* 261–265.

Menon, V., & Desmond, J. E. (2001). Left superior parietal cortex involvement in writing: Integrating fMRI with lesion evidence. *Cognitive Brain Research, 12,* 337–340.

Menon, V., Mackenzie, K., Rivera, S., & Reiss, A. (2002). Prefrontal cortex involvement in processing incorrect arithmetic equations: Evidence from event-related fMRI. *Human Brain Mapping, 16,* 119–130.

Menon, V., Rivera, S. M., White, C. D., Eliez, S., Glover, G. H., & Reiss, A. L. (2000). Dissociating prefrontal and parietal cortex activation during arithmetic processing. *NeuroImage, 12,* 357–365.

Mercer, C. D. (1997). *Students with learning disabilities* (5th ed.). Upper Saddle River, NJ: Merrill/Prentice Hall.

Mercer, C. D., & Mercer, A. R. (2001). *Teaching students with learning problems* (6th ed.). Upper Saddle River, NJ: Merrill/Prentice-Hall.

Mercer, C. D., & Miller, S. P. (1991–1993). *Strategic math series.* Lawrence, KS: Edge Enterprises.

Merrell, K. W. (1999). *Behavioral, social, and emotional assessment of children and adolescents.* Mahwah, NJ: Erlbaum.

Meyer, J. A., & Minshew, N. J. (2002). An update on neurocognitive profiles in Asperger syndrome and high functioning autism. *Focus on Autism and Other Developmental Disabilities, 17,* 152–160.

Meyer, M. S., & Felton, R. H. (1999). Repeated reading to enhance fluency: Old approaches and new directions. *Annals of Dyslexia, 49,* 283–306.

Meyers, J., & Meyers, K. (1995). *The Meyers scoring system for the Rey-Osterrieth Complex Figure and Recognition trial*. Odessa, FL: Psychological Assessment Resources.

Michael, E. B., Keller, T. A., Carpenter, P. A., & Just, M. A. (2001). fMRI investigation of sentence comprehension by eye and by ear: Modality fingerprints on cognitive processes. *Human Brain Mapping, 13*, 239–252.

Michel, F., Henaff, M. A., & Intrilligator, J. (1996). Two different readers in the same brain after a posterior callosal lesion. *NeuroReport, 7*, 786–788.

Middleton, F. A., & Strick, P. L. (2000). Basal ganglia output and cognition: Evidence from anatomical, behavioral, and clinical studies. *Brain and Cognition, 42*, 183–200.

Milberg, W. P., Hebben, N., & Kaplan, E. (1986). The Boston process approach to neuropsychological assessment. In I. Grant & K. M. Adams (Eds.), *Neuropsychological assessment of neuropsychiatric disorders* (pp. 58–80). New York: Oxford University Press.

Milich, R., Balentine, A. C., & Lyman, D. R. (2001). ADHD combined type and ADHD predominantly inattentive type are distinct and unrelated disorders. *Clinical Psychology: Science and Practice, 8*, 463–488.

Miller, J. N., & Ozonoff, S. (2000). The external validity of Asperger disorder: Lack of evidence from the domain of neuropsychology. *Journal of Abnormal Psychology, 109*, 227–238.

Miller, S. L., & Tallal, P. (1995). A behavioral neuroscience approach to developmental language disorders: Evidence for a rapid temporal processing deficit. In D. Cicchetti & D. J. Cohen (Eds.), *Developmental psychopathology: Vol. 2. Risk, disorder, and adaptation* (pp. 274–298). New York: Wiley.

Miller, S. P., Butler, F. M., & Kit-hung, L. (1998). Validated practices for teaching mathematics to students with learning disabilities: A review of literature. *Focus on Exceptional Children, 30*, 1–16.

Milner, A. D. (1995). Aspects of human frontal lobe function. *Advances in Neurology, 66*, 67–84.

Milner, A. D., & Goodale, M. A. (1995). *The visual brain in action*. New York: Oxford University Press.

Minshew, N. J., Goldstein, G., & Siegal, D. J. (1997). Neuropsychologic functioning in autism: Profile of a complex information processing disorder. *Journal of the International Neuropsychological Society, 3*, 303–316.

Mirsky, A. F. (1996). Disorders of attention. In G. R. Lyon & N. A. Krasnegor (Eds.), *Attention, memory, and executive function* (pp. 71–95). Baltimore: Brookes.

Moffitt, T. E. (1993). The neurobiology of conduct disorder. *Development and Psychopathology, 5*, 135–151.

Moffitt, T. E., Lynam, D. R., & Silva, P. A. (1994). Neuropsychological tests predicting persistent male delinquency. *Criminology, 32*, 277–300.

Molfese, D. L. (2000). Predicting dyslexia at 8 years of age using neonatal brain responses. *Brain and Language, 72*, 238–245.

Molfese, D. L., & Molfese, V. J. (1997). Discrimination of langauge skills at five years of age using event related potentials recorded at birth. *Developmental Neuropsychology, 13*, 135–156.

Molfese, D. L., Morse, P. A., & Peters, C. J. (1990). Auditory evoked responses to names for different objects: Cross-modal processing as a basis for infant language acquisition. *Developmental Psychology, 26*, 780–795.

Molfese, V. J., Molfese, D. L., & Modgline, A. A. (2001). Newborn and preschool predictors of second-grade reading scores: An evaluation of categorical and continuous scores. *Journal of Learning Disabilities, 34*, 245–254.

Moll, J., de Oliveira-Souza, R., Passman, L. J., Cunha, F. C., Souza-Lima, F., & Andreiuolo, P. A. (2000). Functional MRI correlates of read and imagined tool use pantomimes. *Neurology, 54*, 1331–1336.

Montague, M. (1992). The effects of cognitive and metacognitive strategy instruction on the mathematical problem solving of middle school students with learning disabilities. *Journal of Learning Disabilities, 25*, 230–248.

Montague, M., & Bos, C. (1986). The effect of cognitive strategy training on verbal math problem solving performance of learning disabled adolescents. *Journal of Learning Disabilities, 19*, 26–33.

Moretti, R., Torre, P., Antonello, R. M., Ukmar, M., & Cazzato, G. (2001). Writing and praxis: What is new? *European Journal of Neurology, 8*, 91.

Morris, R. D. (1996). Relationships and distinctions among the concepts of attention, memory, and executive function: A developmental perspective. In G. R. Lyon & N. A. Krasnegor (Eds.), *Attention, memory, and executive function* (pp. 11–16). Baltimore: Brookes.

Morris, R. D., Stuebing, K. K., Fletcher, J. M., Shaywitz, S. E., Lyon, G. R., & Shankweiler, D. P. (1998). Subtypes of reading disability: Variability around the phonological core. *Journal of Educational Psychology, 90*, 347–373.

Mulick, J. A., & Hale, J. B. (1996). Communicating assessment results in mental retardation. In J. J. Jacobson & J. A. Mulick (Eds.), *Manual of diagnosis and professional practice in mental retardation* (pp. 257–263). Washington, DC: American Psychological Association.

Muller, R., Kleinhans, N., Pierce, K., Kemmotsu, N., & Courchesne, E. (2002). Functional MRI of motor sequence acquisition effects of learning stage and performance. *Cognitive Brain Research, 14*, 277–293.

Murphy, F. C., & Sahakian, B. J. (2001). Neuropsychology of bipolar disorder. *British Journal of Psychiatry, 178,* S120–S127.

Myers, P. S. (1993). Narrative expressive deficits associated with right hemisphere damage. In H. H. Brownwell & Y. Joanette (Eds.), *Narrative discourse in neurologically-impaired and normal aging adults* (pp. 279–298). San Diego, CA: Singular.

Naglieri, J. A., & Das, J. P. (1997). *Das–Naglieri Cognitive Assessment System administration and scoring manual.* Itasca, IL: Riverside.

Naglieri, J. A., & Gottling, S. H. (1995). A study of planning and mathematics instruction for students with learning disabilities. *Psychological Reports, 76*(3, Pt. 2), 1343–1354.

Naglieri, J. A., & Gottling, S. H. (1997). Mathematics instruction and PASS cognitive processes: An intervention study. *Journal of Learning Disabilities, 30,* 513–520.

Naglieri, J. A., & Johnson, D. (2000). Effectiveness of a cognitive strategy intervention in improving arithmetic computation based on the PASS theory. *Journal of Learning Disabilities, 33,* 591–597.

National Center for Education Statistics. (2002). *Digest of education statistics* [Online]. Retrieved from *http://nces.ed.gov*

National Information Center for Children and Youth with Disabilities (NICHCY). (1994). "Guidance response" from the U. S. Department of Education Office of Special Education and Rehabilitation Services (OSERS) in 1994. Retrieved from *http://www.wrightslaw.com/info/lre.faqs.inclusion.htm*

Neisser, U., Boodoo, G., Bouchard, T. J., Jr., Boykin, A. W., Brody, N., Ceci, S. J., et al. (1996). Intelligence: Knowns and unknowns. *American Psychologist, 51,* 77–101.

Newcomer, P. L., & Barenbaum, E. M. (1991). The written composing ability of children with learning disabilities: A review of the literature from 1980 to 1990. *Journal of Learning Disabilities, 24,* 578–593.

Newcomer, P. L., & Hammill, D. D. (1997). *Test of Language Development—Intermediate: Third Edition.* Austin, TX: PRO-ED.

Newman, S. D., & Tweig, D. (2001). Differences in auditory processing of words and pseudowords: An fMRI study. *Human Brain Mapping, 14,* 39–47.

Nichelli, P., Grafman, J., Pietrini, P., Clark, K., Lee, K. Y., & Miletich, R. (1995). Where the brain appreciates the moral of the story. *NeuroReport, 6,* 2309–2313.

Nicholson, R. I., & Fawcett, A. J. (2001). Dyslexia, learning and the cerebellum. In M. Wolf (Ed.), *Dyslexia, fluency, and the brain* (pp. 159–188). Timonium, MD: York Press.

Nicholson, R. I., Fawcett, A. J., & Dean, P. (1995). Time estimation deficits in developmental dyslexia: Eviddence of cerebellar involvement. *Proceedings of the Royal Society of London, Series B: Biological Sciences, 259,* 43–47.

Nicholson, R. I., Fawcett, A. J., & Dean, P. (2001). Developmental dyslexia: The cerebellar deficit hypothesis. *Trends in Neuroscience, 24,* 508–511.

Nigg, J. T., Blaskey, L. G., Huang-Pollock, C. L., & Rappley, M. D. (2002). Neuropsychological executive functions and DSM-IV ADHD subtypes. *Journal of the American Academy of Child and Adolescent Psychiatry, 41,* 59–66.

Nigg, J. T., Hinshaw, S. P., Carte, E. T., & Treuting, J. J. (1998). Neuropsychological correlates of childhood attention-deficit/hyperactivity disorder: Explainable by comorbid disruptive behavior or reading problems? *Journal of Abnormal Psychology, 107,* 468–480.

Nobre, A. C., Allison, T., & McCarthy G. (1998). Modulation of human extrastriate visual processing by selective attention to colours and words. *Brain, 121,* 1357–1368.

Novak, G. P., Solanto, M., & Abikoff, H. (1995). Spatial orienting and focused attention in attention deficit hyperactivity disorder. *Psychophysiology, 32,* 546–559.

Nussbaum, N. L., & Bigler, E. D. (1986). Neuropsychological and behavioral profiles of empirically derived subgroups of learning disabled children. *International Journal of Clinical Neuropsychology, 8,* 82–89.

Nussbaum, N. L., & Bigler, E. D. (1997). Halstead–Reitan Neuropsychological Test Batteries for children.. In C. R. Reynolds & E. Fletcher-Janzen (Eds.), *Handbook of clinical child neuropsychology* (2nd ed., pp. 219–236). New York: Plenum Press.

Nussbaum, N. L., Bigler, E. D., & Koch, W. (1986). Neuropsychologically derived subgroups of learning disabled children: Personality/behavioral dimensions. *Journal of Research and Development in Education, 19,* 57–68.

Nussbaum, N. L., Bigler, E. D., Koch, W. R., & Ingram, J. W. (1988). Personality/behavioral characteristics in children: Differential effects of putative anterior versus posterior cerebral asymmetry. *Archives of Clinical Neuropsychology, 3,* 127–135.

O'Driscoll, G. A., Wolff, A. V., Benkelfat, C., Florencio, P. S., Lal, S., & Evans, A. C. (2000). Functional neuroanatomy of smooth pursuit and predictive saccades. *NeuroReport, 11,* 1335–1340.

O'Neill, A. M. (1995). *Clinical inference: How to draw meaningful conclusions from tests*. Brandon, VT: Clinical Psychology.

O'Neill, R. E., Horner, R. H., Albin, R. W., Sprague, J. R., Storey, K., & Newton, J. S. (1997). *Functional assessment and program development for problem behavior: A practical handbook* (2nd ed.). Pacific Grove, CA: Brooks/ Cole.

Obrzut, J. E., & Hynd, G. W. (Eds.). (1986). *Child neuropsychology: Vol. 2. Clinical practice*. Orlando, FL: Academic Press.

Ogbu, J. U. (2002). Cultural amplifiers of intelligence: IQ and minority status in cross-cultural perspective. In J. M. Fish (Ed.), *Race and intelligence: Separating science from myth* (pp. 241–278). Mahwah, NJ: Erlbaum.

Ogden, J. A. (1996). Phonological dyslexia and phonological dysgraphia following left and right hemispherectomy. *Neuropsychologia, 34*, 905–918.

Olson, R., Forsberg, H., Wise, B., & Rack, J. (1994). Measurement of word recognition, orthographic, and phonological skills. In G. R. Lyon (Ed.), *Frames of reference for the assessment of learning disabilities* (pp. 243–277). Baltimore: Brookes.

Orton, S. (1937). *Reading, writing, and speech problems in children*. New York: Norton.

Orton-Gillingham, A., & Stillman, B. (1973). *Remedial training for children with specific disability in reading, spelling, and penmanship* (7th ed.). Cambridge, MA: Educators.

Owen, A. M., Lee, A. C. H., & Williams, E. J. (2000). Dissociating aspects of verbal working memory within the human frontal lobe: Further evidence for a "process-specific" model of human lateralization. *Psychobiology, 28*, 146–155.

Palinscar, A. S., & Brown, A. L. (1988). Teaching and practicing thinking skills to promote comprehension in the context of group problem solving. *Remedial and Special Education, 9*, 53–59.

Pallier, G., Roberts, R. D., & Stankov, L. (2000). Biological versus psychometric intelligence: Halstead's (1947) distinction revisited. *Archives of Clinical Neuropsychology, 15*, 205–226.

Papolos, D. F., & Papolos, J. (2000). *The bipolar child: The comprehensive and reassuring guide to childhood's most misunderstood disorder*. New York: Broadway Books.

Pasternack, R. H. (2002). *The demise of IQ testing for children with learning disabilities*. Paper presented at the annual convention of the National Association of School Psychologists, Chicago.

Patterson, K., Vargha-Khadem, F., & Polkey, C. (1989). Reading with one hemisphere. *Brain, 112*, 39–63.

Paulesu, E., Frith, C. D., & Frackowiak, R. S. J. (1993). The neural correlates of the verbal component of working memory. *Nature, 362*, 342–345.

Pearson, E. S. (1986). Summing it all up: Pre-1900 algorithms. *The Arithmetic Teacher, 33*, 38–41.

Pena, L. M., Megargee, E. I., & Brody, E. (1996). MMPI-A patterns of male juvenile delinquents. *Psychological Assessment, 8*, 388–397.

Pennington, B. F. (1991). *Diagnosing learning disorders: A neuropsychological framework*. New York: Guilford Press.

Pennington, B. F., Groisser, D., & Welsh, M. C. (1993). Contrasting cognitive deficits in attention deficit hyperactivity disorder versus reading disability. *Developmental Psychology, 29*, 511–523.

Pennington, B. F., & Ozonoff, S. (1996). Executive functions and developmental psychopathology. *Journal of Child Psychology and Psychiatry, 37*, 51–87.

Peretz, I. (1990). Processing of local and global musical information by unilateral brain-damaged patients. *Brain, 113*, 1185–1205.

Perugini, E. M., Harvey, E. A., Lovejoy, D. W., Sandstrom, K., & Webb, A. H. (2000). The predictive power of combined neuropsychological measures for attention-deficit/hyperactivity disorder in children. *Child Neuropsychology, 6*, 101–114.

Petersen, S. E., Fox, P. T., Posner, M. I., Mintun, M., & Raichle, M. E. (1989). Positron emission tomographic studies of the processing of single words. *Journal of Cognitive Neuroscience, 1*, 153–170.

Petersen, S. E., Fox, P. T., Snyder, A., & Raichle, M. E. (1990). Activation of the extrastriate and frontal cortical areas by visual words and word-like stimuli. *Science, 249*, 1041–1044.

Petersen, S. E., van Mier, H., Fiez, J. A., & Raichle, M. E. (1998). The effects of practice on the functional anatomy of task performance. *Proceedings of the National Academy of Science, 95*, 853–860.

Peterson, B. S. (1995). Neuroimaging in child and adolescent psychiatric disorders. *Journal of the American Academy of Child and Adolescent Psychiatry, 34*, 1560–1574.

Pfeiffer, S. I., Reddy, L. A., Kletzel, J. E., Schmelzer, E. R., & Boyer, L. M. (2000). The practitioner's view of IQ testing and profile analysis. *School Psychology Quarterly, 15*, 376–385.

Phelps-Terasaki, D., & Phelps-Gunn, T. (2000). *Teaching competence in written language* (2nd ed.). Austin, TX: PRO-ED.

Piaget, J. (1965). *The child's conception of number.* New York: Norton.

Pirozzolo, F. J., & Papanicolaou, A. C. (1986). Plasticity and recovery of function in the central nervous system. In J. E. Obrzut & G. W. Hynd (Eds.), *Child neuropsychology: Vol. 1. Theory and research* (pp. 141–154). Orlando, FL: Academic Press.

Pisecco, S. Baker, D. B., Silva, P. A., & Brooke, M. (2001). Boys with reading disabilities and/or ADHD: Distinctions in early childhood. *Journal of Learning Disabilities, 34,* 98–106.

Pliszka, S. R. (1999). The psychobiology of oppositional defiant disorder and conduct disorder. In H. C. Quay & A. E. Hogan (Eds.), *Handbook of disruptive behavior disorders* (pp. 371–395). New York: Kluwer Academic.

Pliszka, S. R., Carlson, C. L., & Swanson, J. M. (1999). *ADHD with comorbid disorders: Clinical assessment and management.* New York: Guilford Press.

Plomin, R., Price, T. S., Eley, T. C., Dale, P. S., & Stevenson, J. (2002). Associations between behaviour problems and verbal and nonverbal cognitive abilities and disabilities in early childhood. *Journal of Child Psychology and Psychiatry, 43,* 619–633.

Poizner, H., Klima, E. S., & Bellugi, U. (1987). *What the hands reveal about the brain.* Cambridge, MA: MIT Press.

Poldrack, R. A. (2001). A structural basis for developmental dyslexia: Evidence from diffusion tensor imaging. In M. Wolf (Ed.), *Dyslexia, fluency, and the brain* (pp. 213–234). Timonium, MD: York Press.

Polloway, E. A., Patton, J., & Cohen, S. (1981). Written language for mildly handicapped children. *Focus on Exceptional Children, 14,* 1–16.

Polloway, E. A., & Smith, T. E. C. (1999). *Language instruction for students with disabilities* (2nd ed.). Denver, CO: Love.

Posner, M. I. (1994). Neglect and spatial attention. *Neuropsychological Rehabilitation, 4,* 183–187.

Posner, M. I., & Petersen, S. E. (1990). The attention system of the human brain. *Annual Review of Neuroscience, 13,* 25–42.

Posner, M. I., & Raichle, M. (1994). *Images of mind.* New York: Scientific American Library.

Postle, B. R., & D'Esposito, M. (2000). Evaluating models of the topographical organization of working memory function in frontal cortex with event-related MRI. *Psychobiology, 28,* 132–145.

Prabhakaran, V. Rypma, B., & Gabrieli, J. D. E. (2001). Neural substrates of mathematical reasoning: A functional magnetic resonance image study of neocortical activation during performance of the necessary arithmetic operations test. *Neuropsychology, 15,* 115–127.

Price, C. J., Wise, R. J. S., & Frackowiak, R. S. J. (1996). Demonstrating the implicit processing of visually presented words and pseudowords. *Cerebral Cortex, 6,* 62–70.

Price, C. J., Wise, R. J. S., Watson, J. D. G., Patterson, K. E., Howard, D., & Frackowiak, R. S. J. (1994). Brain activity during reading: The effects of exposure duration and task. *Brain, 117,* 1255–1269.

Prifitera, A., & Dersh, J. (1993). Base rates of WISC-III diagnostic subtest patterns among normal, learning-disabled, and ADHD samples. *Journal of Psychoeducational Assessment (WISC-III Monograph),* 43–55.

Prifitera, A., Weiss, L. G., & Saklofske, D. H. (1998). The WISC-III in context. In A. Prifitera & D. H. Saklofske (Eds.), *WISC-III clinical use and interpretation: Scientist-practitioner perspectives* (pp. 1–38). San Diego, CA: Academic Press.

Pring, L., Hermelin, B., & Heavey, L. (1995). Savants, segments, art, and autism. *Journal of Child Psychology and Psychiatry, 31,* 1065–1076.

Prior, M., Smart, D., Sanson, A., & Oberklaid, F. (1999). Relationships between learning difficulties and psychological problems in preadolescent children from a longitudinal sample. *Journal of the American Academy of Child and Adolescent Psychiatry, 38,* 429–436.

Pugh, K. R., Mencl, W. E., Shaywitz, B. A., Shaywitz, S. E., Fulbright, R. K., Constable, R. T., et al. (2000). The angular gyrus in developmental dyslexia: Task-specific difference in functional connectivity within posterior cortex. *Psychological Science, 11,* 51–56.

Pugh, K., Shaywitz, B., Shaywitz, S., Shakweiler, D., Katz, L., Fletcher, J., et al. (1997). Predicting reading performance through neuroimaging profiles: The cerebral basis of phonological effects in printed word identification. *Journal of Experimental Psychology: Human Perception and Performance, 23,* 299–318.

Purdie, N., Hattie, J., & Carroll, A. (2002). A review of the research on interventions for attention deficit hyperactivity disorder: What works best? *Review of Educational Research, 72,* 61–99.

Purvis, K. L., & Tannock, R. (2000). Phonological processing, not inhibitory control, differentiates ADHD and reading disability. *Journal of the American Academy of Child and Adolescent Psychiatry, 39,* 485–494.

Quraishi, S., & Frangou, S. (2002). Neuropsychology of bipolar disorder: A review. *Journal of Affective Disorders, 72,* 209–226.

Raichle, M. E., Fiez, J. A., Videen, T. O., MacLeod, A. M., Pardo, J. V., Fox, P. T., et al. (1994). Practice-related changes in human brain functional anatomy during nonmotor learning. *Cerebral Cortex, 4,* 8–26.

Raine, A. (1993). *The psychopathology of crime: Criminal behavior as a clinical disorder.* San Diego, CA: Academic Press.

Raine, A. (2002). Annotation: The role of prefrontal deficits, low autonomic arousal, and early health factors in the development of antisocial and aggressive behavior in children. *Journal of Child Psychology and Psychiatry, 43,* 417–434.

Raine, A., Park, S., Lencz, T., Bihrle, S., Lacasse, L., Widom, C. S., et al. (2001). Reduced right hemisphere activation in severely abused violent offenders during a working memory task as indicated by fMRI. *Aggressive Behavior, 27,* 111–129.

Raine, A., Yaralian, P. S., Reynolds, C., Venables, P. H., & Mednick, S. A. (2002). Spatial but not verbal cognitive deficits at age 3 years in persistently antisocial individuals. *Development and Psychopathology, 14,* 25–44.

Rammsayer, T. H., Hennig, J., Haag, A., & Lange, N. (2001). Effects of noradrenergic activityon temporal information processing in humans. *Quarterly Journal of Experimental Psychology, 54B,* 247–258.

Ramus, F. (2001). Talk of two theories. *Nature, 412,* 393–395.

Ramus, F., Pidgeon, E., & Frith, U. (2003). The relationship between motor control and phonology in dyslexic children. *Journal of Child Psychology and Psychiatry, 44,* 712–722.

Ranganath, C., & Paller, K. A. (1999). Neural correlates of memory retrieval and evaluation. *Cognitive Brain Research, 9,* 209–222.

Rapin, I., & Katzman, R. (1998). Neurobiology of autism. *Annals of Neurology, 43,* 7–14.

Rapoport, M. D., van Reekum, R., & Mayberg, H. (2000). The role of the cerebellum in cognition and behavior. *Journal of Neuropsychiatry, 12,* 193–198.

Rapp, B. (Ed.). (2001). *The handbook of cognitive neuropsychology: What deficits reveal about the human mind.* Philadelphia: Psychology Press.

Rapp, B., & Caramazza, A. (1997). From graphemes to abstract letter shapes: Levels of representation in written spelling. *Journal of Experimental Psychology, 23,* 1130–1152.

Rathvon, N. (1999). *Effective school interventions: Strategies for enhancing academic achievement and social competence.* New York: Guilford Press.

Rayner, K., & Pollatsek, A. (1989). *The psychology of reading.* Englewood Cliffs, NJ: Prentice-Hall.

Read Naturally. (1997). St. Paul, MN: Turman.

Rehabilitation Act (RA), 20 U.S.C. § 794 [statute] (1973a).

Rehabilitation Act (RA), 34 C.F.R. § 104 [regulations] (1973b).

Reisman, R. K. (1977). *Diagnostic teaching of elementary school mathematics: Methods and content.* Chicago: Rand McNally.

Reitan, R. M. (1974). Psychological effects of cerebral lesions in children of early school age. In R. M. Reitan & L. A. Davidson (Eds.), *Clinical neuropsychology: Current status and applications.* Washington, DC: Winston.

Reitan, R. M., & Wolfson, D. (1985). *Neuroanatomy and neuropathology: A clinical guide for neuropsychologists.* Tucson, AZ: Neuropsychology Press.

Reitan, R. M., & Wolfson, D. (1993). *The Halstead–Reitan Neuropsychological Test Battery: Theory and clinical interpretation* (2nd ed.). Tucson, AZ: Neuropsychology Press.

Reschly, D. J., & Gresham, F. (1989). Current neuropsychological diagnosis of learning problems: A leap of faith. In C. R. Reynolds & E. Fletcher-Janzen (Eds.), *Child neuropsychological techniques in diagnosis and treatment* (pp. 503–519). New York: Plenum Press.

Reynolds, C. R. (1985). Measuring the aptitude–achievement discrepancy in learning disability diagnosis. *Remedial and Special Education, 6,* 37–48.

Reynolds, C. R. (1988). Putting the individual into aptitude–treatment interaction. *Exceptional Children, 54,* 324–331.

Reynolds, C. R. (1997). Measurement and statistical problems in neuropsychological assessment of children. In C. R. Reynolds & E. Fletcher-Janzen (Eds.), *Handbook of clinical child neuropsychology* (2nd ed., pp. 180–203). New York: Plenum Press.

Reynolds, C. R. (2002). *Comprehensive Trail-Making Test.* Point Roberts, WA: M.D. Angus & Associates.

Reynolds, C. R., & Bigler, E. D. (1994). *Test of Memory and Learning.* Austin, TX: PRO-ED.

Reynolds, C. R., & Fletcher-Janzen, E. (Eds.). (1997). *Handbook of clinical child neuropsychology* (2nd ed.). New York: Plenum Press.

Reynolds, C. R., & Kamphaus, R. W. (1992). *Behavior Assessment System for Children*. Circle Pines, MN: American Guidance Service.

Reynolds, C. R., Kamphaus, R. W., Rosenthal, B. L., & Hiemenz, J. R. (1997). Applications of the Kaufman Assessment Battery for Children (K-ABC) in neuropsychological assessment. In C. R. Reynolds & E. Fletcher-Janzen (Eds.), *Handbook of clinical child neuropsychology* (2nd ed., pp. 252–269). New York: Plenum Press.

Reynolds, C. R., & Mayfield, J. W. (1999). Neuropsychological assessment in genetically linked neurodevelopmental disorders. In S. Goldstein & C. R. Reynolds (Eds.), *Handbook of neurodevelopmental and genetic disorders in children* (pp. 9–37). New York: Guilford Press.

Reynolds, C. R., Sanchez, S., & Wilson, V. L. (1998). Normative tables for calculating the WISC-III Performance and Full Scale IQs when Symbol Search is substituted for Coding. *Psychological Assessment, 8*, 378–382.

Riccio, C. A., & Hynd, G. W. (2000). Measurable biological substrates to Verbal–Performance differences in Wechsler scores. *School Psychology Quarterly, 15*, 386–399.

Rice, M. L. (1993). Social consequences of specific language impairment. In H. Grimm & H. Skowronek (Eds.), *Language acquisition problems and reading disorders: Aspects of diagnosis and intervention* (pp. 111–128). New York: de Gruyter.

Richards, L., & Chiarello, C. (1997). Activation without selection: Parallel right hemisphere roles in language and intentional movement? *Brain and Language, 57*, 151–178.

Richek, M., Caldwell, J., Jennings, J., & Lerner, J. (1996). *Reading problems: Assessment and teaching strategies* (3rd ed.). Boston: Allyn & Bacon.

Rickard, T. C., Romero, S. G., Basso, G.,. Wharton, C., Flitman, S., & Grafman, J. (2000). The calculating brain: An fMRI study. *Neuropsychologia, 38*, 325–335.

Rico, G. L. (1983). *Writing the natural way*. Boston: Houghton Mifflin.

Riddick, B. (2000). An examination of the relationship between labeling and stimatisation with special reference to dyslexia. *Disability and Society, 15*, 653–667.

Riley-Tillman, T. C., & Chafouleas, S. M. (2002). *Using interventions that exist in the natural environment as a way to enhance social influence and treatment integrity*. Manuscript in preparation.

Rinehart, N. J., Bradshaw, J. L., Brereton, A. V., & Tonge, B. J. (2002). A clinical and neurobehavioural review of high-functioning autism and Asperger's disorder. *Australian and New Zealand Journal of Psychiatry, 36*, 762–770.

Rippon, G., & Brunswick, N. (2000). Trait and state EEG indices of information processing in developmental dyslexia. *International Journal of Psychophysiology, 36*, 251–265.

Rivera, D. M., & Bryant, B. R. (1992). Mathematics instruction for students with special needs. *Intervention in School and Clinic, 28*, 71–86.

Roberts, B. W., & DelVecchio, W. E. (2000). The rank-order consistency of personality traits from childhood to old age: A quantitative review of longitudinal studies. *Psychological Bulletin, 126*, 3–25.

Roberts, R. D., Goff, G. N., Anjoul, F., Kyllonen, P. C., Pallier, G., & Stankov, L. (2000). The Armed Services Vocational Aptitude Battery (ASVAB): Little more than acculturated learning (*Gc*)!? *Learning and Individual Differences, 12*, 81–103.

Robinson, F. P. (1961). *Effective study*. New York: Harper & Row.

Robinson, R. G., Kubos, K. L., Starr, L. B., Rao, K., & Price, T. R. (1984). Mood disorders in stroke patients. Importance of location of lesion. *Brain, 107*, 81–93.

Roeltgen, D. (1985). Agraphia. In K. M. Heilman & E. Valenstein (Eds.), *Clinical neuropsychology* (pp. 75–96). New York: Oxford University Press.

Roid, G. (2003). *Stanford–Binet Intelligence Scale: Fifth Edition*. Itasca, IL: Riverside.

Rojahn, J., & Tasse, M. J. (1996). Psychopathology in mental retardation. In J. W. Jacobson & J. A. Mulick (Eds.), *Manual of diagnosis and professional practice in mental retardation* (pp. 147–156). Washington, DC. American Psychological Association.

Roland, P. E., & Friberg, L. (1985). Localization of cortical areas activated by thinking. *Journal of Neurophysiology, 53*, 1219–1243.

Rosenthal, R., & Jacobson, L. (1968). *Pygmalion in the classroom*. New York: Holt, Rinehart & Winston.

Ross, R. P. (1995). Implementing intervention assistance teams. In A. Thomas & J. Grimes (Eds.), *Best practices in school psychology III* (pp. 227–238). Washington, DC: National Association of School Psychologists.

Rosselli, M., & Ardila, A. (1989). Calculation deficit in patients with right and left hemisphere damage. *Neuropsychologia, 27*, 607–617.

Rourke, B. P. (1987). Syndrome of nonverbal learning disabilities: The final common pathway of white-matter disease/dysfunction? *The Clinical Neuropsychologist, 1*, 209–234.

Rourke, B. P. (1988). The syndrome of nonverbal learning disabilities: Developmental manifestations in neurological disease, disorder, and dysfunction. *The Clinical Neuropsychologist, 2,* 293–330.

Rourke, B. P. (1989). *Nonverbal learning disabilities: The syndrome and the model.* New York: Guilford Press.

Rourke, B. P. (1993). Arithmetic learning disabilities, specific and otherwise: A neuropsychological perspective.
Journal of Learning Disabilities, 26, 214–226.

Rourke, B. P. (1994). Neuropsychological assessment of children with learning disabilities. In G. R. Lyon (Ed.),
Frames of reference for the assessment of learning disabilities (pp.475–509). Baltimore, MD: Brookes.

Rourke, B. P. (2000). Neuropsychological and psychosocial subtyping: A review of investigations within the University of Windsor laboratory. *Canadian Psychology, 41,* 34–51.

Rourke, B. P., & Fuerst, D. R. (1991). *Learning disabilities and psychosocial functioning: A neuropsychological perspective.* New York: Guilford Press.

Rourke, B. P., & Fuerst, D. R. (1996). Psychological dimensions of learning disability subtypes. *Assessment, 3,* 277–
290.

Ruais, R. W. (1978). A low-stress algorithm for fractions. *Mathematics Teacher, 71,* 258–260.

Rubia, K. (2002). The dynamic approach to neurodevelopmental psychiatric disorders: Use of fMRI combined
with neuropsychology to elucidate the dynamics of psychiatric disorders, exemplified in ADHD and schizophrenia. *Behavioural Brain Research, 130,* 47–56.

Rubia, K., Overmeyer, S. O., Taylor, E., Brammer, M., Williams, S. C. R., Simmons, A., et al. (1999). Hypofrontality
in attention deficit hyperactivity disorder during higher order motor control: A study with functional MRI.
American Journal of Psychiatry, 156, 891–896.

Rucklidge, J. J., & Tannock, R. (2002). Neuropsychological profiles of adolescents with ADHD: Effects of reading
difficulties and gender. *Journal of Child Psychology and Psychiatry, 43,* 988–1003.

Rueckert, L., Appollonio, I., Grafman, J., Jezzard, P., Johnson, R., Le Bihan, D., et al. (1994). Magnetic resonance
imaging functional activation of left frontal cortex during covert word production. *Journal of Neuroimaging,
4,* 67–70.

Rueckert, L., Lange, N., Partiot, A., Appollonio, I., Litvan, I., Le Bihan, D., et al. (1996). Visualizing cortical activation during mental calculation with functional MRI. *Neuroimage, 3,* 97–103.

Rumsey, J. M., Andreason, P., Zametkin, A. J., Aquino, T., King, A. C., Hamburger, S. D., et al. (1992). Failure to activate the left temporoparietal cortex in dyslexia: An oxygen 15 positron emission tomographic study. *Archives of Neurology, 49,* 527–534.

Rumsey, J. M., Horwitz, B., Donohue, B. C., Nace, K. L., Maisong, J. M., & Andreason, P. (1997). Phonologic and
orthographic components of word recognition: A PET-rCBF study. *Brain, 120,* 739–759.

Rumsey, J. M., Horwitz, B., Donohue, B. C., Nace, K. L., Maisong, J. M., & Andreason, P. (1999). A functional lesion in developmental dyslexia: Left and angular gyral blood flow predicts severity. *Brain and Language, 70,*
187–204.

Rumsey, J. M., Zametkin, A. J., Andreason, P., Hanahan, A. P., Hamburger, S. D., King, A. D., et al. (1994). Normal
activation of frontotemporal language cortex in dyslexia, as measured with oxygen 15 positron emission tomography. *Archives of Neurology, 51,* 27–38.

Rushworth, M. F. S., Paus, T., & Sipila, P. K. (2001). Attention systems and the organization of the human parietal
cortex. *Journal of Neuroscience, 21,* 5262–5271.

Rye, J. (1982). *Cloze procedure and the teaching of reading.* London: Heinemann.

Sachs, A. (1983). The effects of three prereading activities on learning disabled students' reading comprehension.
Learning Disability Quarterly, 6, 248–251.

Sackheim, H. A., Decina, P., & Malitz, S. (1982). Functional brain asymmetry and affective disorders. *Adolescent
Psychiatry, 10,* 320–335.

Samuels, S. J. (1979). The method of repeated readings. *Reading Teacher, 32,* 403–408.

Samuelsson, S. (2000). Converging evidence for the role of occiptal regions in orthographic processing: A case of
developmental surface dyslexia. *Neuropsychologia, 38,* 351–362.

Sandler, A. D., Watson, T. E., Footo, M., Levine, M. D., Coleman, W. L., & Hooper, S. R. (1992). Neurodevelopmental study of writing disorders in middle childhood. *Journal of Developmental and Behavioral Pediatrics, 13,* 17–23.

Sattler, J. M. (2001). *Assessment of children: Cognitive applications.* La Mesa, CA: Author.

Sattler, J. M. (2002). *Assessment of children: Behavioral and clinical applications.* La Mesa, CA: Author.

Saudargas, R. A., & Lentz, J. (1986). Estimating percentage of time and rate via direct observation: A suggested
observational procedure and format. *School Psychology Review, 15*(1), 36–48.

Sbordone, R. J. (2000). The assessment interview in clinical neuropsychology. In G. Groth-Marnat (Ed.), *Neuropsychological assessment in clinical practice* (pp. 94–128). New York: Wiley.

Sbordone, R. J., & Purisch, A. D. (1996). Hazards of blind analysis of neuropsychological test data in assessing cognitive disability: The role of confounding factors. *Neurorehabilitation, 1*, 15–26.

Scarborough, H. S., & Domgaard, R. M. (1998). *An exploration of the relationship between reading and rapid serial naming.* Paper presented at the meeting of the Society for the Scientific Study of Reading, San Diego, CA.

Scheres, A., Oosterlaan, J., & Sergeant, J. A. (2001). Response execution and inhibition in children with AD/HD and other disruptive disorders: The role of behavioural activation. *Journal of Child Psychology and Psychiatry, 42*, 347–357.

Schneider, F., Gur, R. E., Alavi, A., Seligman, M. E. P., Mozley, L. H., Smith, R. J., et al. (1996). Cerebral blood flow changes in limbic regions induced by unsolvable anagram tasks. *American Journal of Psychiatry, 153*, 206–212.

Schubotz, R. I., & von Cramon, D. Y. (2001). Functional organization of the lateral premotor cortex: fMRI reveals different regions activated by anticipation of object properties, location and speed. *Cognitive Brain Research, 11*, 97–112.

Schultz, R. T., Gauthier, I., Klin, A., Fulbright, R. K., Anderson, A. W., Volkmar, F., et al. (2000). Abnormal ventral temporal cortical activity during face discrimination among individuals with autism and Asperger syndrome. *Archives of General Psychiatry, 57*, 331–340.

Schumaker, J. B., Deshler, D. D., Alley, G. R., Warner, M. M., & Denton, P. H. (1982). Multipass: A learning strategy for improving reading comprehension. *Learning Disability Quarterly, 5*, 295–304.

Schumaker, J. B., Deshler, D. D., & Denton, P. (1984). *The learning strategies curriculum: The paraphrasing strategy.* Lawrence: University of Kansas, Center for Research on Learning.

Schumaker, J. B., Nolan, S. M., & Deshler, D. D. (1985). *Learning strategies curriculum: The error monitoring strategy.* Lawrence: University of Kansas, Center for Research on Learning.

Schumaker, J. B., & Sheldon, J. (1985). *The sentence writing strategy.* Lawrence: University of Kansas, Center for Research on Learning.

Schwartz, S., & Baldo, J. (2001). Distinct patterns of word retrieval in right and left frontal lobe patients: A multidimensional perspective. *Neuropsychologia, 39*, 1209–1217.

Seguin, J. R., Pihl, R. O., Harden, P. W., Tremblay, R. E., & Boulerice, B. (1995). Cognitive and neuropsychological characteristics of physically aggressive boys. *Journal of Abnormal Child Psychology, 104*, 614–625.

Seidman, L. J., Biederman, J., Faraone, S. V., Weber, W., & Ouellette, C. (1997). Toward defining a neuropsychology of attention deficit-hyperactivity disorder: Performance of children and adolescents from a large clinically referred sample. *Journal of Consulting and Clinical Psychology, 65*, 150–160.

Seidman, L. J., Biederman, J., Monuteauz, M. C., Doyle, A. E., & Faraone, S. V. (2001). Learning disabilities and executive dysfunction in boys with attention-deficit/hyperactivity disorder. *Neuropsychology, 15*, 544–556.

Semel, E., Wiig, E. H., & Secord, W. (2003). *Clinical Evaluation of Language Fundamentals—Fourth Edition.* San Antonio, TX: Psychological Corporation.

Semrud-Clikeman, M., Filipek, P. A., Biederman, J., Steingard, R., Kennedy, D., Renshaw, P., et al. (1994). Attention-deficit hyperactivity disorder: Magnetic resonance imaging morphometric analysis of the corpus callosum. *Journal of the American Academy of Child and Adolescent Psychiatry, 33*, 875–881.

Semrud-Clikeman, M., & Hynd, G. W. (1990). Right hemisphere dysfunction in nonverbal learning disabilities: Social, academic, and adaptive functioning in adults and children. *Psychological Bulletin, 107*, 196–209.

Semrud-Clikeman, M., Steingard, R. J., Filipek, P., Biederman, J., Bekken, K., & Renshaw, P. F. (2000). Using MRI to examine brain–behavior relationships in males with attention deficit disorder with hyperactivity. *Journal of the American Academy of Child and Adolescent Psychiatry, 39*, 477–484.

Sergeant, J. A., Geurts, H., & Oosterlaan, J. (2002). How specific is a deficit in executive functioning for attention-deficit/hyperactivity disorder? *Behavioural Brain Research, 130*, 3–28.

Sergent, J. (1995). Hemispheric contribution to face processing: Patterns of convergence and divergence. In R. J. Davidson & K. Hugdahl (Eds.), *Brain asymmetry* (pp. 157–181). Cambridge, MA: MIT Press.

Sergent, J., Zuck, E., Terriah, S., & MacDonald, B. (1992). Distributed neural network underlying musical sight-reading and keyboard performance. *Science, 257*, 106–109.

Seron, X., & Fayol, M. (1994). Number transcoding in children: A functional analysis. *British Journal of Developmental Psychology, 12*, 281–300.

Shadmehr, R., & Holcomb, H. H. (1997). Neural correlates of motor memory consolidation. *Science, 277*, 821–825.

Shaffer, D., Schonfeld, L. O'Conner, P. A., Stokman, C., Trautman, P., Shafer, S., et al. (1985). Neurological soft signs. *Archives of General Psychology, 42*, 342–351.

Shalev, R. S., Manor, O., Amir, N., Wertman-Elad, R., & Gross-Tsur, V. (1995). Developmental dyscalculia and brain laterality. *Cortex, 31*, 357–365.

Shallice, T. (1982). Specific impairment in planning. *Philosophical Transactions of the Royal Society of London, 298*, 199–209.

Shallice, T. (1989). *From neuropsychology to mental structure*. New York: Cambridge University Press.

Shallice, T., Marzocchi, G. M., Coser, S., Del Savio, M., Meuter, R. F., & Rumiati, R. I. (2002). Executive function profile of children with attention deficit hyperactivity disorder. *Developmental Neuropsychology, 21*, 43–71.

Shanker, J. L., & Ekwall, E. E. (1998). *Locating and correcting reading difficulties* (7th ed.). Upper Saddle River, NJ: Prentice-Hall.

Shaywitz, B. A., Fletcher, J. M., Holahan, J. M., & Shaywitz, S. E. (1992). Discrepancy compared to low achievement definitions of reading disability: Results from the Connecticut Longitudinal Study. *Journal of Learning Disabilities, 25*, 639–648.

Shaywitz, B. A., Fletcher, J. M., & Shaywitz, S. E. (1995). Defining and classifying learning disabilities and attention-deficit/hyperactivity disorder. *Journal of Child Neurology, 10*, 50–57.

Shaywitz, B. A., Shaywitz, S. E., Pugh, K. R., Mencl, W. E., Fulbright, R. K., Skuldlarski, P., et al. (2002). Disruption of posterior brain systems for reading in children with developmental dyslexia. *Biological Psychiatry, 53*, 101–110.

Shaywitz, S. E., Escobar, M. D., Shaywitz, B. A., Fletcher, J. M., & Makuch, R. (1992). Evidence that dyslexia may represent the lower tail of a normal distribution of reading ability. *New England Journal of Medicine, 326*, 145–150.

Shaywitz, S. E., Fletcher, J. M., & Shaywitz, B. A. (1994). Issues in the defintion and classification of attention deficit disorder. *Topics in Language Disorders, 14*, 1–25.

Shaywitz, S. E., Shaywitz, B. A., Fulbright, R. K., Skudlarski, P., Mencl, W. E., Constable, R. T., et al. (2003). Neural systems for compensation and persistence: Young adult outcome of childhood reading disability. *Biological Psychiatry, 54*, 25–33.

Shaywitz, S. E., Shaywitz, B. A., Pugh, K. R., Fulbright, R. K., Constable, R. T., Mencl, W. E., et al. (1998). Functional disruption in the organization of the brain for reading in dyslexia. *Proceedings of the National Academy of Sciences USA, 95*, 2636–2641.

Shenal, B. V., Harrison, D. W., & Demaree, H. A. (2003). The neuropsychology of depression: A literature review and preliminary model. *Neuropsychology Review, 13*, 33–42.

Sheridan, S. M., & Gutkin, T. B. (2000). The ecology of school psychology: Examining and changing our paradigm for the 21st century. *School Psychology Review, 29*, 485–502.

Sheslow, D., & Adams, W. (1990). *Wide Range Assessment of Memory and Learning*. Wilmington, DE: Jastak Associates.

Shimamura, A. P. (2000). The role of the prefrontal cortex in dynamic filtering. *Psychobiology, 28*, 207–218.

Shinn, M. R. (Ed.). (1989). *Curriculum-based measurement: Assessing special children*. New York: Guilford Press.

Shuren, J. E. Maher, L. M., & Heilman, K. M. (1996). The role of visual imagery in spelling. *Brain and Language, 52*, 365–372.

Siebner, H. R., Limmer, C., Peinemann, A., Bartenstein, P., Drzezga, A., & Conrad, B. (2001). Brain correlates of fast and slow handwriting in humans: A PET–performance correlation analysis. *European Journal of Neuroscience, 14*, 726–736.

Siegel, L. S. (1992). Dyslexic vs. poor readers: Is there a difference? *Journal of Learning Disabilities, 25*, 618–629.

Siegel, L. S. (1993). Phonological processing deficits as the basis of a reading disability. *Developmental Review, 13*, 246–257.

Silbert, J., Carnine, D., & Stein, M. (1990). *Direct instruction mathematics* (2nd ed.). Columbus, OH: Merrill.

Silka, V. R., & Hauser, M. J. (1997). Psychiatric assessment of the person with mental retardation. *Psychiatric Annals, 27*, 162–169.

Silver, L. B. (1990). ADHD: Is it a learning disability or related disorder? *Journal of Learning Disabilities, 23*, 394–397.

Simmonds, E. P. M. (1992). The effects of teacher training and implementation of two methods of improving the comprehension skills of students with learning disabilities. *Learning Disabilities Research and Practice, 7*, 194–198.

Simmons, D. C., Chard, D., & Kame'enui, E. J. (1996). Translating research into basal reading programs: Applications of curriculum design. *LD Forum, 20*, 9–13.

Simmons, D. C., Gunn, B., Smith, S. B., & Kame'enui, E. J. (1995). Phonological awareness: Applications of instructional design. *LD Forum, 19*, 7–9.

Simos, P. G., & Molfese, D. L. (1997). Electrophysiological responses from a temporal order continuum in the newborn infant. *Neuropsychologia, 35*, 89–98.

Sinatra, R. C., Berg, D., & Dunn, R. (1985). Semantic mapping improves reading comprehension of learning disabled students. *Teaching Exceptional Children, 17*, 310–314.

Singer, B. D. (1995). Written language development and disorders: Selected principles, patterns, and intervention possibilities. *Topics in Language Disorders, 16*, 83–98.

Singer, H. S., Reiss, A. L., Brown, J. E., Aylward, E. H., Shih, B., Chee, E., et al. (1993). Volumetric MRI changes in basal ganglia of children with Tourette's syndrome. *Neurology, 43*, 950–956.

Sirigu, A., Cohen, L., Zalla, T., Pradat-Dichl, P., Van Eeckhout, P., Grafman, J., et al. (1998). Distinct frontal regions for processing sentence syntax and story grammar. *Cortex, 34*, 771–778.

Skinner, B. F. (1966). What is the experimental analysis of behavior? *Journal of the Experimental Analysis of Behavior, 9*(3), 213–218.

Slattery, M. J., Garvey, M. A., & Swedo, S. E. (2001). Frontal–subcortical circuits: A functional developmental approach. In D. G. Lichter & J. L. Cummings (Eds.), *Frontal–subcortical circuits in psychiatric and neurological disorders* (pp. 314–333). New York: Guilford Press.

Smart, D., Sanson, A., & Prior, M. (1996). Connections between reading disability and behavior problems: Testing temporal and causal hypotheses. *Journal of Abnormal Child Psychology, 24*, 363–383.

Smith, C. R. (1998). *Learning disabilities: The interaction of learner, task, and setting* (4th ed.). Boston: Allyn & Bacon.

Smith, D. D. (1981). *Teaching the learning disabled.* Englewood Cliffs, NJ: Prentice-Hall.

Smith, E. E. & Jonides, J. (1999). Storage and executive processes in the frontal lobes. *Science, 283*, 1657–1661.

Sofie, C. A., & Riccio, C. A. (2002). A comparison of multiple methods for the identification of children with reading disabilities. *Journal of Learning Disabilities, 35*, 234–244.

Sonuga-Barke, E. J. S. (1998). Categorical model in child psychopathology: A conceptual and empirical analysis. *Journal of Child Psychology and Psychiatry, 39*, 115–133.

Sosniak, L. A., & Ethington, C. A. (1994). When teaching problem solving proceeds successfully in U. S. eighth-grade classrooms. In I. Westbury, C. A. Ethington, L. A. Sosniak, & D. P. Baker (Eds.), *In search of more effective mathematics education* (pp. 33–60). Norwood, NJ: Ablex.

Spearman, C. (1904). "General intelligence," objectively determined and measured. *American Journal of Psychology, 15*, 201–293.

Speece, D. L. (1990). Aptitude–treatment interactions: Bad rap or bad idea? *Journal of Special Education, 24*, 139–149.

Spreen, O. (1989). The relationship between learning disability, emotional disorders, and neuropsychology: Some results and observations. *Journal of Clinical and Experimental Neuropsychology, 11*, 117–140.

Spreen, O. (2001). Learning disabilities and their neurological foundations, theories, and subtypes. In A. S. Kaufman & N. L. Kaufman (Eds.), *Specific learning disabilities and difficulties in children and adolescents: Psychological assessment and evaluation* (pp. 283–308). New York: Cambridge University Press.

Spreen, O., & Benton, A. L. (1977). *Neurosensory Center Comprehensive Examination for Aphasia (NCCEA).* Victoria, British Columbia, Canada: University of Victoria Neuropsychology Laboratory.

Spreen, O., Risser, A. H., & Edgell, D. (1995). *Developmental neuropsychology.* New York: Oxford University Press.

Spreen, O., & Strauss, E. (1998). *A compendium of neuropsychological tests: Administration, norms, and commentary* (2nd ed.). New York: Oxford University Press.

Springer, S. P., & Deutsch, G. (1998). *Left brain, right brain: Perspectives from cognitive neuroscience* (5th ed.). New York: Freeman.

St. George, M., Kutas, M., Martinez, A., & Sereno, M. I. (1999). Semantic integration in reading: Engagement of the right hemisphere during discourse processing. *Brain, 122*, 1317–1325.

Staines, W. R., Padilla, M., & Knight, R. T. (2002). Frontal–parietal event-related potential chages associated with practising a novel visuomotor task. *Cognitive Brain Research, 13*, 195–202.

Stanescu-Cosson, R., Pinel, P., van de Moortele, P., Hbihan, D., Cohen, L., & Dehaene, S. (2000). Understanding dissociations in dyscalcuia: A brain imaging study of the impact of number size on the cerebral networks for exact and approximate calculation. *Brain, 123*, 2240–2255.

Stanovich, K. E. (1994). Constructivism in reading education. *Journal of Special Education, 28*, 259–274.

Stanovich, K. E., & Siegel, L. S. (1994). Phenotypic performanc profile of children with reading disability: A regression based test of the phonological–core variable difference model. *Journal of Educational Psychology, 86,* 24–53.

Starkstein, S. E., & Kremer, J. (2001). The disinhibition syndrome and frontal–subcortical circuits. In D. G. Lichter & J. L. Cummings (Eds.), *Frontal–subcortical circuits in psychiatric and neurological disorders* (pp. 163–176). New York: Guilford Press.

Stein, J. F. (2001). The neurobiology of reading difficulties. In M. Wolf (Ed.), *Dyslexia, fluency, and the brain* (pp. 3–22). Timonium, MD: York Press.

Stein, J. F., & McAnally, K. I. (1996). Impaired auditory temporal processing in dyslexics. *Irish Journal of Psychology, 16,* 220–228.

Stein, M. (1983). Finger spelling: A kinesthetic aid to phonetic spelling. *Academic Therapy, 18,* 305–313.

Stemmer, B., & Joanette, Y. (1998). The interpretation of narrative discourse of brain-damaged individuals within a framework of a multilevel discourse model. In M. Beeman & C. Chiarello (Eds.), *Right hemisphere language comprehension: Perspectives from cognitive neuroscience* (pp. 329–348). Mahwah, NJ: Erlbaum.

Stephens, T. M. (1977). *Teaching skills to children with learning and behavior disorders.* Columbus, OH: Merrill.

Sternberg, R. J. (1997). The triarchic theory of intelligence. In D. P. Flanagan, J. L. Genshaft, & P. L. Harrison (Eds.), *Contemporary intellectual assessment: Theories, tests, and issues* (pp. 92–104). New York: Guilford Press.

Sternberg, R. J., Grigorenko, E. L., Ferrari, M., & Clinkenbeard, P. (1999). A triarchic analysis of an aptitude–treatment interaction. *European Journal of Psychological Assessment, 15,* 3–13.

Stevens, D. D., & Englert, C. S. (1993). Making writing strategies work. *Teaching Exceptional Children, 26,* 34–39.

Stewart, S. R., & Cegelka, P. T. (1995). Teaching reading and spelling. In P. T. Cegleka & W. H. Berdine (Eds.), *Effective instruction for students with learning difficulties* (pp. 265–301). Boston: Allyn & Bacon.

Strauss, E., Semenza, C., Hunter, M., Hermann, B., Barr, W., Chelune, G., et al. (2000). Left anterior lobectomy and category-specific naming. *Brain and Cognition, 43,* 403–406.

Stringer, A. Y., & Nadolne, M. J. (2000). Neuropsychological assessment: Contexts for contemporary clinical practice. In G. Groth-Marnat (Ed.), *Neuropsychological assessment in clinical practice: A guide to test interpretation and integration* (pp. 26–47). New York: Wiley.

Stromswold, K., Caplan, D., Alpert, N., & Rauch, S. (1996). Localization of syntactic comprehension by positron emission tomography. *Brain and Language, 52,* 452–473.

Strong, W. (1983). *Sentence combining: A composing book* (2nd ed.). New York: Random House.

Suchan, B., Yagliez, L., Wunderlich, G., Canavan, A. G. M., Herzog, H., Tellmann, L., et al. (2002). Hemispheric dissociation of visual-pattern processing and visual rotation. *Behavioral Brain Research, 136,* 533–544.

Sunderland, A., & Sluman, S. (2000). Ideomotor apraxia, visuomotor control, and the explicit representation of posture. *Neuropsychologia, 38,* 923–934.

Surian, L., & Siegal, M. (2001). Sources of performance on theory of the mind tasks in right hemisphere damaged patients. *Brain and Language, 78,* 224–232.

Sussman, K., & Lewandowski, L. (1990). Left hemisphere dysfunction in autism: What are we measuring? *Archives of Clinical Neuropsychology, 5,* 137–146.

Swanson, H. L., & Alexander, J. E. (1997). Cognitive processes as predictors of word recognition and reading comprehension in learning-disabled and skilled readers: Revisiting the specificity hypothesis. *Journal of Educational Psychology, 89,* 128–158.

Swanson, H. L., & Ashbaker, M. H. (2000). Working memory, short-term memory, speech rate, word recognition, and reading comprehension in learning disabled readers: Does the executive system have a role? *Intelligence, 28,* 1–30.

Swanson, H. L., Hoskyn, M., & Lee, C. (1999). *Interventions for students with learning disabilities: A meta-analysis of treatment outcomes.* New York: Guilford Press.

Swanson, H. L., Mink, J., & Bocian, K. M. (1999). Cognitive processing deficits in poor readers with symptoms of reading disabilities and ADHD: More alike than different? *Journal of Educational Psychology, 91,* 321–333.

Swanson, J. M., Cantwell, D., Lerner, M., McBurnett, K., & Hanna, G. (1991). Effects of stimulant medication on learning in children with ADHD. *Journal of Learning Disabilities, 24,* 219–230.

Swanson, J. M., Castellanos, F. X., Murias, M., LaHoste, G., & Kennedy, J. (1998). Cognitive neuroscience of attention deficit hyperactivity disorder and hyperkinetic disorder. *Current Opinion in Neurobiology, 8,* 263–271.

Szatmari, P., Offord, D. R., Siegel, L. S., Finlayson, M. A. J., & Tuff, L. (1990). The clinical significance of neurocognitive impairments among children with psychiatric disorders: Diagnosis and situational specificity. *Journal of Child Psychology and Psychiatry, 31,* 287–299.

Talcott, J. B., Hansen, P. C., Elikem, L. A., & Stein, J. F. (2000). Visual motion sensitivity in dyslexia: Evidence for temporal and motion energy integration deficits. *Neuropsychologia, 38*, 935–943.

Talcott, J. B., Witton, C., McClean, M. Hansen, P. C. Rees, A., Green, G. R. G., & Stein, J. F. (2000). Visual and auditory transient sensitivity determines decoding skills. *Proceedings of the National Academy of Sciences, 97*, 2952.

Tallal, P., Miller, S., & Fitch, R. H. (1993). Neurobiological basis of speech: A case for the pre-eminence of temporal processing. *Annals of the New York Academy of Sciences, 682*, 27–47.

Tallal, P., Sainburg, R. L., & Jernigan, T. (1991). The neuropathology of developmental dysphasia: Behavioral, morphological, and physiological evidence for a pervasive temporal processing disorder. *Reading and Writing: An Interdisciplinary Journal, 3*, 363–377.

Tannock, R. (1998). Attention deficit hyperactivity disorder: Advances in cognitive, neurobiological, and genetic research. *Journal of Child Psychology and Psychiatry, 39*, 65–99.

Taylor, H. G. (1989). Learning disabilities. In E. J. Mash & R. A. Barkley (Eds.), *Treatment of childhood disorders* (pp. 347–380). New York: Guilford Press.

Taylor, H. G. (1996). Critical issues and future directions in the development of theories, models, and measurements for attention, memory, and executive function. In G. R. Lyon & N. A. Krasnegor (Eds.), *Attention, memory, and executive function* (pp. 399–412). Baltimore: Brookes.

Taylor, H. G., & Fletcher, J. M. (1990). Neuropsychological assessment of children. In G. Goldstein & H. Hersen (Eds.), *Handbook of psychological assessment* (2nd ed., pp. 228–255). New York: Pergamon Press.

Teeter, P. A. (1997). Neurocognitive interventions for childhood and adolescent disorders: A transactional model. In C. R. Reynolds & E. Fletcher-Janzen (Eds.), *Handbook of clinical child neuropsychology* (2nd ed., pp. 387–417). New York: Plenum Press.

Teeter, P. A., & Semrud-Clikeman, M. (1995). Integrating neurobiological, psychosocial, and behavioral paradigms: A transactional model for the study of ADHD. *Archives of Clinical Neuropsychology, 10*, 433–461.

Teichner, G., & Golden, C. J. (2000). The relationship of neuropsychological impairment to conduct disorder in adolescence: A conceptual review. *Aggression and Violent Behavior, 5*, 509–528.

Telzrow, C. F. (1989). Neuropsychological applications of common educational and psychological tests. In C. R. Reynolds, & E. Fletcher-Janzen (Eds.), *Handbook of clinical child neuropsychology* (pp. 227–245). New York: Plenum Press.

Templeton, S. (1986). Synthesis of research on the learning and teaching of spelling. *Educational Leadership, 43*, 73–78.

Terman, L. M. (1916). *The measurement of intelligence.* Boston: Houghton Mifflin.

Teuber, H. L. (1975). Recovery of function after brain injury in man. *Ciba Foundation Symposium, 34*, 159–190.

Teuber, H. L., & Rudel, R. G. (1962). Behavior after cerebral lesions in children and adults. *Developmental Medicine and Child Neurology, 4*, 3–20.

Thatcher, R. W. (1992). Cyclical cortical reorganization during early childhood. *Brain and Cognition, 20*, 24–50.

Thomas, A., & Grimes, J. (Eds.). (2002). *Best practices in school psychology IV* (Vol. 1). Bethesda, MD: National Association of School Psychologists.

Thorndike, R. L., Hagen, E. P., & Sattler, J. M. (1986). *The Stanford–Binet Intelligence Scale: Fourth Edition. Guide for administration and scoring.* Chicago: Riverside.

Thornton, C. A., & Toohey, M. A. (1985). Basic math facts: Guidelines for teaching and learning. *Learning Disabilities Focus, 1*, 44–57.

Thurstone, L. L. (1938). *Primary mental abilities.* Chicago: University of Chicago Press.

Tindal, G., & Parker, R. (1991). Identifying measures for evaluating written expression. *Learning Disabilities Research and Practice, 6*, 211–218.

Tomblin, J. B., Zhang, X., & Buckwalter, P. (2000). The association of reading disability, behavioral disorders, and language impairment among second-grade children. *Journal of Child Psychology and Psychiatry, 41*, 473–482.

Tompkins, G. E. (1998). *Language arts: Content and teaching strategies* (4th ed.). Upper Saddle River, NJ: Merrill/ Prentice Hall.

Tompkins, G. E., & Friend, M. (1985). On your mark, get set, write! *Teaching Exceptional Children, 18*, 82–89.

Torgesen, J. K. (1996). A model of memory from an information processing perspective: The special case of phonological memory. In G. R. Lyon & N. A. Krasnegor (Eds.), *Attention, memory, and executive function* (pp. 157–184). Baltimore: Brookes.

Torgesen, J. K. (2000). Individual differences in response to early interventions in reading: The lingering problem of treatment resisters. *Learning Disabilities Research and Practice, 15*, 55–64.

Torgesen, J. K., Rashotte, C. A., & Alexander, A. W. (2001). Principles of fluency instruction in reading: Relationship with established empirical outcomes. In M. Wolf (Ed.), *Dyslexia, fluency, and the brain* (pp. 333–356). Timonium, MD: York Press.

Torgesen, J. K., Wagner, R. K., & Rashotte, C. A. (1994). Longitudinal studies of phonological processing and reading. *Journal of Learning Disabilities, 27*, 276–286.

Torgesen, J. K., Wagner, R. K., Rashotte, C. A., Burgess, S., & Hecht, S. (1997). Contributions of phonological awareness and rapid automatic naming ability to the growth of word-readng skills in second- to fifth-grade children. *Scientific Studies of Reading, 1*, 161–185.

Toupin, J., Dery, M., Pauze, R., Mercier, H., & Fortin, L. (2000). Cognitive and familial contributions to conduct disorder in children. *Journal of Child Psychology and Psychiatry, 41*, 333–344.

Tramontana, M. G., & Hooper, S. R. (1997). Neuropsychology of childhood psychopathology. In C. R. Reynolds & E. Fletcher-Janzen (Eds.), *Handbook of clinical child neuropsychology* (2nd ed., pp. 120–139). New York: Plenum Press.

Tramontana, M. G., Hooper, S. R., & Nardolillo, E. M. (1988). Behavioral manifestations of neuropsychological impairments in children with psychiatric disorders. *Archives of Clinical Neuropsychology, 3*, 369–374.

Treiman, R., Cassar, M., & Zukowski, A. (1994). What types of linguistic information do children use in spelling?: The case of flaps. *Child Development, 65*, 1318–1337.

Tsai, L. (1992). Diagnostic issues in high-functioning autism. In E. Schopler & G. B Mesibov (Eds.), *High-functioning individuals with autism* (pp. 11–40). New York: Plenum Press.

Tulving, E., Kapur, S., Craik, F. I. M., Moscovitch, M., & Houle, S. (1994). Hemispheric encoding/retrieval asymmetry in episodic memory: Positron emission tomography findings. *Proceeedings of the National Academy of Sciences USA, 91*, 2016–2020.

Tulving, E., & Markowitsch, H. J. (1997). Memory beyond the hippocampus. *Current Opinion in Neurobiology, 7*, 209–216.

Underhill, R. G., Uprichard, A. E., & Heddens, J. W. (1980). *Diagnosing mathematical difficulties*. Columbus, OH: Merrill.

Ungerleider, L. G., & Mishkin, M. (1982). Two cortical visual systems. In D. J. Engle, M. A. Goodale, & R. J. Mansfield (Eds.), *Analysis of visual behavior* (pp. 549–586). Cambridge, MA: MIT Press.

Vaidya, C. J., Austin, G., Kirkorian, G., Ridlehuber, H. W., Desmond, J. E., Glover, G. H., et al. (1998). Selective effects of methylphenidate in attention deficit hyperactivity disorder: A functional magnetic resonance study. *Proceedings of the National Academy of Sciences USA, 95*, 14494–14499.

Vandenberghe, R., Price, C., Wise, R., Josephs, O., & Frackowiak, R. S. (1996). Functional anatomy of a common semantic system for words and pictures. *Nature, 383*, 254–256.

Vanderwood, M. L., McGrew, K. S., Flanagan, D. P., & Keith, T. Z. (2001). The contribution of general and specific cognitive abilities to reading achievement. *Learning and Individual Differences, 13*, 159–188.

Van Lancker, D. (1997). Rags to riches: Our increasing appreciation of cognitive and communicative abilities of the right hemisphere. *Brain and Language, 57*, 1–11.

van Mier, H., Tempel, L. W., Perlmutter, J. S., Raichle, M. E., & Petersen, S. E. (1998). Changes in brain activity during motor learning measured with PET: Effects of hand of performance and practice. *Journal of Neurophysiology, 80*, 2177–2199.

Vaughn, S., & Wilson, C. (1994). Mathematics assessment for students with learning disabilities. In G. R. Lyon (Ed.), *Frames of reference for the assessment of learning disabilities* (pp. 459–472). Baltimore: Brookes.

Vellutino, F. R., Scanlon, D. M., & Tanzman, M. S. (1994). Components of reading ability: Issues and problems in operationalizing word identification, phonological coding, and orthographic coding. In G. R. Lyon (Ed.), *Frames of reference for the assessment of learning disabilities* (pp. 279–332). Baltimore: Brookes.

Vicari, S., Marotta, L., Menghini, D., Molinari, M., & Petrosini, D. (2003). Implicit learning deficit in children with developmental dyslexia. *Neuropsychologia, 41*, 108–114.

Vitiello, B. (2001). Psychopharmacology for young children: Clinical needs and research opportunities. *Pediatrics, 108*, 983–989.

Voeller, K. K. S. (1986). Right hemisphere deficit syndrome in children. *American Journal of Psychiatry, 143*, 1004–1009.

Voeller, K. K. S. (1994). Techniques for measuring social competence in children. In G. R. Lyon (Ed.), *Frames of reference for the assessment of learning disabilities* (pp. 523–554). Baltimore: Brookes.

Voeller, K. K. S. (2001). Attention-deficit/hyperactivity disorder as a frontal–subcortical disorder. In D. G. Lichter & J. L. Cummings (Eds.), *Frontal–subcortical circuits in psychiatric and neurological disorders* (pp. 334–371). New York: Guilford Press.

Volkmar, F. R., Klin, A., Schultz, R. T., Rubin, E., & Bronen, R. (2000). Asperger's disorder. *American Journal of Psychiatry, 157,* 262–267.

Waber, D. P., Weiler, M. D., Wolff, P. H., Bellinger, D., Marcus, D. J., Ariel, R., et al. (2001). Processing of rapid auditory stimuli in school-age children referred for evaluation of learning disorders. *Child Development, 72,* 37–49.

Wagner, R. K., Torgesen, J. K., & Rashotte, C. A. (1999). *Comprehensive Test of Phonological Processing*. Austin, TX: PRO-ED.

Walsh, A., Petee, T. A., & Beyer, J. A. (1987). Intellectual imbalance and delinquency: Comparing high Verbal and high Performance IQ delinquents. *Criminal Justice and Behavior, 14,* 370–379.

Warner, M. M., Alley, G. R., Schumaker, J. B., Deshler, D. D., & Clark, F. L. (1980). *An epidemiological study of learning disabled adolescents in secondary schools: Achievement and ability, socioeconomic status, and school experiences*. Lawrence: University of Kansas Center for Research on Learning.

Watanabe, A. (1991). *The effects of a mathematical word problem solving strategy on problem solving performance by middle school students with mild disabilities*. Unpublished doctoral dissertation, University of Florida.

Weber-Fox, C., & Neville, H. J. (1996). Maturational constraints on functional specializations for language processing: ERP and behavioral evidence in bilingual speakers. *Journal of Cognitive Neuroscience, 8,* 231–256.

Wechsler, D. (1939). *Measurement of adult intelligence*. Baltimore: Williams & Wilkins.

Wechsler, D. (1991). *Wechsler Intelligence Scale for Children—Third Edition*. San Antonio, TX: Psychological Corporation.

Wechsler, D. (2003). *Wechsler Intelligence Scale for Children—Fourth Edition*. San Antonio, TX: Psychological Corporation.

Weekes, B., Coltheart, M., & Gordon, E. (1997). Deep dyslexia and right hemisphere reading: A regional cerebral blood flow study. *Aphasiology, 11,* 1139–1158.

Weiler, M. D., Bernstein, J. H., Bellinger, D. C., & Waber, D. P. (2000). Processing speed in children with attention deficit/hyperactivity disorder, inattentive type. *Child Neuropsychology, 6,* 218–234.

Weisenberg, T. H., & McBride, K. E. (1935). *Aphasia: A clinical and psychological study*. New York: Commonwealth Fund.

Welch, M. (1992). The PLEASE strategy: A metacognitive learning strategy for improving the paragraph writing of students with mild learning disabilities. *Learning Disability Quarterly, 15,* 119–128.

Welsh, M. C., Pennington, B. F., & Groisser, D. B. (1991). A normative-developmental study of executive function: A window on prefrontal function in children. *Developmental Neuropsychology, 7,* 131–149.

Wepman, J. M., & Reynolds, W. M. (1987). *Wepman Auditory Discrimination Test—Second Edition*. Los Angeles: Western Psychological Services.

Werner, H., & Strauss, A. (1940). Causal factors in low performance. *American Journal of Mental Deficiency, 45,* 213–218.

Whalen, J., McCloskey, M., Lesser, R. P., & Gordon, B. (1997). Localizing arithmetic processes in the brain: Evidence from a transient deficit during cortical stimulation. *Journal of Cognitive Neuroscience, 9,* 409–417.

Wheeler, M. A., Stuss, D. T., & Tulving, E. (1995). Frontal damage produces episodic memory impairment. *Journal of the International Neuropsychological Society, 1,* 525–536.

Whelan, T. B. (1999). Integrative developmental neuropsychology: A general systems and social-ecological approach to the neuropsychology of children with neurogenetic disorders. In S. Goldstein & C. R. Reynolds (Eds.), *Handbook of neurodevelopmental disorders in children* (pp. 84–98). New York: Guilford Press.

Whitaker, H. A., Bub, D., & Leventer, S. (1981). Neurolinguistic aspects of language acquisition and bilingualism. *Annals of the New York Academy of Sciences, 379,* 59–74.

White, J. L., Moffitt, T. E., Caspi, A., Bartusch, D. J., Needles, D. J., & Stouthamer-Loeber, M. (1994). Measuring impulsivity and examining its relationship to delinquency. *Journal of Abnormal Psychology, 103,* 192–205.

White, J. L., Moffitt, T. E., & Silva, P. A. (1992). Neuropsychological and socio-emotional correlates of specific arithmetic disability. *Archives of Clinical Neuropsychology, 7,* 1–16.

Whitehurst, G. J., & Fischel, J. E. (1994). Early developmental language delay: What, if anything, should the clinician do about it? *Journal of Child Psychology and Psychiatry, 35,* 613–648.

Wickstrom, K. F., Jones, K. M., LaFleur, L. H., & Witt, J. C. (1998). An analysis of treatment integrity in school-based behavioral consultation. *School Psychology Quarterly, 13*(2), 141–154.

Wiggs, C. L., Weisberg, J., & Martin, A. (1999). Neural correlates of semantic and episodic memory retrieval. *Neuropsychologia, 37,* 103–118.

Wilczynski, S. M., Mandal, R. L., & Fusilier, I. (2000). Bridges and barriers in behavioral consultation. *Psychology in the Schools, 37*(6), 495–504.

Willcutt, E. G., & Pennington, B. F. (2000). Comorbidity of reading disability and attention-deficit/hyperactivity disorder: Differences by gender and subtype. *Journal of Learning Disabilities, 33,* 179–191.

Williams, J. P. (1980). Teaching decoding with an emphasis on phoneme analysis and blending. *Journal of Educational Psychology, 72,* 1–15.

Williams, J. P., Lauer, K. D., Hall, K. M., Lord, K. M., Gugga, S. S., Bak, S., et al. (2002). Teaching elementary school students to identify story themes. *Journal of Educational Psychology, 94,* 235–248.

Williams, K. T. (1997). *Expressive Vocabulary Test.* Circle Pines, MN: American Guidance Service.

Willis, W. G. (1986). Actuarial and clinical approaches to neuropsychological diagnosis: Applied considerations. In J. E. Obrzut & G. W. Hynd (Eds.), *Child neuropsychology: Vol. 2. Clinical practice.* Orlando, FL: Academic Press.

Wilson, B. M., & Proctor, A. (2000). Oral and written discourse in adolescents with closed head injury. *Brain and Cognition, 43,* 425–429.

Wilson, M. (1993). DSM-III and the transformation of American psychiatry: A history. *American Journal of Psychiatry, 150,* 399–410.

Wilson, P. H., & McKenzie, B. E. (1998). Information processing deficits associated with developmental coordination disorder: A meta-analysis of research findings. *Journal of Child Psychology and Psychiatry, 39,* 829–840.

Wing, L. (1998). The history of Asperger syndrome. In E. Schopler, G. B Mesibov, & L. J. Kunce (Eds.), *Asperger syndrome or high-functioning autism?: Current issues in autism* (pp. 11–28). New York: Plenum Press.

Wirtz, C. L., Gardner, R., III, Weber, K., & Bullara, D. (1996). Using self-correction to improve the spelling performance of low-achieving third graders. *Remedial and Special Education, 17,* 48–58.

Wise, P. S. (1995). Communicating with parents. In A. Thomas & J. Grimes (Eds.), *Best practices in school psychology III* (pp. 279–288). Washington, DC: National Association of School Psychologists.

Witton, C., Stein, J. F., Stoodley, C. J., Rosner, B. S., & Talcott, J. B. (2002). Separate influences of acoustic AM and FM sensitivity on the phonological decoding skills of impaired and normal readers. *Journal of Cognitive Neuroscience, 14,* 866–874.

Wolf, M. (Ed.). (2001). *Dyslexia, fluency, and the brain.* Timonium, MD: York Press.

Wolf, M., & Bowers, P. G. (1999). The double-deficit hypothesis for the developmental dyslexias. *Journal of Educational Psychology, 91,* 415–438.

Wolf, M., Miller, L., & Donnelly, K. (2000). Retrieval, automaticity, vocabulary elaboration, orthography (RAVE-O): A comprehensive, fluency-based reading intervention program. *Journal of Learning Disabilities, 33,* 375–386.

Wong, B. Y. L. (1986). A cognitive approach to teaching spelling. *Exceptional Children, 53,* 169–173.

Wong, B. Y. L. (1991). On cognitive process-based instruction: An introduction. *Journal of Learning Disabilities, 25,* 150–152, 172.

Wong, B. Y. L. (1996). *The ABCs of learning disabilities.* San Diego, CA: Academic Press.

Wong, B. Y. L., Butler, D. L., Ficzere, S. A., & Kuperts, S. (1996). Teaching low achievers and students with learning disabilities to plan, write, and revise opinion essays. *Journal of Learning Disabilities, 29,* 197–212.

Wong, B. Y. L., & Jones, W. (1982). Increasing metacomprehension in learning disabled and normally achieving students through self-questioning. *Learning Disability Quarterly, 5,* 228–240.

Wood, F. B., Flowers, D. L., & Grigorenko, E. (2001). The functional neuroanatomy of fluency or why walking is just as important to reading as talking is. In M. Wolf (Ed.), *Dyslexia, fluency, and the brain* (pp. 235–244). Timonium: York Press.

Wood, F. B., & Grigorenko, E. L. (2001). Emerging issues in the genetics of dyslexia: A methodological preview. *Journal of Learning Disabilities, 34,* 503–511.

Woodcock, R. W., McGrew, K. S., & Mather, N. (2001). *Woodcock–Johnson III.* Itasca, IL: Riverside.

Wright, C. E., & Lindemann, P. (1993, November). *Effector independence in hierarchically-structured motor programs for handwriting.* Paper presented at the 34th annual convention of the Psychonomic Society, Washington, DC.

Ysseldyke, J. (2001). Reflections on a research career: Generalizations from 25 years of research on assessment and instructional decision making. *Exceptional Children, 67*(3), 295–309.

Ysseldyke, J. E., & Sabatino, D. A. (1973). Toward validation of the diagnostic-prescriptive model. *Academic Therapy, 8,* 415–422.

Ysseldyke, J. E., & Salvia, J. (1974). Diagnostic–prescriptive teaching: Two models. *Exceptional Children,* 181–185.

Zametkin, A. J., Liebenauer, L., Fitzgerald, G. A., King, A. C., Minkunas, D. V., Herscovitch, P., et al. (1993). Brain metabolism in teenagers with attention-deficit hyperactivity disorder. *Archives of General Psychiatry, 50,* 333–340.

Zatorre, R. J. (1984). Musical perception and cerebral function: A critical review. *Music Perception, 2,* 196–221.

Zawaiza, T. R. W., & Gerber, M. M. (1993). Effects of explicit instruction on math word-problem solving by community college students with learning disabilities. *Learning Disability Quarterly, 16,* 64–79.

Zentall, S. S. (1990). Fact-retrieval automatization and math problem solving by learning disabled, attention-disordered, and normal adolescents. *Journal of Educational Psychology, 82,* 856–865.

Zentall, S. S., & Smith, Y. N. (1993). Mathematical performance and behaviour of children with hyperactivity with and without coexisting aggression. *Behaviour Research and Therapy, 31,* 701–710.

Zentall, S. S., Smith, Y. N., Yung-bin, B. L., & Wieczorek, C. (1994). Mathematical outcomes of attention-deficit hyperactivity disorder. *Journal of Learning Disabilities, 27,* 510–519.

Ziatas, K., Durkin, K., & Pratt, C. (1998). Belief term development in children with autism, Asperger syndrome, specific language impairment, and normal development: Links to theory of mind development. *Journal of Child Psychology and Psychiatry, 39,* 755–763.

Index